Medical Progress through Technology

VOLUME 12

Medical engineering in Japan
Research and development

guest editors:
Kazuhiko Atsumi and Fumihiko Kajiya
(Tokyo) (Kurashiki)

Associate guest editors:
Takayuki Tsuji and Katushiko Tsujioka
(Tokyo) (Kurashiki)

1987 **MARTINUS NIJHOFF PUBLISHERS**
a member of the KLUWER ACADEMIC PUBLISHERS GROUP
BOSTON / DORDRECHT / LANCASTER

Preface

The complete volume 12 of *Medical Progress through Technology* is devoted to the work of colleagues in Japan. Additionally, whole authority and responsibility both for the election of topics and for the reviewing procedure had been delegated to Guest Editors from Japan.

What are the objectives of this special issue and why has Japan been elected to present itself in this way?

International journals such as *Medical Progress through Technology* usually contain papers from authors all over the world. Such issues provide a rather comprehensive survey on different scientific projects but do not reflect the standard and extent of medical technology in a certain country. I think that issues like the present one give far better information on the actual state of research and development in a country than an irregular sequence of scientific reports. It is not intended that all future issues of *Medical Progress through Technology* will concern only national issues. The present issue is an exception. However, if the readers appreciate such an approach, then other national issues may be published.

There are several reasons in favor of Japan preparing the first national issues. We all admire the history, tradition and culture of this country, but we are also impressed by the high standard of research, development and technical realisation achieved in nearly all high technology fields. There is no doubt, that Japan is among the leading nations in the field of medical technology. However, foreigners find it extremely difficult to keep informed of the progress in Japan due to unfamiliarity with the language. This issue may help to supply you with relevant information and to prepare you for 1991, when Japan will be the organiser of the XVI International Conference on Medical and Biological Engineering. I am convinced that this meeting in the wonderful old city of Kyoto will become an outstanding one.

I gratefully acknowledge the excellent work of my Japanese friends and colleagues in preparing this issue. Professor Atsumi and Professor Kajiya have overtaken full responsibility as Guest-Editors assisted by Dr. Tsuji and Dr. Tsujioka as Associate Guest Editors. Furthermore, I would like to thank all authors of papers in this issue for their invaluable cooperation.

H. Hutten
(Mainz)

Medical Progress through Technology 12 (1987) 5–16

Research and development on total artificial heart in University of Tokyo

Kazuhiko Atsumi, I. Fujimasa, K. Imachi, M. Nakajima, K. Mabuchi, S. Tsukagoshi, T. Chinzei & Y. Abe
Institute of Medical Electronics, University of Tokyo, 7-3-1 Hongo, Bunkyo-ku, Tokyo, 113, Japan

Abstract

The research and development on the total artificial heart (TAH) in the University of Tokyo can be divided chronologically into the three stages, i.e., the first stage (1959–1970); trial and error stage to find appropriate hardwares, the second stage (1970–1985); software stage to find how to control pneumatic TAH and to manage the animals, and the third stage (1985–); final goal to develop implantable TAH for animal and human.

This paper reviews the process of research and development in each stage.

1. Introduction

In 1959, research and development on total artificial heart (TAH) was started in the University of Tokyo. Many kinds of blood pumps, driving mechanisms, sensors and control systems have been constructed and tested in the mock circulatory models and also in the animal experiments. Since 1970, pneumatic units with sac type blood pumps have been used as the most convenient system for TAH animal experiments. After many years' experiences using various animals, goat has been selected as the most appropriate and been used mostly in our animal experiments since 1971. In 1983, the longest survival (344 days) of the TAH goat was obtained by use of the pneumatic unit.

In 1980, the sac type blood pump was modified and the pneumatic driving unit was miniaturized and they were used for clinical cases of left or right ventricular assist devices. In 1983, an electric wheel-chair type of pneumatic driving unit by which an AH patient can move around, has been developed and tested in the animal experiments. Recently, a newly designed implantable TAH, mechanically driven, of which blood pump has free diaphragm and has no compliance chamber, has been under investigation in vitro and in vivo experiments.

The research and development on the TAH in the University of Tokyo can be divided chronologically into the three stages: the first stage (1959–1970); trial and error stage to find appropriate hardwares, the second stage (1970–1985); software stage to find how to control pneumatic TAH and to manage the animals, and the third stage (1985–); final goal to develop implantable TAH for animal and human.

2. The first stage of the TAH R & D in the University of Tokyo

The research and development (R & D) projects on TAH in the University of Tokyo started in 1959 and have continued until now. In 1959, hydraulic driven unit was constructed which is composed of two blood pumps and driving and control unit. The blood pump is cylindrical in shape with two door type valves and the material of the inner sac is made of purified natural rubber specially cured by use of peroxide. In the hydraulic mechanism, the two metal bellows were used to move the special cams which can produce pulse flow curves of water pressures. In 1960, the TAH animal experiment to use the hydraulic unit was tried in dogs. A dog could survive for two hours with spontaneous respiration by the AH unit. In 1961, roller pumps driven by micromotor, a non-pulsatile AH unit, was con-

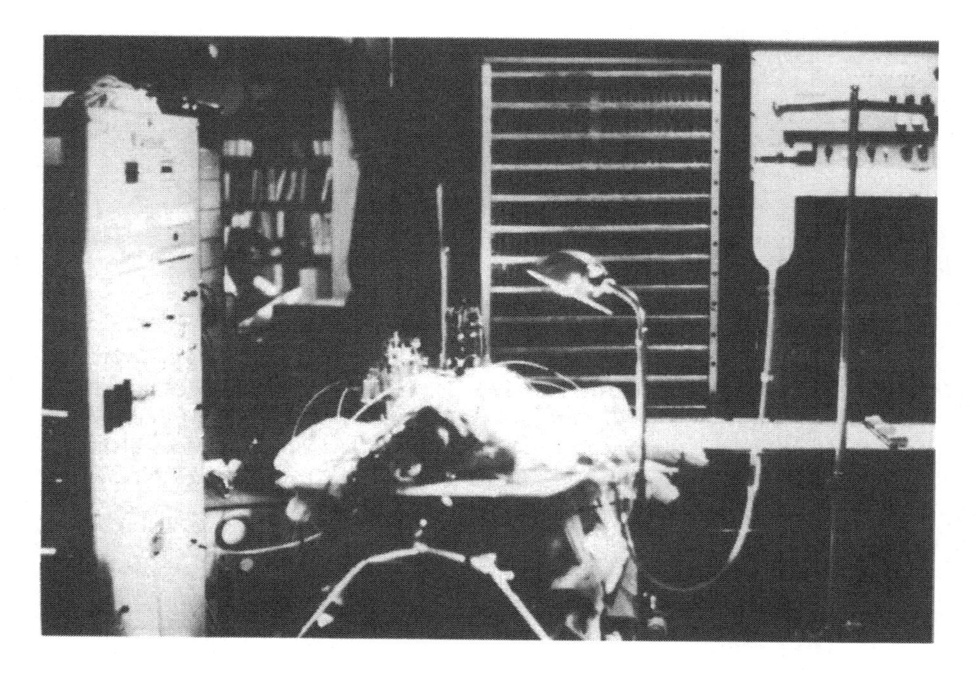

Fig. 1. Automatic control of TAH by digital computer. A dog survived for 24 hours.

structed and a dog survived for 13 hours when its natural heart was replaced by the AH unit. In 1963, the implantable TAH unit was constructed which is driven by the polyethylene micro-bellows with cams. The TAH unit was incorporated into a dog's thoracic cavity to replace natural heart under deep hypothermia. The dog could survive for 7 hours with spontaneous respiration. After the trials and errors in the TAH animal experiments, air driven mechanism was considered as the appropriate driving unit. Many kinds of animals – dog, rabbit, calf, sheep – were used for TAH experiments and goat is selected as the most suitable animal and has been used until now in our laboratory.

According with the accumulation of the experimental data on TAH, automatic control was required for TAH driving. Therefore, the digital computer was applied to control the pressure wave form in the pneumatic unit (1964–1965). The software is based on the regulation of pulmonary and aortic pressures within normal range. A TAH dog could survive for 24 hours under the computer control (Fig. 1). At that time, digital computers were so bulky that, in order to miniaturize the driving unit, a fluid amplifier element was to apply into the pneumatic unit. This element has unique advantage to provide miniaturization of the hardware and also performance of automatic control without mechanical parts. Utilizing the portable unit of fluid amplifier driving, a goat with left ventricular assist device can walk out of doors (Fig. 2). However, in spite of many advantages, fluid amplifier element was given up to use for TAH driving, because the unit could not control positive and negative pressure independently.

In the first stage, many kinds of driving units were constructed to try various mechanisms and they were used in the animal experiments. However, the TAH animals could not survive more than two days because the level of practical engineering, biomaterial and knowledge for artificial blood circulation were too poor and too premature to be used.

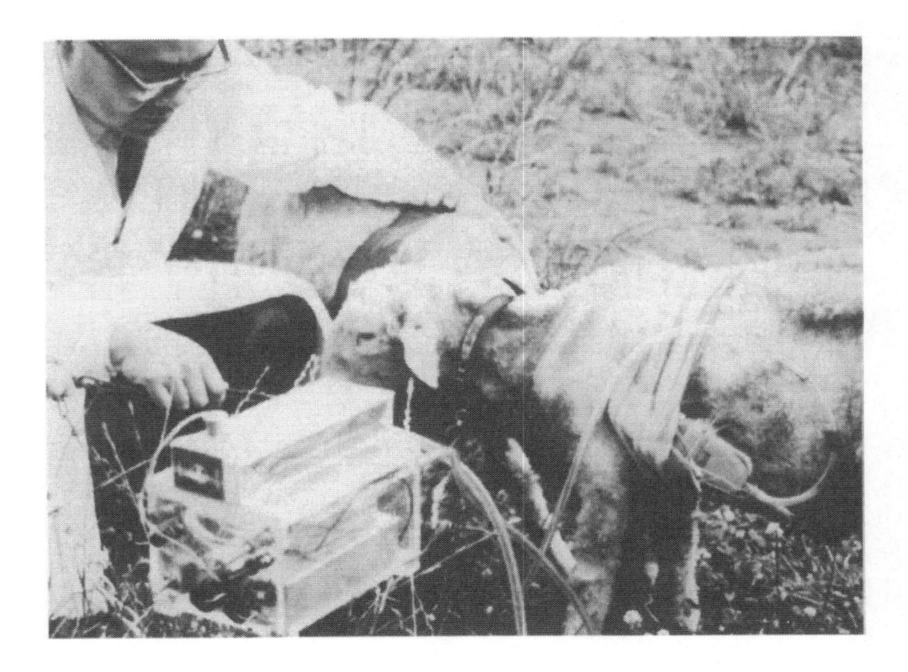

Fig. 2. A goat with left ventricular assist device by fluid amplifier driving could walk out of doors.

3. The second stage of TAH R & D in the University of Tokyo

From the in vitro and in vivo experiments on TAH during the first stage, pneumatic driven type was considered as an appropriate mechanism to be applied. Therefore, in the second stage, the animal experiments concentrated on studying thoroughly the pneumatic driven unit.

In our laboratory, in order to replace the natural heart functions, several kinds of surgical operations to connect the blood pumps with the experimental animals have been studied. Our methods are different from those which have been utilized by the other TAH researchers in the world to remove natural heart and to incorporate the blood pump inside the animal's thoracic cavity. Our definition of TAH is an artificial system which substitutes the biological cardiac functions completely without consideration of the original shape, size and installed position.

In the 2nd stage, three types of pneumatic TAH were studied: FTAH, HTAH and TRAH with paracorporeal pumps. Fig. 3 shows the scheme of the three types. In FTAH, two bypass pumps were connected and then, the natural heart was fibrillated electrically. In HTAH, two bypass pumps were connected and then, the both outflows of the natural heart were occluded by ligation of main pulmonary artery and ascending aorta. Thirdly, the project of TRAH was started in which the animal's natural heart is removed by use of pump oxygenator, special atrial cuffs are sutured to the margin of the both remaining atria at the position of the atrioventricular ring. Then the AH blood pumps (right and left) are connected with the cuffs and are fitted paracorporeally outside the body.

The research and development on TAH in the second stage clarified the following essential problems.

1. The possibility of surviving with TAH: Utilizing the TRAH method, the 344 days survival of TAH goat was experienced in our laboratory in 1984 which is the longest survival of TAH animal in the world (Fig. 4).

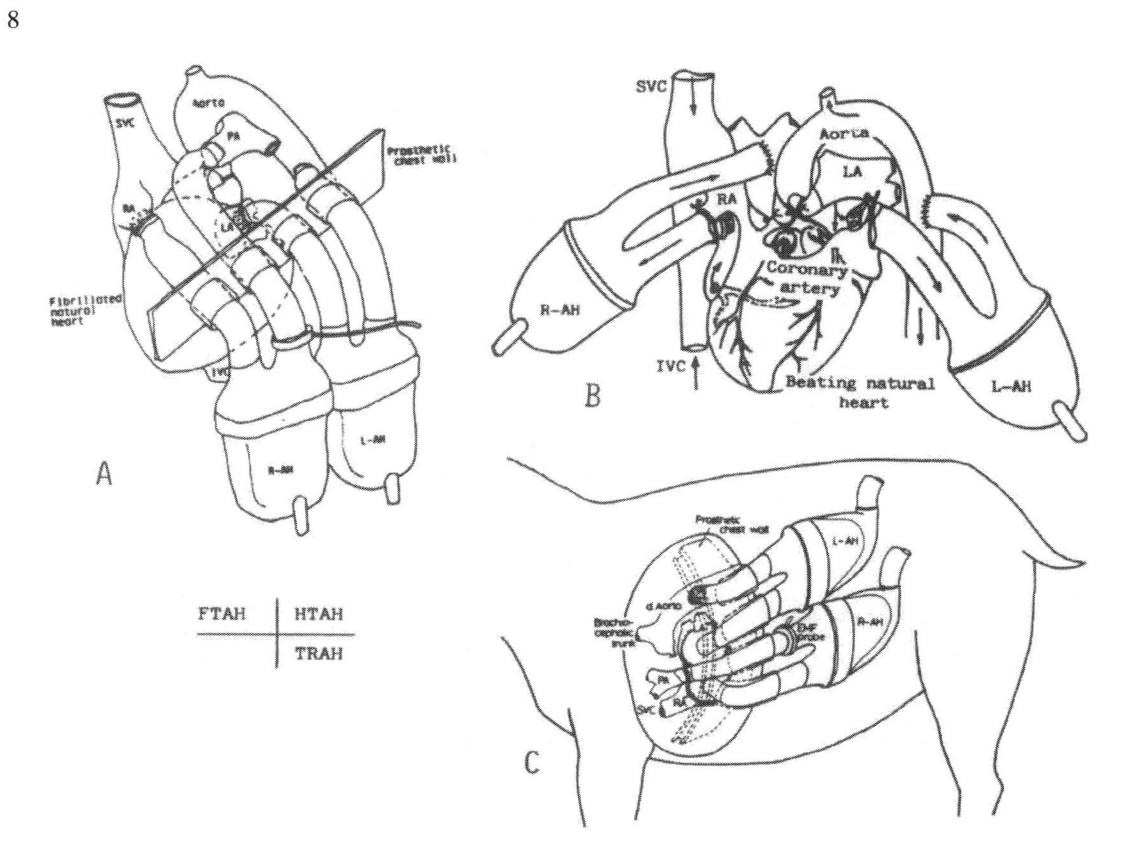

Fig. 3. Three types of TAH in the University of Tokyo, A: FTAH, B: HTAH and C: TRAH.

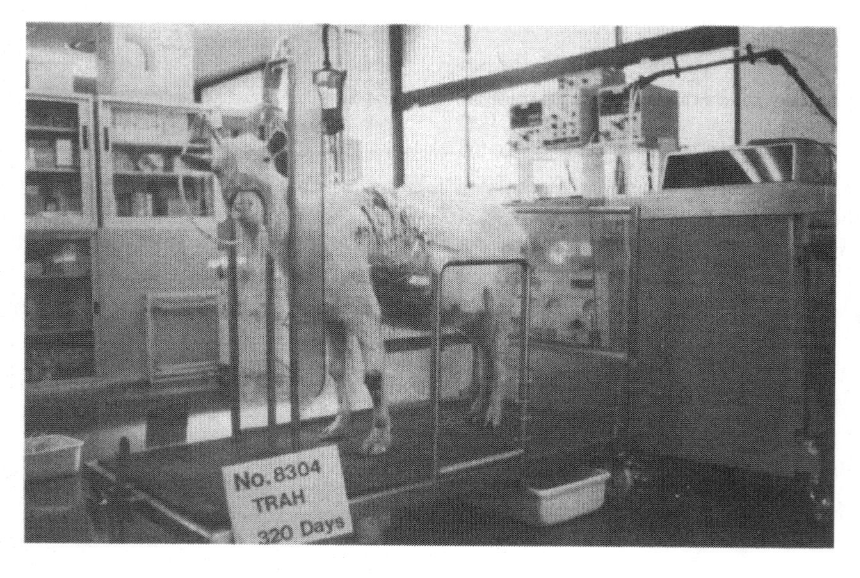

Fig. 4. A TAH goat survived for 344 days by pneumatic driving unit.

2. The basic control method of TAH: The basic control principle established was to regulate the cardiac output of right AH within normal range and suck up the whole blood returned to the left atrium and push out it as the left cardiac output.

3. The material surface and blood flow rate influences on thrombus formation: The material of the inner sac of the blood pump was made of polyvinylchloride coated by Cardiothane (block copolymer of polyurethane and polydimethylsiloxane) and the surface was smooth which is considered preferable for antithrombogenecity. The pump design was aimed to reduce flow stagnation inside the sac.

4. The durability of driving system: It was approved that the routine overhaul on driving unit can maintain the durability of continuous driving for one year.

5. The pathophysiology in TAH: During the last 25 years, a lot of animal experiments on TAH have been carried out by many investigators. As a result, in the main facilities of the TAH research in the world, the 18 cases of over 6 months survivals could be obtained until now as shown in the Table 1. In

Table 1. TAH animals survived over 6 months in the world (May, 1984).

Facility	Animal	Survival days	Blood pump		Cause of death
			Type	Material	
1 Tokyo Univ.	Goat	344	Sac	Cardiothane - PVC	Lung embolism, Anemia
2 Utah Univ.	Sheep	297	J_7	Biomer	B-S valve, rupture
3 Tokyo Univ.	Goat	288	Sac	Polyurethane	Human accident
4 Hershey Med. Center	Calf	270	Diaphragm	Biomer	
5 Utah Univ.	Calf	268	J_5	Biomer	Left heart failure
6 Tokyo Univ.	Goat	243	Sac	Avcothane - PVC	Pannus, Reoperation
7 Tokyo Univ.	Goat	232	Sac	Polyurethane	Peripheral circulatory insufficiency
8 Kyoto Univ.	Calf	226	Diaphragm	Polyurethane	
9 Hershey Med. Center	Calf	222	Diaphragm (DC motor driven)	Biomer	Electronic component failure
10 Utah Univ.	Calf	221	J_7	Biomer	Pannus, GI-bleeding
11 Hershey Med. Center	Calf	220	Diahragm	Biomer	
12 Utah Univ.	Calf	217	J_5	Biomer	Ecchymotic hemorrhage serosa
13 Utah Univ.	Calf	210	J_5	Avcothane	Sepsis, Pannus
14 Berlin Univ.	Calf	210	Diaphragm	Pellethane (?)	
15 Berlin Univ.	Calf	194	Diaphragm	Pellethane	Rupture of blood pump
16 Hershey Med. Center	Calf	190	Diaphragm	Biomer	
17 Utah Univ.	Calf	184	J_5	Biomer	Pannus, Reoperation
18 Utah Univ.	Calf	183	J_5	Avcothane	Lung edema, Hemiplegia, Pannus (Accident)

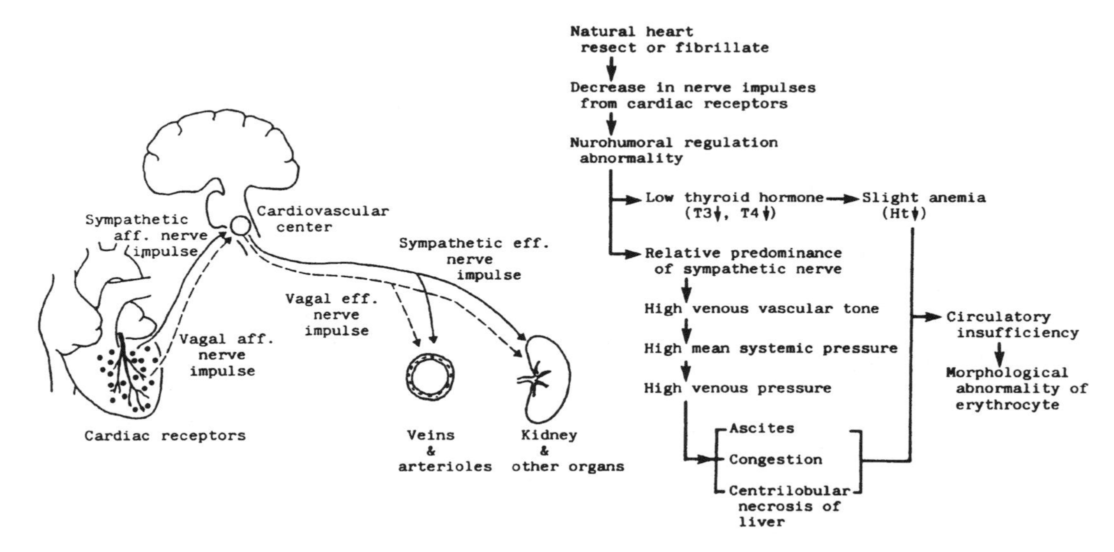

Fig. 5. The generation mechanism of pathophysiological abnormality with cardiac receptor hypothesis.

analyzing their causes of death, one third are considered to be related with pannus formation, clotting and embolie, one third are with disorder of AH hardwares and the others are with infection, peripheral circulatory insufficiency and unknown factors. The experimental data and the autopsy findings have been indicating that the living conditions of the long surviving TAH animals were not normal conditions but were unphysiological states such as arterial hypertension, high central venous pressure, mild anemia, liver tissue damages, low thyroid hormone, etc. Some experimental data on TAH animals show gradual and continuous increasing of arterial pressure and right atrial pressure. However, in these cases, vasoconstrictors were not concerned with these results because the values of renin and angiotensin did not increase significantly. The loss of feedback loop of autonomic regulations by the removal of the natural heart are suspected of the causes of these unphysiological conditions. The disorder of ANP (atrial natriuretic polypeptide) should be also investigated.

6. The importance of natural heart beating: In spite of reduction of hematocrit (Ht) and thyroid hormone level (THL) in FTAH and TRAH, Ht and THL in HTAH did not show as significant a

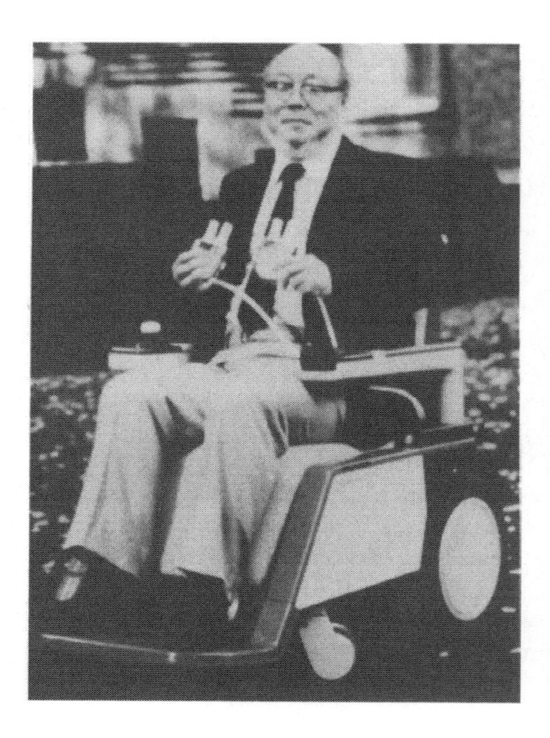

Fig. 6. An electric wheel-chair unit by which the TAH patient can move easily. Pneumatic driving, control and monitoring units and energy sources are incorporated inside the chair.

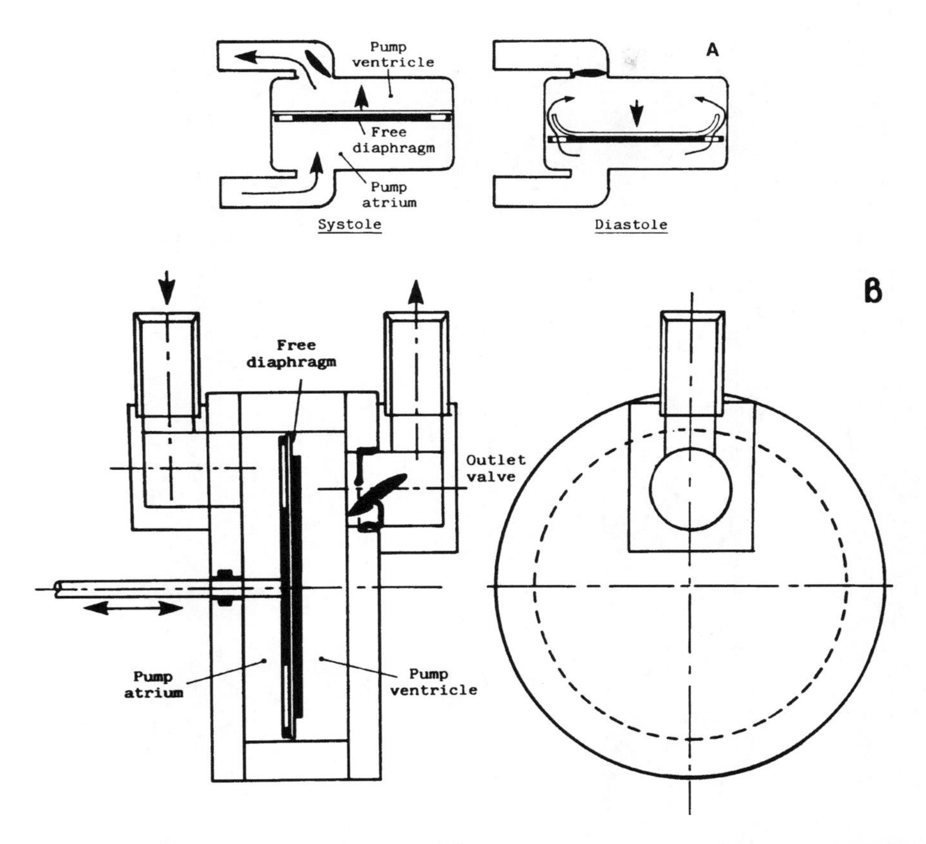

Fig. 7. Mechanism and design of blood pump of implantable TAH in University of Tokyo. (A) Mechanism of free diaphragm blood pump for implantable TAH. (B) Design of free diaphragm blood pump for implantable TAH.

reduction. In our hypothesis, the natural heart beating has significant meaning for systemic circulation, especially for its neurohumoral regulation. Therefore, the deficiency of nerve impulse from cardiac receptors of the beating natural heart may cause many pathophysiological abnormalities in TAH animals (Fig. 5).

7. Necessity of neural control in TAH: By electrical stimulation instead of nerve impulses from cardiac receptors, some of the pathophysiological abnormalities were improved in FTAH and TRAH experiments. The results suggest that the other abnormalities will be able to be solved by further study of neural control. And now, the next TRAH project has been started in which AH blood pump is implanted into the animal's thorax. At the present state, the goat with TRAH replacement could survive for two weeks.

4. Miniaturization of TAH driving and control units

Generally speaking, at the present time, pneumatic TAH has many advantages in practical use, if it would be compared with hydraulic and mechanical TAH units. Therefore, miniaturization of the driving and control units was studied. Two types were developed – one is a portable unit and the other is an electric wheel chair type.

4.1 Portable driving unit

If the TAH patient who is confined to bed because of driving air tubes wants to move, a portable driving unit is indispensably necessary. For this purpose, CORART 301 was constructed and the standard specification is shown as follows;

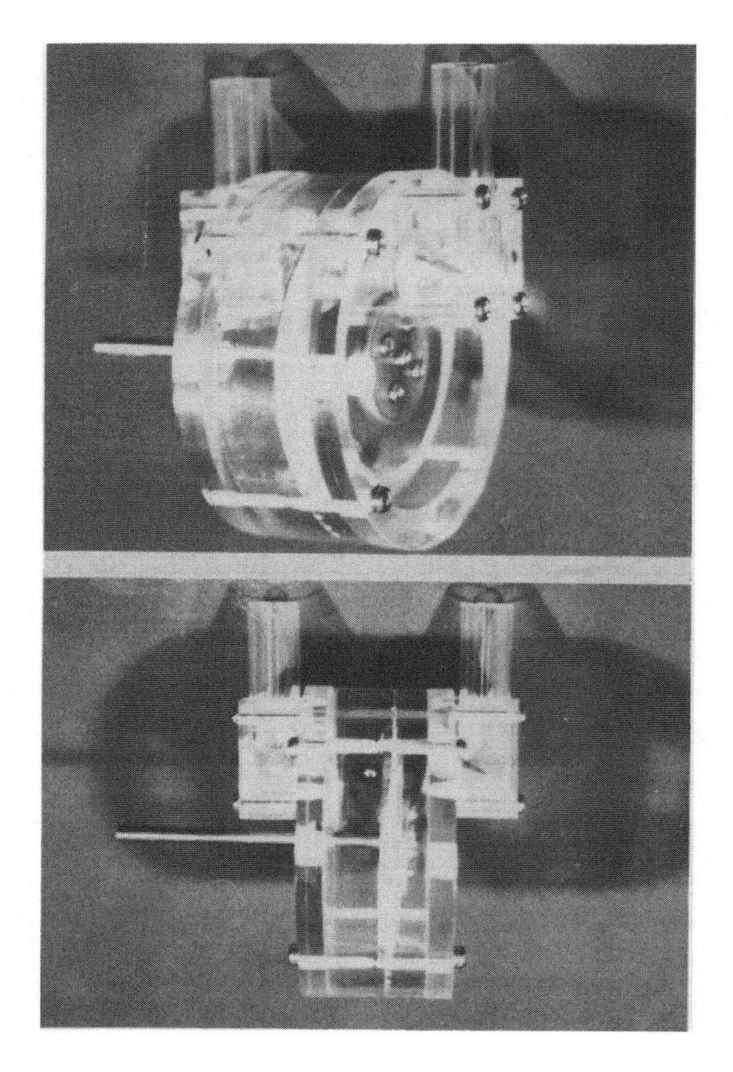

Fig. 8. Diaphragm type of the blood pumps of the implantable TAH. Upper is front view and lower is side view.

pneumatic pressure : −150 ∼ +300 mmHg
Pulse rate : Max., 250/min.
Power supply : 24 V (Battery)
Synchronization : ECG and External
Weight (Kg) : 36
Size (mm) : 680(H) × 225 (W) ×510 (D)

4.2 Electric wheel chair unit

Pneumatic sources of positive and negative pressures, monitoring & control and energy sources are incorporated in the electric wheel-chair unit by which the TAH patient can move easily (Fig. 6). The standard specification of the unit is shown as follows:

Max. pump output : 6.5 L/min. (180 mmHg, −60 mmHg, 100 beat/min)
Operating duration by battery (24 V) : 30 min.
Remote control
Weight (Kg) : 145
Size (cm) : 112(L) × 60 (W) × 96 (H)

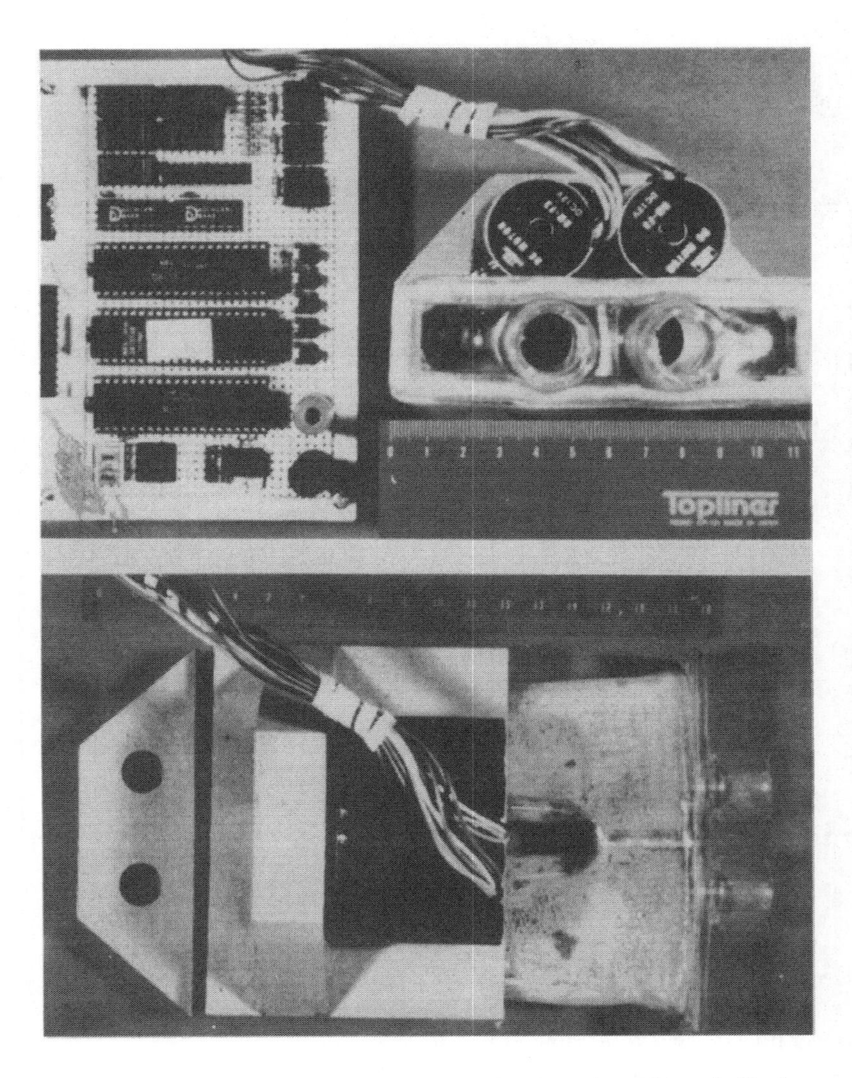

Fig. 9. Prototype model of the driving system of the implantable TAH. Upper is up view and lower is side view.

5. The third stage of the TAH project in the University of Tokyo

In the third stage our final goal is to construct implantable TAH and to implant it in the human thorax. In order to have a cushion to make a driving pressure balance, a compliance chamber is usually required to develop implantable TAH. Therefore, the research was started on the new idea of saving the space of the compliance chamber inside the body.

5.1 Blood pump

A newly designed blood pump was constructed in which the atrio-ventricular septal wall can be moved resulting in pumping power. A valve is inserted into the septum between the atrium and the ventricle as a inflow valve and another valve is installed in the ouflow conduit. In basis on this idea, two prototype models – sac type and diaphragm type – were constructed and evaluated in vitro testing (Figs. 7, 8).

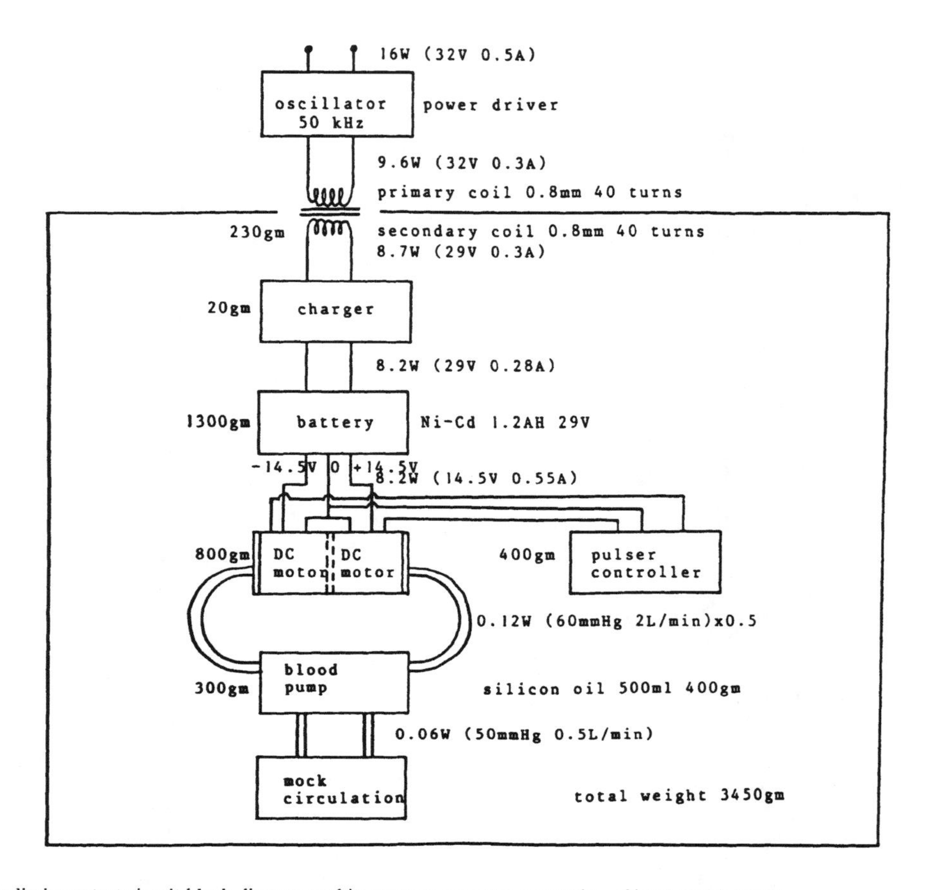

Fig. 10. Preliminary test circuit block diagram and its average power consumption of implantable TAH.

5.2 Driving mechanism

As a driving power transmission, a hydraulic driven system with centrifugal pump and some kinds of DC motors were evaluated. Two centrifugal pumps immersed in a silicone oil tank can push the two blood sac pumps alternatively for systolic and diastolic duration (Fig. 9).

5.3 Energy transmission

Electromagnetic energy transmission by wireless coupling has been investigated. Actually, power transmission of 20 W with 50 KHz of frequency is available to drive the implantable TAH (Fig. 10). However, further studies are necessary to improve enhancement of efficiency and to reduce heating.

5.4 Automatic control logics

Multi-data processing modules have been developing which can process cardiac outputs, aortic & pulmonary arterial pressures, right atrial pressure and driving pressures simultaneously with the softwares of artificial intelligence (Fig. 11).

5.5 Biocompatible and antithrombogenic materials

The longest surviving TAH goat of 344 days showed thrombus formation and calcification on the Cardiothane surface of the blood pumps. In

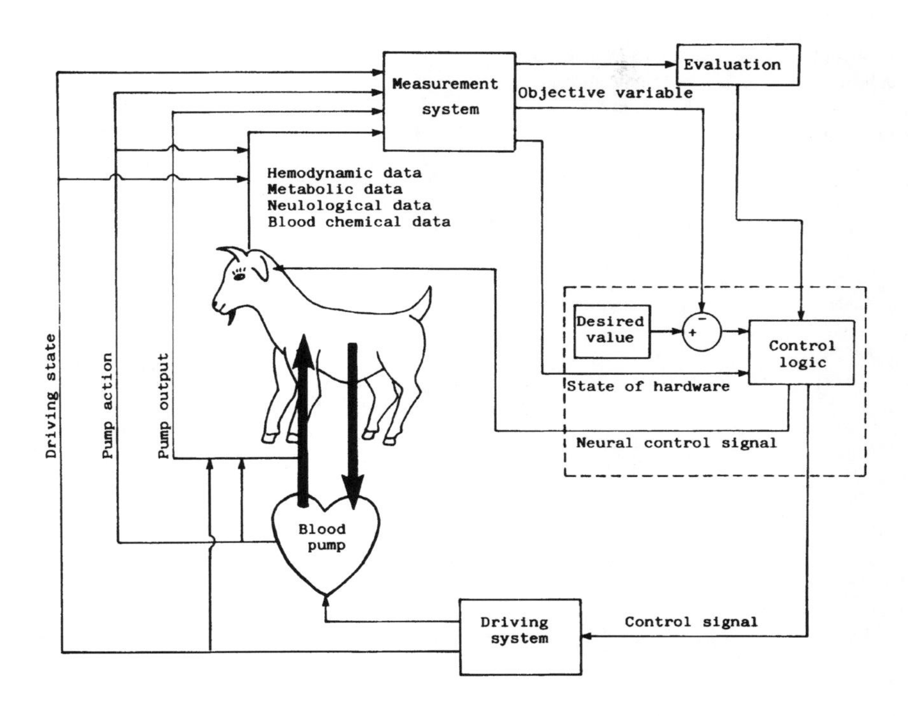

Fig. 11. The block diagram of TAH control in University of Tokyo.

order to evaluate the blood compatibility of multiple materials simultaneously in the same condition, in vivo, the new method was developed to attach the objective materials on the inner surface of blood pump which are evaluated with SEM after AH pumping for several weeks.

6. Conclusion

The R & D on TAH of the University of Tokyo was started in 1959 and has been continued until now. The R & D process can be divided into the three stages. In the first stage, many kinds of hardwares were investigated and pneumatic driving unit was selected as the appropriate hardware for TAH. In the second stage, the software to control TAH unit and to manage the TAH animals were studied by using air driven units and a TAH goat survival of 344 days was experienced. The third stage to develop implantable TAH has been started since 1985. This is the final goal for R & D on TAH. For the implantable TAH, newly designed TAH pumps without a compliance chamber has been under investigation.

References

1. Atsumi K, Hori M, Ikeda S, Sakurai Y, Fujimori Y, Kimoto S: Artificial heart incorporated in the chest. Trans Am Soc Artif Intern Organs 9: 292–298, 1963.
2. Atsumi K, Sakurai Y, Fujimasa I, Imachi K, Nishizaka T, Mano I, Ohmichi H, Mori J, Iwai N, Kouno A: Hemodynamic analysis on prolonged survival cases (30 days and 20 days) of artificial total heart replacement. Trans Am Soc Artif Intern Organs 21: 545–554, 1975.
3. Atsumi K, Fujimasa I, Imachi K, Miyake H, Takido N, Nakajima M, Kouno A, Ono T, Yuasa Y, Mori S, Nagaoka S, Kawase S, Kikuchi T: Three goats survived for 288 days, 243 days, and 232 days with hybrid total artificial heart (HTAH). Trans Am Soc Intern Organs 27: 77–83, 1981.
4. Imachi K, Fujimasa I, Nakajima M, Mabuchi K, Tsukagoshi S, Motomura K, Miyamoto A, Takido N, Inou N, Kouno A, Ono T, Atsumi K: Overall analysis of the causes of pathophysiological problems in total artificial heart in analysis by cardiac receptor by pathesis. Trans Am Soc Artif Intern Organs 30: 591–596, 1984.

5. Atsumi K, Fujimasa I, Imachi K, Nakajima M: How can the total artificial heart (TAH) patient be mobile and enjoy his life with an air driven system? Trans Am Soc Artif Intern Organs 30: 86–91, 1984.

Address for offprints:
K. Atsumi
Institute of Medical Electronics
University of Tokyo
7-3-1 Hongo, Bunkyo-ku
Tokyo 113, Japan

Medical Progress through Technology 12 (1987) 17–24

Hepatic assist device, using membrane plasma separator and dialyzer

Zenya Yamazaki[1] & Noboru Inoue[2]
[1] 2nd Department of Surgery, University of Tokyo and [2] National Oji Hospital, Japan

Key words: hepatic assist, membrane plasma separator, plasma exchange, hepatic failure

Abstract

Our hepatic assist device is composed of a membrane plasma separator, blood and plasma pumps, hemodialyzer and controller. Using this device, the patients plasma is replaced with fresh donor plasma in a 5000 ml amount daily. This procedure of plasma exchange takes place in the intensive care unit, until the patient recovers conciousness or cerebral death is confirmed. In the initial results of this plasma exchange, 5 out of 10 patients with fulminant hepatic failure survived. Even with fatal cases, prolongation of survival time was observed.

Our hepatic assist device, performing an easy and safe procedure for plasma exchange, appears to be the most promising method of providing long-term hepatic support for acute liver failure at the present time.

1. Introduction

To prevent the complications accompanying direct hemoperfusion over encapsulated adsorbent, where the blood cells contact the adsorbent, a plasma perfusion detoxication system was developed, using a membrane plasma separator of cellulose acetate hollow fiber [1]. When the system was applied to a patient with acute hepatic failure, however, it did not give us better results than the direct hemoperfusion. This may be due to the insufficient removal of protein-bound or macromolecular toxins and a lack of supplementation for essential factors, such as coagulation factors and necessary nutrients, synthesized in the normal liver. Therefore, our latest hepatic assist device, performing plasma exchange easily and safely with the use of the membrane plasma separator and dialyzer, has been developed and satisfactorily applied to patients with acute hepatic failure.

2. Materials and methods

2.1 Membrane plasma separator

Membrane plasma separator, a cellulose acetate hollow fiber (CAHF), (PF-01), filter Plasmaflo was originally developed for the treatment of intractable ascites [2, 3] and then utilized in the hepatic support system [1] or plasma exchange for acute hepatic failure [4]. Thereafter, Plasmaflo has been widely used in renal, liver and immune diseases [5, 6] not only to remove toxic macromolecular substances but also to supply necessary nutrients. Moreover, membrane donor plasmapheresis has been recently investigated [7, 8, 9]. Also our research team has endeavoured to improve the efficiency and biocompatibility of CAHF filter and developed a new module of an improved CAHF (PF-02) and recently succeeded in developing an innovative, surfactant-free polyolefine membrane plasma separator with an excellent efficiency and biocompatibility [10].

Following our Plasmaflo, other modules, made of various synthetic polymer membranes, have

Table 1. Specification of membrane plasma separator.

Trade name	Plasmaflo (Hi-05)	Plasmax (PS-05H)	Plasmacure (SA)	Plasma separator (MPS)	Plasma separator (TP50)	(PS-4000)	Plasma separator (PEX-50)	Kawasumi plasma separator	Plasmaflux (PS-500)	(CPS-10)	TPE Plasma separator
Material	Cellulose-di-acetate (CDA)	Polymethyl metacrylate (PMMA)	Polyvinyl alcohol (PVA)	Polyethylene (PE)	Polymeralloy	Cellulose acetate (CA)	Cellulose triacetate (CTA)	Polypropy-lene (PP)	Polypropy-lene (PP)	Polypropy-lene (PP)	Polyvinyl-chloride (PVC) with F-68 polyol
Style	HF	HF	HF	HF	HF	Sheet	HF	HF	HF	HF	Sheet
Surface area	0.5 m^2	0.5 m^2	0.6 m^2	0.6 m^2	0.5 m^2	0.5 m^2	0.5 m^2	0.4 m^2	0.5 m^2	0.17 m^2	
Max. Pore Size	0.2 μm	0.5 μm	0.4 μm		0.2 μm	0.46 μm	0.4 μm	0.6 μm	0.5 μm	0.55 μm	0.6 μm
Wall Thickness	60 μm	90 μm	125 μm	60 μm	75 μm	170 μm	72 μm	140 μm	140 μm	150 μm	
ID of HF	360 μm	300 μm	330 μm	270 μm	330 μm		285 μm	330 μm	330 μm	320 μm	
Sterilization	EOG	χ ray	Autoclave	2% Formalin	EOG	EOG	EOG	Steam	EOG	EOG	EOG
Manufacturer	Asahi M.	Toray	Kurare	Mitsubishi	Teijin	Terumo	Nipro	Kawasumi	Fresenius	Travenol	Cobe Lab.

HF: Hollow Fiber. EOG: Ethlene Oxide Gas. ID: Inner Diameter.

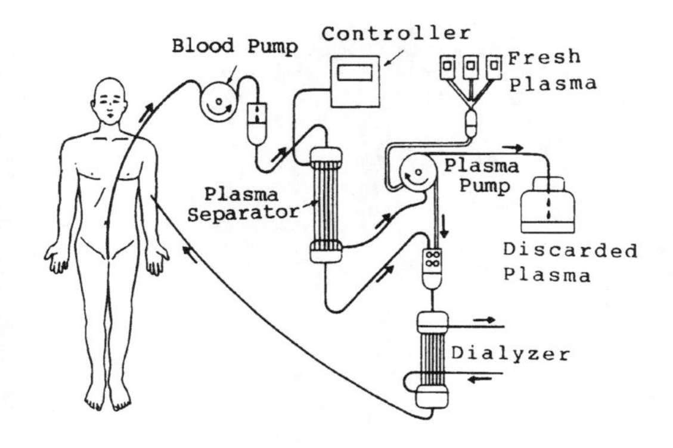

Fig. 1. Illustration of Extracorporeal hepatic assist device.

been developed and are available for practical use with almost the same efficiency and biocompatibility. These membrane separators are indicated in Table 1.

2.2 Composition of the hepatic assist device

Our extracorporeal hepatic assist system is composed of a membrane plasma separator (Plasmaflo AP05), blood and plasma pumps, hemodialyzer and controller, as illustrated in Fig. 1.

2.3 Plasma exchange regimen

All patients were treated with full supportive measures, including intravenous infusions of 10% glucose, correction of electrolytes and acid-base disturbances, intragastric administrations of lactulose and antiacids, and intravenous injections of cimetidine. Respiratory assist was preformed when necessary. In acute cases, where hepatic encephalopathy appeared within 10 days after the onset of fulminant hepatic failure, we started plasma exchange when the patient showed a grade III coma. For the subacute cases of fulminant hepatic failure, where encephalopathy occurred more than 11 days after the initiation of the diseases, we started plasma exchange when the patient was in a grade II coma.

Another form of acute or chronic hepatic coma was treated with plasma exchange when patients fell into grade II or III coma, where they had a fairly good hepatic reserve before their coma began, the inducing cause of their coma could be removed quickly, and their encephalopathy was refractory to conventional treatment modality.

About 5 liters of patients plasma was replaced with fresh frozen plasma or fresh plasma from a donor over 3 hours of 60–100 ml/min extracorporeal perfusion, and transmembrane pressure was kept less than 50 mm Hg during the procedure. The procedure was repeated once daily until the patient regained conciousness or cerebral death was confirmed by the continuation of flat EEG wave and loss of the vestibulooccular reflex.

A picture taken during the procedure is shown in Fig. 2.

3. Results

3.1 Fulminant hepatic failure

Ten patients with fulminant hepatic failure were treated with intensive plasma exchange. On the survivors, encephalopathy appeared within two weeks after the onset of liver dysfunction. After several plasma exchanges, the levels of conciousness were improved and there was a general rapid recovery. The concentration of amino acids was less than 100 mg/dl. Fig. 3 shows the clinical course and the laboratory data in a representative case.

In most of the fatal cases, encephalopathy appeared more than two weeks after the onset of liver dysfunction. The level of consciousness was improved by repeated plasma exchanges, but it deteriorated again. The prothrombin time, plasma concentration of bile acids, most of coagulation factors, and rapid turnover protein were maintained within acceptable range by daily repeated plasma exchanges. However, the plasma levels of amino acids and bilirubin remained elevated or at the pretreatment level on the day following plasma exchange, despite a decrease in the treated plasma. In most of the fatal cases, the continuation of the flat EEG wave and disappearance of oculovestibular reflex indicated cerebral death and so the

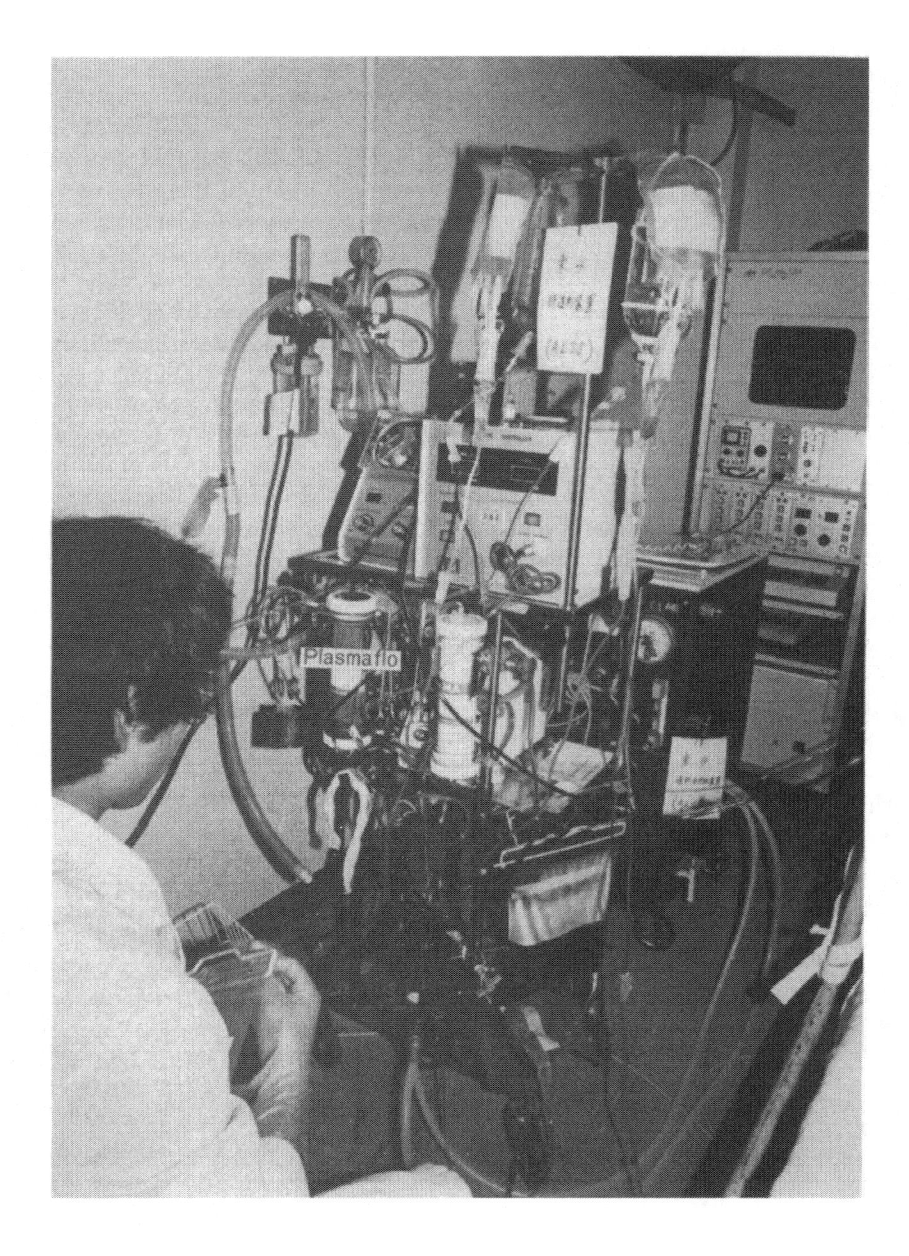

Fig. 2. A picture taken during the hepatic assist procedure.

plasma exchange was stopped. Fig. 4 shows the clinical course of such a patient. Table 2 shows the results of 10 patients with fulminant hepatic failure, treated with the plasma exchange.

3.2 Acute decompensation in chronic hepatic failure

Table 3 shows our results of 10 acute onsets of hepatic encephalopathies in the patients with chronic liver diseases. Although all the patients

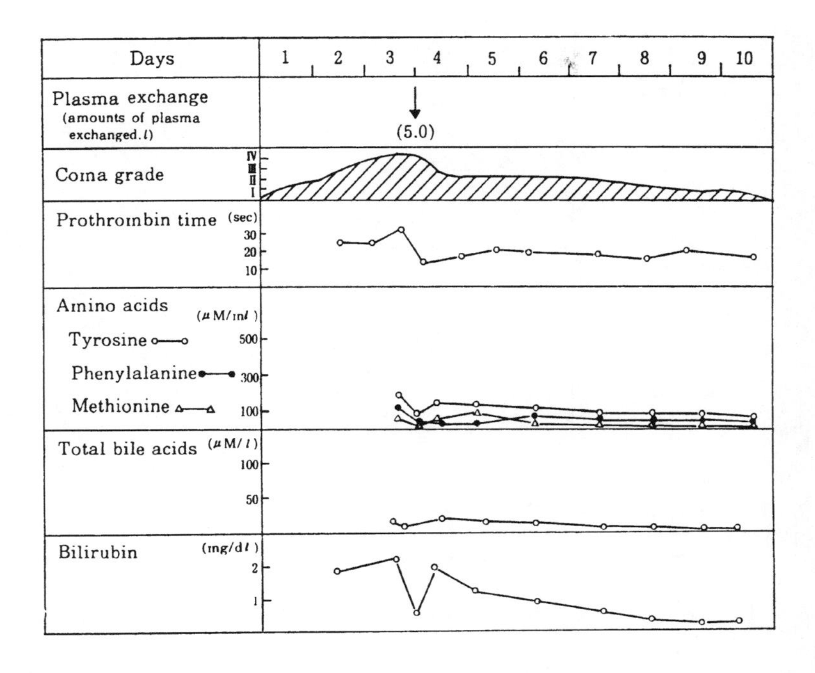

Fig. 3. Clinical course and changes in laboratory data in a patient with fulminant hepatic failure, treated with the hepatic assist device (survivor).

Table 2. Patients with fulminant hepatic failure, treated with the hepatic assist device.

Patient	Age/sex	Diagnosis	Grade	Coma recovery	Plasma exchange No.	Exchange volume (ml)	Outcome
1.	60/F	FHF Viral, non B	IV	Yes Partial	16	78600	Died Brain death
2.	25/M	FHF Viral, B	IV	Yes	6	29800	Recovered
3.	62/F	FHF Viral, non B	IV	Yes	1	6300	Recovered
4.	47/F	FHF Viral, non B	IV	No	5	23800	Died Brain death
5.	43/F	FHF Viral, non B	IV	No	3	14400	Died Brain death
6.	15/F	FHF Viral, non B	IV	No	8	38400	Died Brain death
7.	69/M	FHF Viral, non B	IV	Yes	1	5010	Recovered
8.	43/M	FHF Viral, B	IV	Yes	20	96000	Recovered
9.	25/F	FHF Viral, non B	III	Yes	3	14000	Recovered
10.	27/M	FHF Viral, B	IV	No	8	38400	Died Brain death

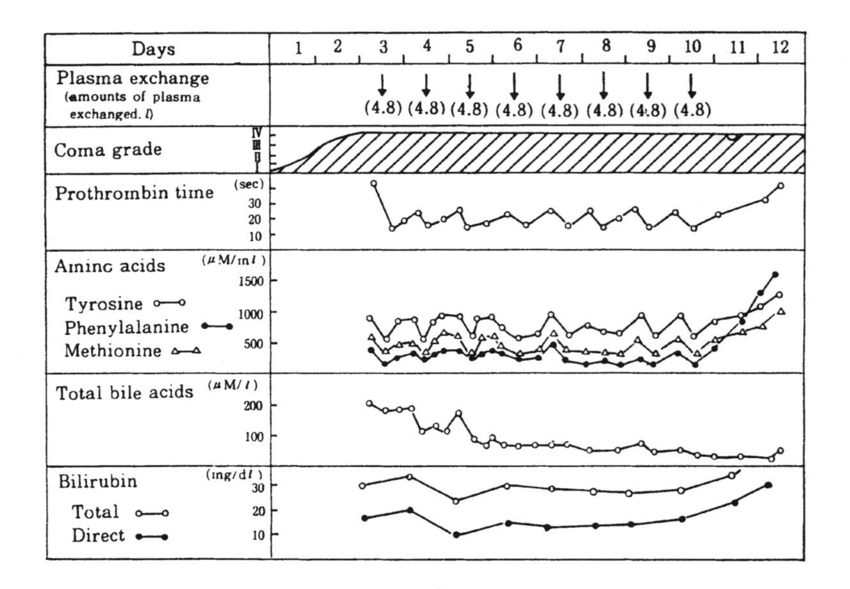

Fig. 4. Clinical course and changes in laboratory data in a patient with fulminant hepatic failure, treated with the hepatic assist device (non-survivor).

regained consciousness using plasma exchange, they eventually showed poor prognosis due to other complications such as primary liver tumor, infection, and gastrointestinal bleeding.

3.3 A case of acute hepatic failure after surgery

A twenty six year old female patient with mitral and aortic insufficiency.

After replacement of the mitral and aortic valves she developed acute renal failure complications of

Table 3. Patients with acute on chronic liver failure, treated with the hepatic assist device.

Patient	Age/sex	Diagnosis	Grade	Coma recovery	Plasma exchange No.	Exchange volume (ml)	Outcome
1.	64/F	Liver cirrhosis	IV	Yes	1	4200	Recovered
2.	64/F	Liver cirrhosis	IV	Yes	2	8300	Recovered
3.	51/M	Liver cirrhosis	IV	Yes	1	4200	Recovered
4.	49/F	Liver cirrhosis	III	Yes	1	1ps4800	Recovered
5.	56/F	Liver cirrhosis	III	Yes	1	4700	Recovered
6.	53/M	Liver cirrhosis	III	Yes	3	14400	Recovered
7.	52/M	Liver cirrhosis	II	Yes	10	46400	Died Respiratory insufficiency
8.	60/M	Liver cirrhosis	III	Yes	3	14400	Died Renal failure
9.	61/F	Liver cirrhosis	III	Yes	2	9600	Died Renal failure
10.	69/F	Liver cirrhosis	III	Yes	1	4800	Recovered

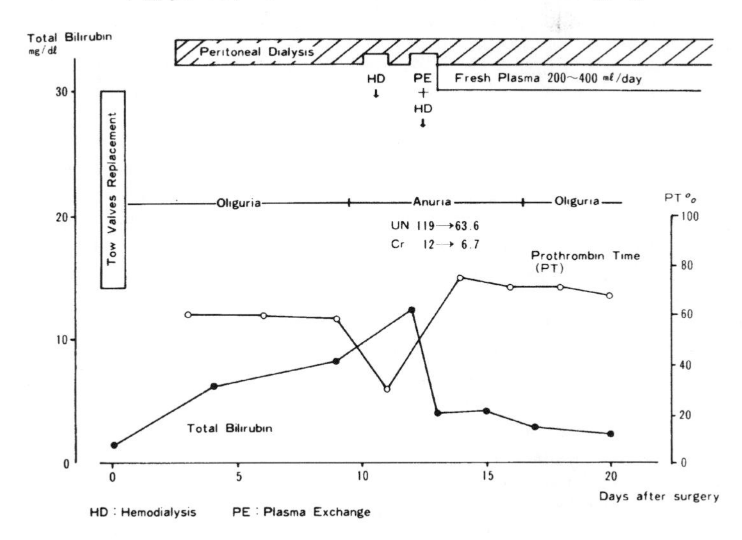

Fig. 5. Clinical course and changes in laboratory data in a patient with acute hepatic failure after cardiac surgery, treated with the hepatic assist device.

oliguria or anuria; and thus, the continued peritoneal dialysis had little effect, so hemodialysis was performed on the 10th day after surgery, giving only a little effect. Her serum bilirubin level was elevated and prothrombin time decreased to 40% due to hepatic insufficiency. Therefore, our hepatic support, including plasma exchange and hemodialysis, was applied succesfully to the patient on the 12th postoperative day. Thereafter, she showed a remarkable improvement and recovered from hepatorenal failure with the aid of peritoneal dialysis and the supplementation of fresh plasma, as shown in Fig. 5.

3.4 National survey of the effect of plasma exchange on fulminant hepatic failure

A national survey of patients with fulminant hepatic failure in 1984, revealed that the survival rate of patients treated with plasma exchange was 34.1% (15/45), while that of the patients untreated with plasma exchange was 14.3% (5/35). The difference was statistically significant.

4. Discussion and conclusion

The present therapeutic strategy for treating an acute hepatic failure consists of three essential parts: 1) removal of toxic metabolites; 2) supplementation of hepatic synthetic defects; and 3) management of the complications involving multiorgan systems. Plasma exchange is able to remove all toxins from the patients blood, as well as to supply the necessary substances deficient due to hepatic failure. Thus the supplementation of hepatic synthetic functions was considerably improved, even in fatal cases, by daily repeated plasma exchange. However, purification of substances with a large pool size, such as amino acids and bilirubin, was temporary. Moreover, plasma exchange requires a large amount of fresh plasma which occasionally induces hepatitis and/or allergies, and the detoxication of the patients plasma was insufficient in severe cases. To overcome these problems, specific adsorption [11] of hepatic toxins and a combined therapy of blood purification with plasma exchange will be studied further.

Presently, our hepatic assist device, performing an easy and safe procedure for plasma exchange, appears to be a tool required for such studies as well as for providing the most promising hepatic support for acute liver failure.

References

1. Yamazaki Z, Fujimori Y, Sanjo K, Sugiura M, Wada T, Inoue N, Sakai T, Oda T, Kominami N, Fujisaki U, Kataoka K: New artificial liver support system (plasma perfusion detoxication) for hepatic coma. Artificial Organs 2: 273–276, 1978.
2. Inoue N, Yamazai Z, Oda T, Sugiura M, Wada T, Fujisaki Y, Hayano Y: Treatment of intractable ascites by continuous reinfusion of sterilized, cell-free and concentrated ascitic fluid. Trans Am Soc Inter Organs 23: 698–02, 1977.
3. Yamazaki Z, Inoue N, Wada T, Oda K, Atsumi K, Kataoka K, Fujisaki Y: Use of AR-1 resin column to reduce bilirubinlevel in modified ascitic fluid. Trans Am Soc Inter Organs 25: 480–486, 1979.
4. Inoue N, Yamazaki Z, Yoshiba M, Okada K, Sanjo K, Oda T, Wada T: Membrane plasmapheresis with plasma exchange in treatent of acute liver failure. In: Oda T (ed) Therapeutic plasmapheresis. Schattauer-Verlag, Stuttgart, New York, 1981, pp 57–63.
5. Samtleben W, Blumenstein M, Liebel L, Gurland HJ: Membrane plasma separation for treatment of immunologically mediated diseases. Trans Am Soc Artif Intern Organs 26: 12–16, 1980.
6. Samtleben W, Bensinger VA, Toyka V, Fateh-Moghadam A, Brehm G, Gurland HJ: Plasma separation in myasthenia gravis: new method of rapid plasma exchange. Klin Wschr 58: 47, 1980.
7. Yamazaki Z, Fujimori Y, Iizuka I, Takahama T, Kanai F, Yabe K, Inoue N, Sonoda T, Wada T: Simultaneous plasma collection and exchange between donor dogs and dogs with galactosamine-induced hepatic failure. In: Nose T, Malchensky PS, Smith JW (eds) Plasmapheresis: Therapeutic application and new techniques. Raven Press, New York, 1983, pp 421–425.
8. Yamazaki Z, Iizuka I, Kanai F, Wada T, Idezuki Y, Ichikawa K, Ichikawa H, Inoue N, Fujimori Y, Takahama T, Asano K: Automatic plasma collection by membrane plasmapheresis through single venous blood access. In: Nose Y, Malchensky PS, Smith JW (eds) Therapeutic aphresis a critical look. ISAO Press, Cleveland, 1984, pp 193–196.
9. Lysaght MJ, Samtleben W, Schmidt B, Stoffner D, Gurland HJ: Simultaneous membrane plasmapheresis. Trans Am Soc Artif Inter Organs 29: 506–510, 1983.
10. Yamazaki Z, Takahama T, Fujimori Y, Kanai F, Ohnishi K, Hiraishi M, Idezuki U, Asano K, Inoue N, Morioka M, Kazama M, Abe T, Takenaka Y, Kamata H, Hagiwara T, Umegae M, Fukumi H: Efficiency and biocompatibility of a surfactant-free polyolfin (polyethylene) membrane plasma separator. In: Nose Y, Kjellstrand C, Ivanovich P (eds) Progress in Artificial Organs – 1985. ISAO Press, Cleveland, 1986 (in press).
11. Yamazaki Z, Fujimori Y, Iizuka I, Kanai F, Idezuki Y, Takahama T, Asano K, Takahashi K, Ogita T, Miyamoto Y, Yamawaki N, Yoshizawa H, Inagaki K, Tsuda N: Effect of immunoadsorption on patients with rheumatoid arthritis. Trans Am Soc Artif Intern Organs 30: 216–216, 1984.

Address for offprints:
Z. Yamazaki
2nd Department of Surgery
University of Tokyo
7-3-1 Hongo, Bunkyo-ku
Tokyo 113, Japan

Medical Progress through Technology 12 (1987) 25–38

Patient monitoring during and after open heart surgery by an improved deep body thermometer

Takayuki Tsuji
Institute for Medical and Dental Engineering, Tokyo Medical and Dental University

Key words: deep body thermometer, forehead tissue temperature, sole tissue temperature, patient monitoring, dynamic thermometry

Abstract

The deep body thermometer developed by Fox was improved by Togawa by thermal insulation of the probe. The present status of medical progress in clinical thermometry through the improved deep body thermometer was reviewed from the view point of cardiac surgery.

The forehead and sole temperatures obtained by this improved thermometer were monitored and recorded by a multipotentiometric recorder continuously up to 12 days in the patients admitted to the ICU who underwent open heart surgery. The forehead tissue temperature measured by this thermometer is slightly lower than and parallel to the rectal temperature, being close to the pulmonary arterial blood temperature. On the other hand, the sole tissue temperature fluctuates from room temperature to the forehead tissue temperature, sometimes showing rhythmic changes. The former seems to be the core temperature and the latter, the shell temperature.

The dissociation when the two temperatures are more than 7° C apart from each other suggests that the hemodynamical condition is worse than in the convergence when they remain within 2° C. A state of shock can be diagnosed when the arterial systolic pressure is less than 90 mmHg and the urine output less than 1 ml/min/mg in addition to the dissociation. The effect of treatment and the prognosis for the patient are predictable according to the trends of the two temperatures as divergent or convergent.

The dynamic thermometry by this thermometer is very informative and the procedure is noninvasive without discomfort to the patient.

1. Introduction

The deep body thermometer which is not instantly influenced by an ambient temperature change was developed by Fox and Solman [10, 24] in 1970 for measuring noninvasively the tissue temperature. The present status of medical progress in clinical thermometry through the deep body thermometer is reviewed from the view point of cardiac surgery.

2. The deep body thermometer

2.1 Principle

Deep tissue temperature can be measured from the skin surface noninvasively with a zero heat flow thermometer [32]. This method is based on the assumption that if heat flow across the skin is reduced to zero, skin surface temperature is equilibrated with tissue temperature, thus allowing the latter to be measured at the surface.

Fox and Solman developed the unit which con-

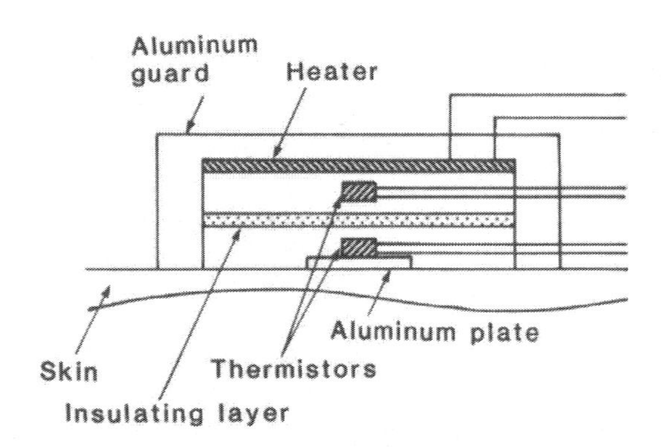

Fig. 1. Schematic diagram of the improved probe of the deep body thermometer.

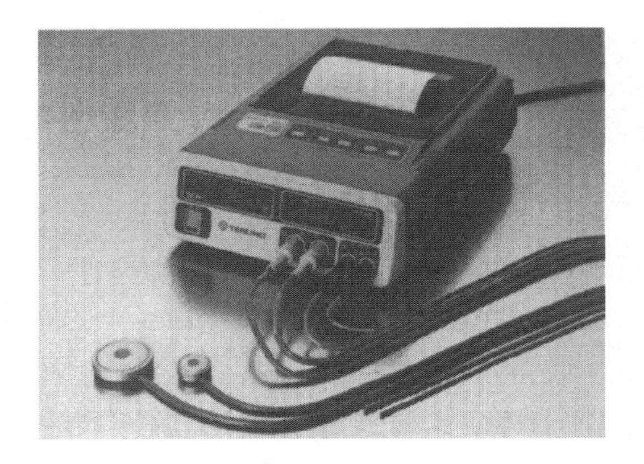

Fig. 2. The deep body thermometer unit (Terumo Corp.).

sists of a probe and the servo-control circuit of the zero heat flow thermometer. A commercial unit has been produced (Deep Body Thermometer Ltd.). The probe of the thermometer is a flat square pad 6 × 6 cm in size. However, its thermal insulation around the peripheral portion is incomplete.

2.2 An improved deep body thermometer

A modified disc probe covered with a thick aluminum guard has been introduced by Togawa [26, 27, 28] to minimize transverse heat flow from the center of the probe to the periphery, as shown schematically in Fig. 1. This modification has been shown to increase the accuracy.

The new probe with the unit equipped with a digital display panel and a multipotentiometric recorder, as shown in Fig. 2 is also commercially available now (Terumo Corp.). We have used this deep body thermometer clinically in cardiac surgery in Japan since 1976 [32, 33, 37] and it has been widely accepted for monitoring patients principally in the intensive care unit (ICU) and operating theater which are air-conditioned at a room temperature of 25° C and a humidity of 60%.

3. Measurement by the deep body thermometer

3.1 Its capability

The disc probe, 4.5 cm in diameter, can measure the deep temperature across a rubber layer 10 mm in thickness with an accuracy of 0.1° C at an ambient temperature of 25° C [28]. Therefore the temperature measured by this probe is the one not in the skin but in the tissue below the skin. The tissue temperature can reflect the tissue blood perfusion while the core temperature, ambient temperature and local heat production remain constant [23, 25] in the patient lying in the supine position.

3.2 Its application to patients

The probe is fixed on the skin surface with adhesive tape as shown in Fig. 3 [35]. It takes about 15 min, depending on the site measured and the ambient temperature, to equilibrate the tissue temperature when the measurement is started. The probe has a thermal switch functioning at 43° C to prevent heat injury to the skin.

Since this method does not cause as much discomfort to the patients as conventional methods [31] which are rectal [20], esophageal [39, 40], and tympanic [4, 5] temperature measurements, the tissue temperature could be recorded up to 12 days

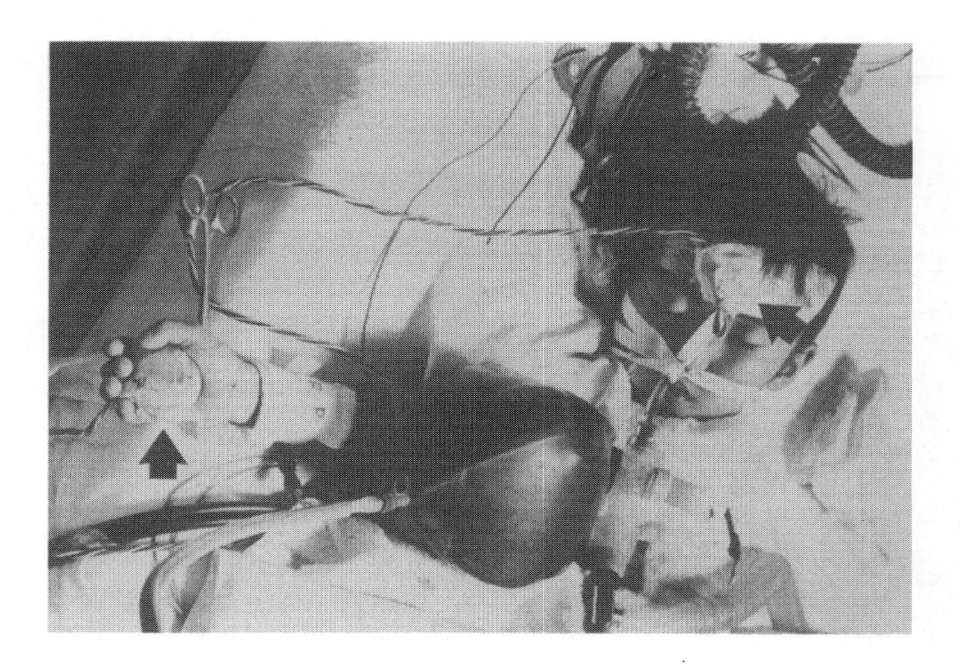

Fig. 3. A patient monitored for forehead and palm tissue temperatures with the improved probes (arrows) in the ICU.

without interruption in a patient in the ICU [29, 30, 34]. However, it constrains the subject near the unit and consumes much electricity because of the zero-heat flow method. If it is improved to become portable, its applicability will be greatly increased.

4. The temperatures measured by the deep body thermometer

4.1 Venous blood temperatures

The temperatures of the venous blood from the head and the liver investigated with a thermistor-mounted catheter in 12 patients during cardiac catheterization were significantly higher than those from the extremities as shown in Table 1 [32]. Therefore the skin surface over the head or abdomen is the proper site for placing the probe for detecting the core temperature.

4.2 Forehead tissue temperature

Many comparative studies of zero heat flow and other conventional temperature measurements have been conducted on the temperatures of various sites of the body [3, 11, 18, 28, 32, 33, 36] as

Table 1. Blood temperatures of blood vessels in various sites (° C).

Internal jugular vein	37.3 ± 0.3	Inferior vena cava (IVC)	37.0 ± 0.3
Axillary vein	36.7 ± 0.4	Hepatic vein	37.3 ± 0.4
Superior vena cava	37.1 ± 0.4	IVC (below kidney)	37.0 ± 0.3
Right atrium	37.1 ± 0.3	Common iliac vein	36.8 ± 0.3
Pulmonary artery	37.1 ± 0.3	External iliac vein	36.6 ± 0.4

Values are means ±SD.

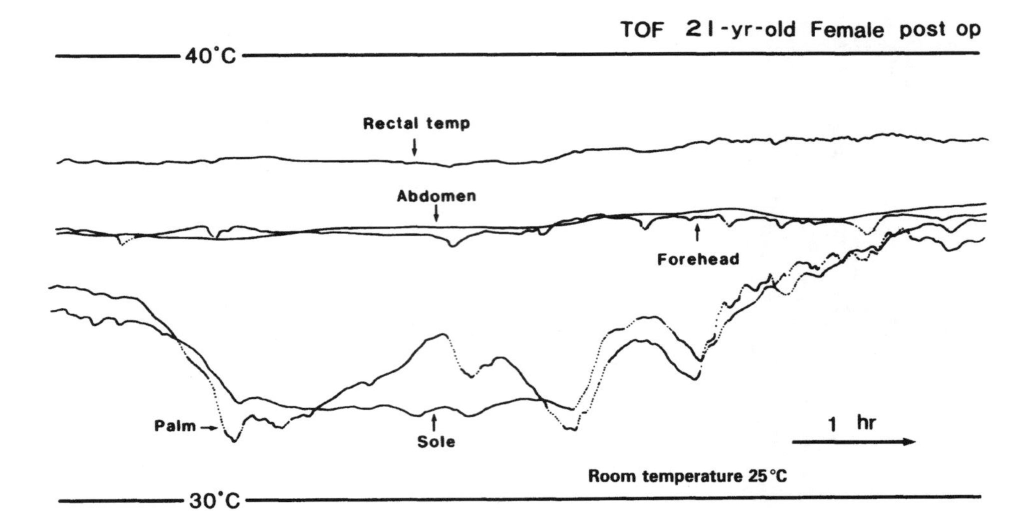

Fig. 4. Postoperative temperature changes in a 21-year-old patient with tetralogy of Fallot (TOF).

shown in Table 2 [30]. The forehead readings with the disc probe, 4.5 cm in diameter, are reported to be close to the pulmonary arterial blood temperature measured with an indwelling Swan-Ganz catheter. Forehead readings are slightly lower than and closely parallel to abdominal readings obtained with the probe 15 cm in diameter and are about 1° C lower than rectal temperature as shown in Fig. 4.

The forehead readings do not seem to vary during defecation while the rectal temperature measurement is interrupted as shown in Fig. 5. The rectal temperature is not restored to the previous value after evacuation suggesting that the rectal temperature is sometimes the accumulated fecal temperature which does not mean the deep body temperature.

During cardiopulmonary bypass in open heart surgery, the forehead tissue temperature (Tf) responded more quickly to the varying blood temperatures in perfusion tubings (Tbpt) than the rectal temperature (Tre) and sole tissue temperature (Ts) as is shown in Fig. 6. The lowest forehead deep temperatures in core cooling were almost the same as the lowest blood temperature in the drainage tubings (Tbdt) in 40 patients with congenital heart disease as is shown in Table 3 [36]. However, the forehead readings obtained with the probe cannot indicate a temperature below room temperature in the patients who have undergone profound hy-

Table 2. Comparison of tissue temperature measurement with the zero-heat-flow probe and by conventional methods.

Measuring site	Temperature reading	No. of cases	Reporters
Over the sternum	0.1 ± 0.4° C below rectal temperature	15	Ball et al. (1973)
Occiput	0.2 ± 0.2° C below rectal temperature	15	Togawa et al. (1976)
Forehead	0.9 ± 0.4° C below rectal temperature	17	Tsuji et al. (1976)
Forehead	0.3 ± 0.3° C below pulmonary arterial blood temperature	7	Tsuji et al. (1976)
Abdomen	0.2 ± 0.2° C below pulmonary temperature (large probe of 100 mm diameter)	22	Tsuji et al. (1976)
Over the biceps	0.14 ± 0.1° C below muscle temperature in exercise	3	Togawa et al. (1976)

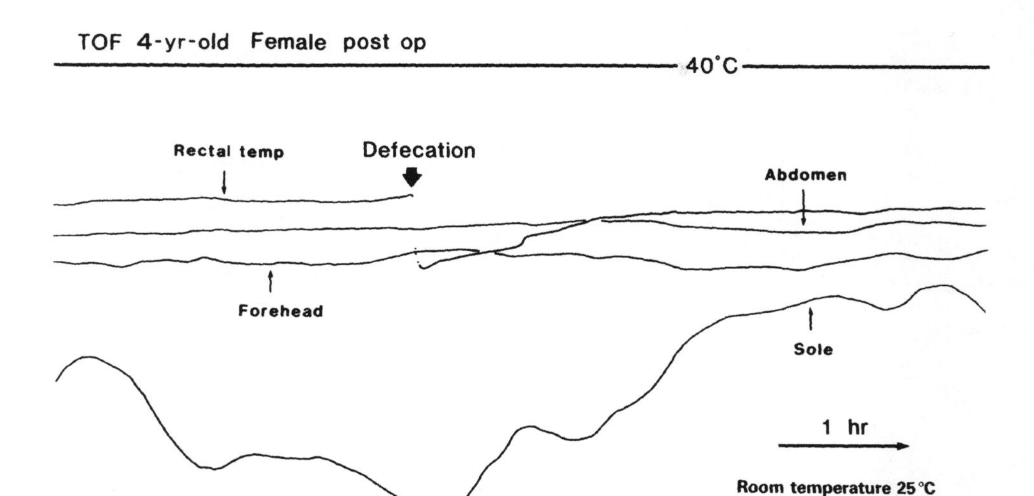

Fig. 5. The rectal temperature changes in defecation. The rectal temperature was decreased after defecation when the forehead tissue temperature remained unchanged.

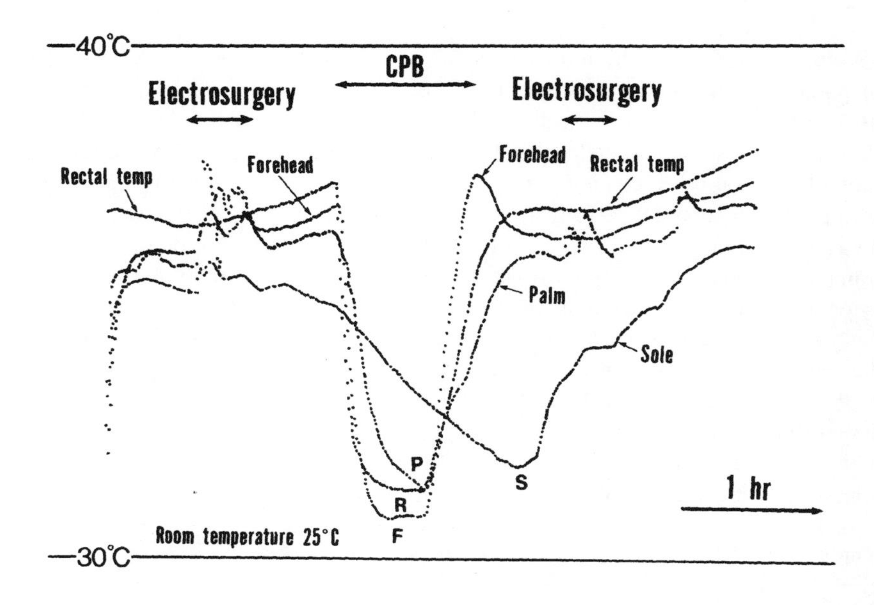

Fig. 6. Temperature changes during cardiopulmonary bypass (CPB). All the temperatures were converging before and after CPB in most cases.

pothermia because the heat flow from the forehead tissue through the probe to the environment cannot take place.

4.3 Sole and palm tissue temperatures

Sole and palm readings indicate lower temperatures than forehead readings and the former fluctuate [7] from close to the forehead temperature to

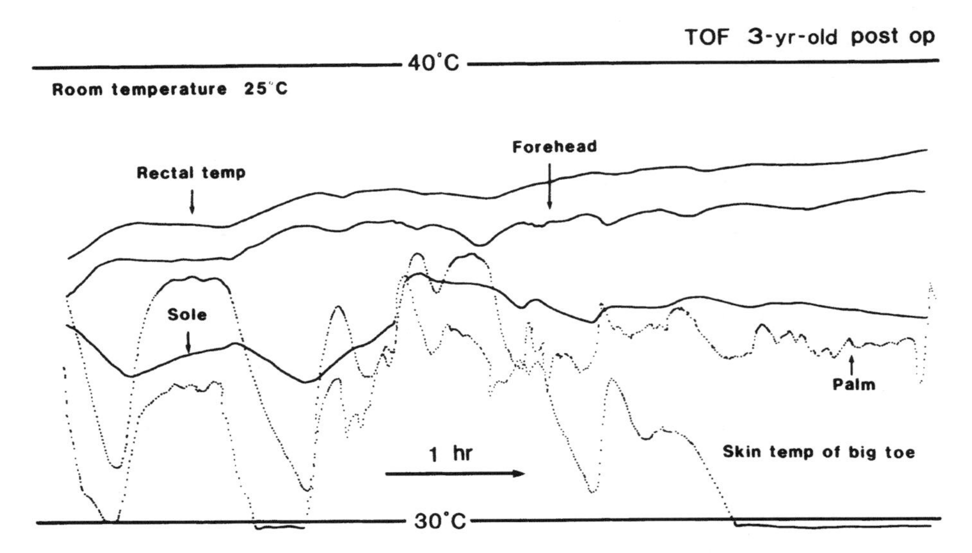

Fig. 7. Tissue temperature changes in the patient in the ICU. The forehead tissue temperature forms a mirror image of the palm and the sole tissue temperatures.

the room temperature. The fluctuation in the recordings of the palm tissue temperature is wider than that of the sole tissue temperature. The direction of rhythmic changes observed in the forehead recordings is completely the reverse of the direction in the palm and the sole recordings. They form a mirror image as is shown in Fig. 7.

A typical example of such recordings is shown in Fig. 8. The temperature differences from the peak to the bottom and vice versa at the marked lines for forehead tissue temperature (Td-f) show a good negative linear correlation (r = 0.99) with that of palm tissue temperature (Td-p) as shown in Fig. 9. This indicates that the palm serves as one of the avenues for arterial heat dissipation [1].

The rhythmic changes in palm recordings frequently observed in infants or in the early phase of sleep are lost in the paralyzed limb. They reappear according to the recovery of the nervous function in a patient suffering from cerebral damage such as an air embolism or hemorrhage. The blood flow in finger skin is known to be very susceptible to sympathetic nervous activity. Palm tissue temperature varies more with the emotional stress than does sole tissue temperature. The former is sometimes reduced to the level of room temperature when the patient is in pain or feels anxiety while the latter is not, and the former shows a quicker response to core cooling and warming than the latter as shown in Fig. 10.

Table 3. Lowest temperatures during cardiopulmonary bypass (°C).

	Tf	Tre	Tbpt	Tbdt
ASD	31.4 ± 0.9	33.0 ± 0.9	30.4 ± 2.1	31.4 ± 1.2
VSD	29.6 ± 1.0	30.8 ± 2.2	28.2 ± 2.0	29.7 ± 2.4
TOF	27.9 ± 1.9	30.9 ± 1.3	27.6 ± 1.6	27.8 ± 1.8

Values are means ±SD.
ASD: Atrial septal defect 15 cases.
VSD: Ventricular septal defect 15 cases.
TOF: Tetralogy of Fallot 20 cases.

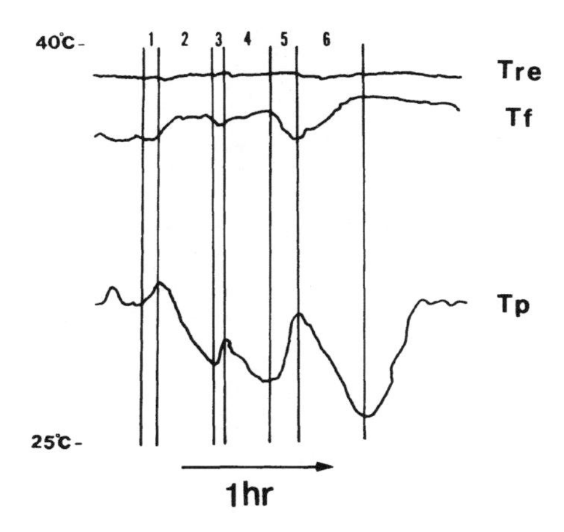

Fig. 8. Postoperative recordings of rectal (Tre), forehead tissue (Tf) and sole tissue (Ts) temperatures in a 5-year-old boy.

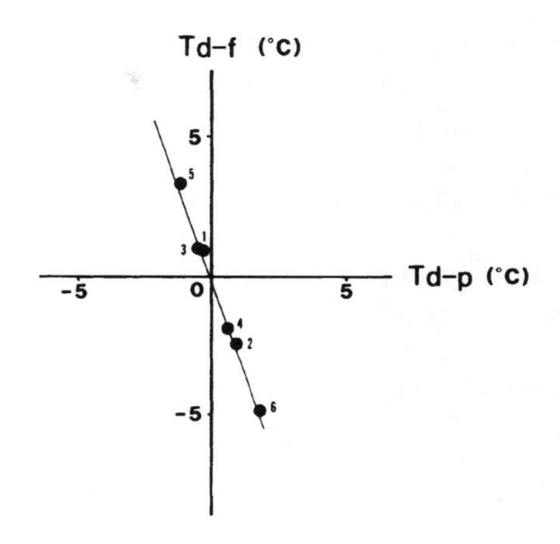

Fig. 9. The relationship between the temperature differences in the forehead (Td-f) and the palm (Td-p) tissue temperatures.

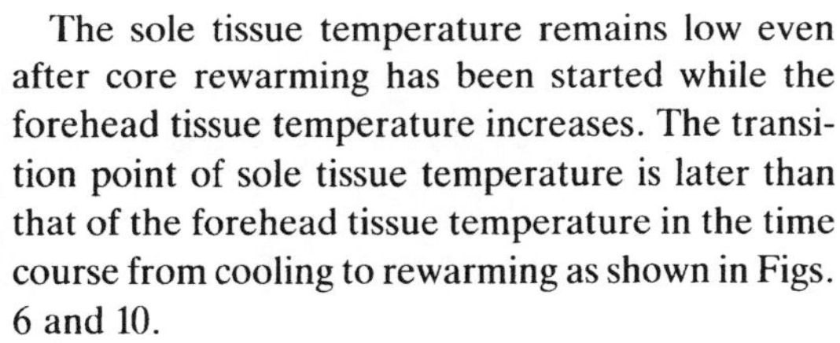

The sole tissue temperature remains low even after core rewarming has been started while the forehead tissue temperature increases. The transition point of sole tissue temperature is later than that of the forehead tissue temperature in the time course from cooling to rewarming as shown in Figs. 6 and 10.

If the artery in the measured side is not stenosed or occluded, the sole tissue temperature is so much more likely to reflect the hemodynamical situation without emotional intervention than the palm tissue temperature that we have been monitoring it as an index of peripheral circulation.

4.4 Core and shell temperatures

As stated above, we can consider that the forehead and the abdominal readings correspond to the core temperature [5], and the sole and the palm readings

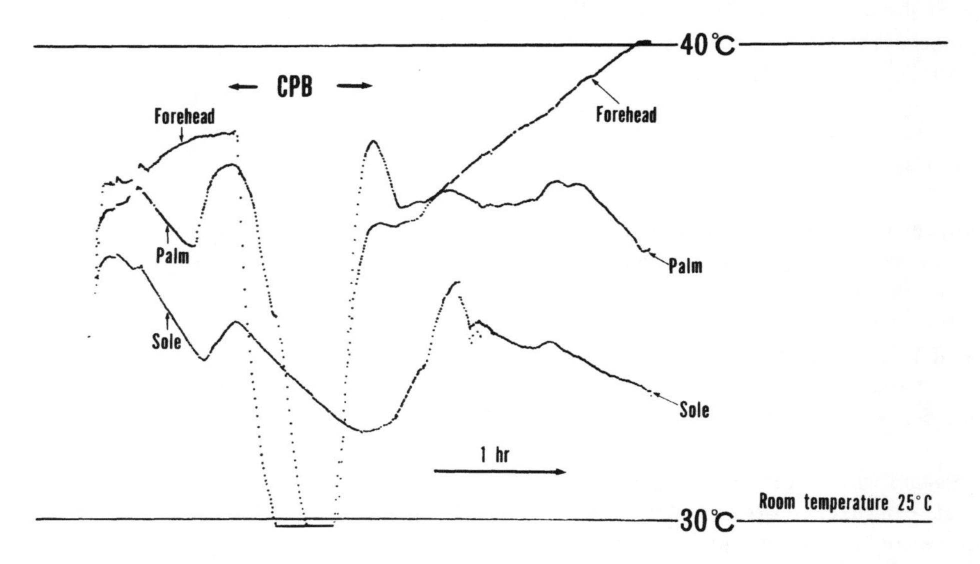

Fig. 10. Temperature changes during CPB. The transition point of the sole tissue temperature is later than that of the forehead tissue temperature when the rewarming is started. The trends of dissociatin were observed before and after CPB in this case.

to the shell temperatures, when the probe of the deep body thermometer is used. The forehead readings with proper fixation of the probe can always indicate the deep body temperature except when the patient is brain dead as will be explained later.

The forehead readings in normothermia might presumably be controlled at 37.0 ± 0.5° C in adults and at 37.5 ± 0.5° C in infants, according to our study [35] in which the forehead and the sole readings were obtained with cardiac output and so on 206 times about every 6 hours during 72 postoperative hours in 32 patients. The sole readings were usually (93%) more than 30° C at the room temperature of 25° C.

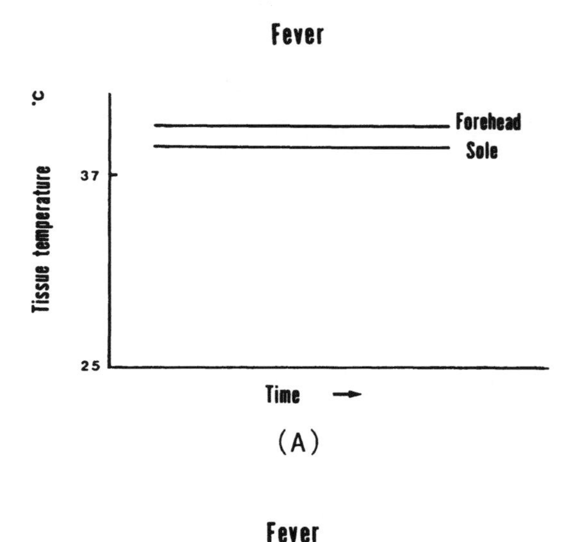

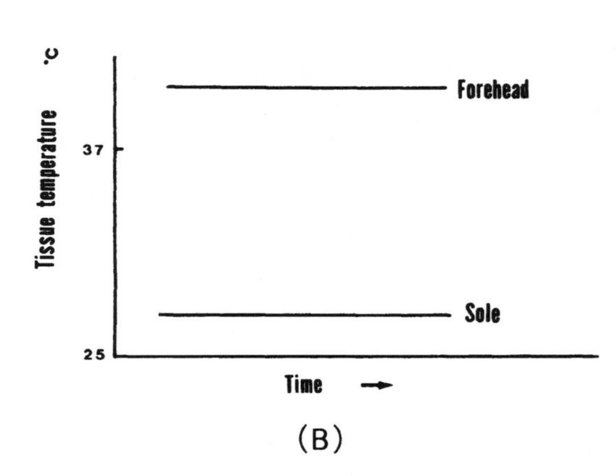

Fig. 11. A schematic diagram of the state of the two tissue temperatures in convergence (A) and dissociation (B).

5. Fever and the deep body thermometer

5.1 Fever monitored by the deep body thermometer

When we touch the forehead or trunk of a patient with fever, it feels hot. However, when we touch the patient's foot at the same time, it can feel either hot or cold. In other words, the sole tissue temperature is either close to the elevated forehead tissue temperature or far apart from it. The two converge in the former case. On the other hand, they diverge in the latter case as shown schematically in the recordings in Fig. 11.

5.2 Fever in convergence

In convergence, the two temperatures are raised together in a narrow range of less than 2° C when the shell is maximally reduced. Rhythmic changes are not observed at that time. This type of fever is common in the postoperative course. The heat dissipation from the body surface is enhanced through a physiological response in hyperthermia induced for any reason. It has to be promoted by removal of bedclothes and with extremities uncovered in the patient not yet awakened from the anesthesia. The treatment is cooling by application of ice-bags to the head and trunk. The sole and the palm tissue temperatures decrease much more than does the forehead tissue temperature by surface cooling applied to the head as shown in Fig. 12.

5.3 Fever in dissociation

In contrast with convergence, the forehead tissue temperature rises to over 38° C while the sole tissue temperature moves in the reverse direction down to the ambient temperature. We call it dissociation when the difference between the two tissue temperatures is more than 7° C. This type of fever was

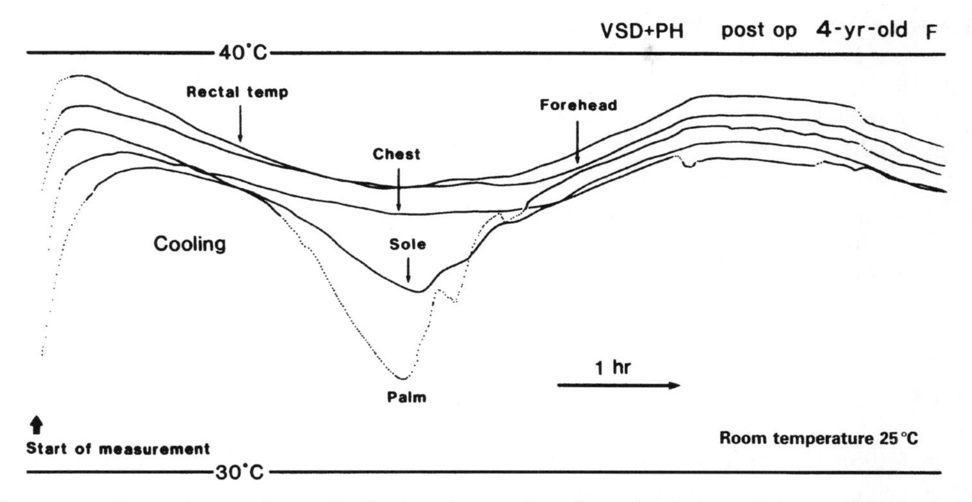

Fig. 12. Temperature changes due to surface cooling for the treatment of fever in a patient with ventricular septal defect associated with pulmonary hypertension.

observed less frequently than that described above.

This fever originates not only in the production of pyrogenic substances [2] but also in markedly depressed heat dissipation. In dissociation, the core temperature seems unable to be adjusted to normal by the shell, which suggests that derangements of homeostasis occur in thermoregulation.

A chilling sensation or shivering are common complaints in the patients with this type of fever. However, the symptom might be easily overlooked in a patient just after open heart surgery because the intubated patient cannot complain of the chilling sensation and shivering does not occur in the patients whose muscles are flaccid owing to residual pharmacological effects in anesthesia. We can detect the masked symptoms early by the trends toward divergence in the recordings.

5.4 Hemodynamics in dissociation

Some hemodynamical parameters are significantly related to the tissue temperature difference between the forehead and the sole (Td-fs). Systolic arterial pressure (APs), cardiac index (CI) and stroke volume index (SVI) were lower and heart rate (HR) was higher when the temperature difference was more than 7° C than when it was less than 7° C in the postoperative patients mentioned above as shown in Table 4 [35]. The systemic pe-

Table 4. Relationships between the forehead and the sole tissue temperature differences and hemodynamic findings.

		$\geqq$ 7°C	< 7°C	P
T_f	(°C)	37.7 ± 0.6	37.4 ± 0.6	<0.05
T_s	(°C)	29.4 ± 1.0	34.9 ± 1.9	<0.001
T_d-f_s	(°C)	8.4 ± 0.8	2.6 ± 1.9	<0.001
HR	(beats/min)	126 ± 21	113 ± 17	<0.01
APs	(mmHg)	113 ± 12	120 ± 16	<0.05
CVP	(cmH_2O)	12 ± 4	12 ± 3	N.S.
CI	(l/min/Øm²)	2.4 ± 0.7	2.8 ± 0.9	<0.05
SVI	(ml/beat/m²)	20 ± 7	32 ± 12	<0.01
SPVR	(PRU)	34 ± 11	32 ± 12	N.S.

Values are means ±SD. N.S., not significant.

ripheral vascular resistance (SPVR) and central venous pressure (CVP) were not related to the temperature difference in our study but those were reported to be related to the temperature difference in other studies [14, 38].

Therefore, the hemodynamical condition in convergence is usually better than that in dissociation. If dissociation is observed in the postoperative patients, the hemodynamical parameters have to be checked.

5.5 Therapy for fever in dissociation

The therapy for this kind of febrile patient is not only surface cooling but also administration of a drug such as indomethacin, a vasodilator, a vasodilator-like drug or a combination of such drugs which promotes heat dissipation from the extremities. Simple surface cooling is insufficient because the shell is widened. The preferential treatment is to widen the core quickly by parenteral administration of drugs. Strong surface cooling should be avoided because it sometimes evokes shivering which changes the patient's condition from serious to very critical.

Surgical hemostasis, drainage of the abscess, mechanical circulatory assistance or mechanical ventilation, respectively should be performed as an emergency in addition to treatment of the fever if the patient has massive bleeding, severe infection, intractable heart failure or respiratory failure.

6. Shock monitoring

6.1 Shock and body temperatures

Methods using differences between big toe skin and ambient temperatures [12, 15, 16, 19], between rectal and big toe skin temperatures [9, 21], and between skin temperatures at two points on the lower limb [22] have been reported for detecting shock but the skin temperatures of the extremities are too sensitive and vary too much with the ambient temperature and emotional stress to be chosen as an index of peripheral circulation.

Marked dissociation between the forehead and the sole tissue temperatures is frequently observed in shock. Both the tissue temperatures at the time of cardiac arrest and the dissociation period preceding cardiac arrest in the patients who died of low cardiac output are shown in Table 5.

6.2 The new criteria of shock

There have been many criteria of shock. We have proposed new criteria for shock based partly on the temperature measured with the deep body ther-

Table 5. Dissociation of the forehead and the sole tissue temperature observed in patients who died of low cardiac output.

Patient	Disease	Age (yr)	Body weight (kg)	Cause of death	POD	Tf (°C)	Ts (°C)	Td-fs (°C)	Dissociation time (hr)
J.N.	ECD+PS	2	10.5	LOS	4	36.4	26.4	10.0	5
Y.O.	TGA	1	8.1	LOS	3	38.1	28.9	9.2	4.5
K.M.	VSD	27	37.5	LOS	1	37.8	30.8	7.0	1.5
S.K.	TOF	21	45.7	LOS	7	35.8	27.1	8.7	8
K.Y.	TOF	4	9.5	LOS	2	37.5	23.6	13.9	6.5
S.E.	ASD	53	37.5	LOS	21	39.8	23.8	16.0	17
A.I.	ECD	1	8	LOS	2	38.5	25.0	13.5	3.5
A.O.	TGA	1	5	LOS	1	37.7	25.1	12.6	3

POD: Postoperative day of death
ECD: Endocardial cushion defect
PS : Pulmonary stenosis
TGA: Transposition of the great vessels
VSD: Ventricular septal defect
TOF: Tetralogy of Fallot
ASD: Atrial septal defect
LOS: Low cardiac output syndrome

mometer. If the following three conditions are observed simultaneously, a state of shock is strongly suspected:

1. Tissue temperature difference between the forehead and the sole measured by the deep body thermometer more than 7° C.
2. Systolic arterial pressure less than 90 mmHg.
3. Urine volume less than 1 ml/kg/hr.

Anti-shock treatment should be started immediately. The trends to convergence or divergence are predictable from the dynamics between two temperatures which is visible on the recording paper. If the treatment is effective, the sole reading rises while the forehead reading decreases and they are approaching each other. On the other hand, the prognosis may be poor when the dissociation is refractory to the treatment as shown in Fig. 13.

Dynamic thermometry by the deep body thermometer unit is useful for judging the effect of the treatment and even for predicting the prognosis for the patient.

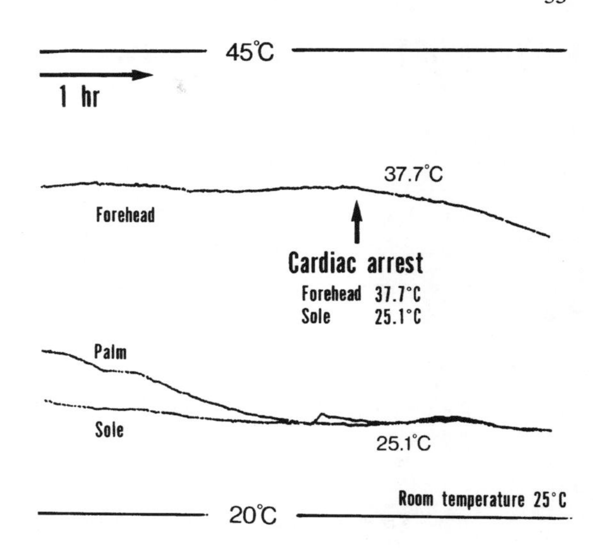

Fig. 13. The dissociation at the time of cardiac arrest. Severe dissociation was observed when the patient died of persisting low cardiac output.

6.3 Limit of this method

This method is informative in that it can give us guide lines for treating the patient but it is sometimes confusing, as described below.

The principle of the method for shock detection through interacting dynamics between the forehead and the sole tissue temperature recordings is the estimation of peripheral circulation controlled mainly by the vasoactive nerve which is stimulated before the shock. Therefore we cannot predict by this method sudden death from arrhythmia or massive hemorrhage from a ruptured ventricle and so on because such a catastrophe is not accompanied by the prodromal dissociation as shown in Fig. 14.

We have to be careful in monitoring the patient administered a strong alpha blocker. Dissociation cannot be observed even in a patient obviously dying of low cardiac output who was administered phenoxybenzamine [8]. On the other hand, dissociation is observed very frequently in the immediate postoperative period in patients who have undergone myocardial revascularizaton surgery even though there is no evidence of circulatory failure [17]. Vasoaction paralyzed by the drug is thought to be the cause in the former case and peripheral vasoconstriction through the sympathoadrenal response evoked by the surgical relief of myocardial ischemia [13] in the latter case. That is why the diagnosis of shock should be made according to the criteria proposed above.

7. Diagnosis of brain death with a deep body thermometer

Convergence of core and shell temperatures is commonly seen in unconscious patients without circulatory failure. However, when the forehead readings which are higher than the sole readings become reversed and lowered more than 2° C below the sole readings by application of ice-bags under and around the head, the patient can be diagnosed as brain dead. Cerebral angiography shows nonfilling in the intracranial region at the time the patient is diagnosed as brain dead from the recordings shown in Fig. 15. This method using the improved deep body thermometer is unique and simple for diagnosis of brain death.

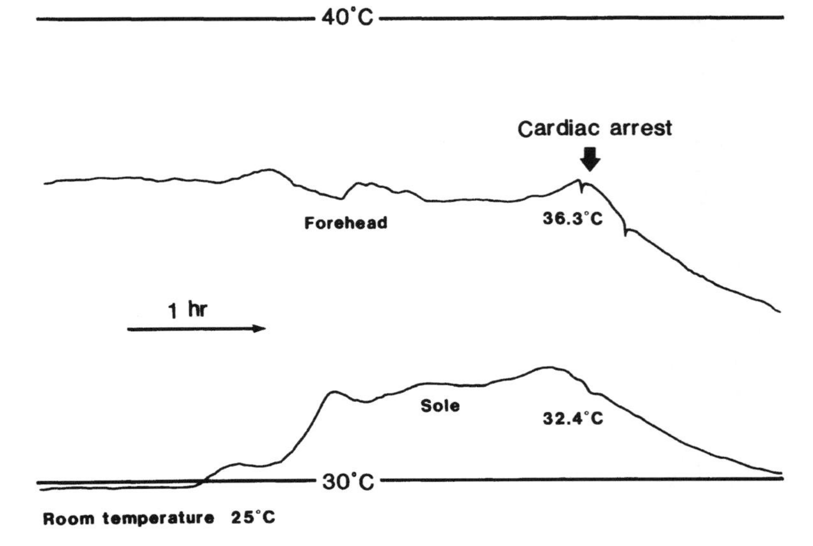

Fig. 14. Dynamics of forehead and sole tissue temperatures in the patient without preceding low cardiac output. Dissociation was not observed in the patient who died of sudden massive hemorrhage because of detachment of the pericardial patch sutured to the right ventricle when she coughed strongly just after extubation.

8. Safety of the measurements

Measurement by the probe is very safe except for occasional complication by contact dermatitis in long-term monitoring. However, reddening of the forehead skin where the aluminum plate for detection of skin temperature is attached was observed in some patients who underwent profound hypothermia by core cooling. Measurements of the tissue temperature which is below room temperature is impossible by this method. Therefore forehead tissue temperature monitoring should be avoided during profound hypothermia.

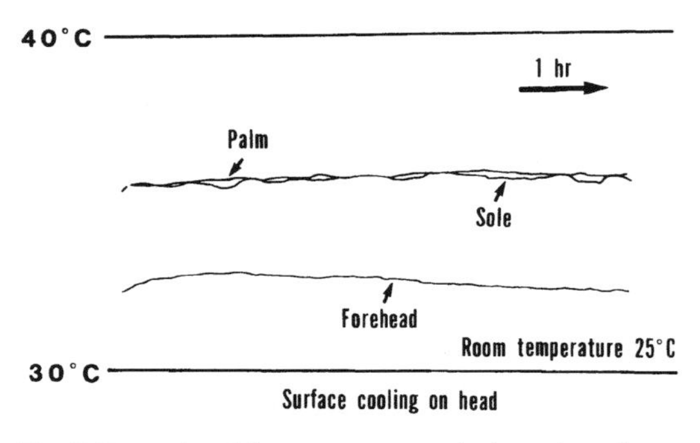

Fig. 15. Dynamics of tissue temperatures in the patient who was brain dead. Lowering of the forehead tissue temperature below the sole temperature during local cooling to the head was observed in the unconscious patient because of cerebral hemorrhage.

9. Conclusion

Continuability of body temperature measurement which can be realized by noninvasive methods is very important. In the improved deep body thermometer, the probe can measure deep body temperature in the forehead and the abdominal tissue. The method gives us information about the patient's circulatory condition through dynamics between the forehead and the sole tissue temperatures with contrasting characteristics, by long-term measurement and recording.

It makes possible easy monitoring of the patient's body temperature and early detection of shock in postoperative patients after open heart surgery with minimum discomfort and maximum safety to the patient.

References

1. Aulick LH, Robinson S, Tzankoff SP: Arm and leg intravascular temperatures of men during submaximal exercise. J Appl Physiol: Respirat Environ Exercise Physiol 51: 1092–1097, 1981.
2. Atkins E, Bodel P: Fever. New Eng J Med 286: 27–34, 1972.
3. Ball SG, Chalmers DMcM, Morgan AG, Solman AJ, Losowsky MS: A critical appraisal of transcutaneous deep body temperature. Biomedicine 18: 290–294, 1973.
4. Benzinger M: Tympanic thermometry in surgery and anesthesia. JAMA 209: 1207–1211, 1969.
5. Benzinger TH: Heat regulation: Homeostasis of central temperature in man. Physiol Rev 49: 671–759, 1969.
6. Benzinger TH: Clinical temperature, new physiological basis. JAMA 209: 1200–1206, 1969.
7. Burton AC, Taylor RM: A study of the adjustment of peripheral vascular tone to the requirements of the regulation of the body temperature. Am J Physiol 129: 565–577, 1940.
8. Eckenhoff JE, Cooperman LH: The clinical application of phenoxybenzamine in shock and vasoconstrictive states. Surg Gynecol Obstet 121: 483–490, 1965.
9. Everhart RC, Trezek GJ: Central and peripheral rewarming patterns in postoperative cardiac patients. Crit Care Med 1: 239–251, 1973.
10. Fox RH, Solman AJ: A new technique for monitoring the deep body temperature in man from the intact skin surface. J Physiol 212: 8–10, 1970.
11. Fox RH, Solman AJ, Fry AJ, MacDonald IC: A new method for monitoring deep body temperature from the skin surfae. Clin Sci 44: 81–86, 1973.
12. Henning RJ, Wiener F, Valdes S, Weil MH: Measurement of toe temperature for assessing the severityof acute circulatory failure. Surg Gynecol Obstet 149: 1–7, 1979.
13. Hoar PF, Hickey RF, Ullypt DJ: Systemic hypertension following myocardial revascularization. A method of treatment using epidural anesthesia. J Thorac Cardiovasc Surg 71: 859–864, 1976.
14. Honda T, Kahata O, Ohmi M, Haneda K, Tabayashi K, Hamada Y, Yokoyama A, Satoh N, Koizumi S, Kagawa Y, Mohri H, Horiuchi T: Measurments of the deep body temperature and hemodynamic changes after open heart surgery. Nippon Kyobu Geka Gakkai Zasshi 27: 148–154, 1979.
15. Ibsen B: Treatment of shock with vasodilators measuring skin temperature on the big toe, ten years' experience in 150 cases. Diseases of the chest 52: 425–429, 1967.
16. Joly HR, Weil MH: Temperature of the great toe as an indication of the severity of shock. Circulation 34: 131–138, 1969.
17. Kawamura T, Itaoka T, Nakata S, Wada J: Measurement of deep body temperature difference after open heart surgery: Correlations with hemodynamics, endogenous catecholamine and renin activity. Nippon Kyobu Geka Gakkai Zasshi 29: 211–217, 1981.
18. Lee DE, Kim YD, MacNamara TE: Noninvasive determination of core temperature during anesthesia. South Med J 75: 1322–1324, 1980.
19. Matthews HR, Meade JB, Evans CC: Peripheral vasoconstriction after open-heart surgery. Thorax 29: 338–342, 1974.
20. Molnar GW, Read RC: Studies during open-heart surgery on the special characteristics of rectal temperature. J App Physiol 36: 333–336, 1974.
21. Ross BA, Borck L, Aynsley-Green A: Observations on central and peripheral temperatures in the understanding and management of shock. Brit J Surg 56: 877–882, 1969.
22. Seki S, Fujii H, Itano T, Murakami T, Teramoto S, Sunada T: Regional changes of skin temperature in the leg after open-heart surgery, their significance in relation to prognosis. J Thorac Cardiovasc Surg 68: 411–418, 1974.
23. Shindo G, Ide H, Miyawaki F, Kotuka Y, Saitou H, Asano K: New thermal parameter for quantitative analysis of the deep body temperature in cases of open heart surgery. Kyobu Geka 38: 24–28, 1985.
24. Solman AJ, Dalton JCP: New thermometers for deep tissue temperature. Biomed Eng 8: 432–434, 1973.
25. Tamura T, Nemoto T, Kamiya A, Togawa T, Tanaka M, Kawakami K: Estimation of regional blood flow from deep tissue temperature. Reports of Institute for Medical & Dental Engineering 13: 27–37, 1979.
26. Togawa T, Nemoto T: Medical thermometer making use of zero-heat-flow method. Reports of Institute for Medical & Dental Engineering 7: 75–83, 1973.
27. Togawa T, Nemoto T, Kobayashi T: An experimental analysis of characteristics of the deep body thermometer. Jap J Med Biol Engng 11: 414–417, 1973.
28. Togawa T, Nemoto T, Yamazaki T, Kobayashi T: A modified internal temperature measurement device. Med Biol Engng 14: 361–364, 1976.
29. Togawa T: Non-invasive deep body temperature measurement. In: Rolf P (ed) Non-invasive physiological Measurement, Vol. 1. Academic Press, London, 1979, p 261–277.
30. Togawa T, Nemoto T, Tsuji T, Suma K: Deep temperature monitoring in intensive care. Resuscitation 7: 53–57, 1979.
31. Togawa T: Body temperature measurement. Clin Phys Physiol Meas 6: 83–108, 1985.
32. Tsuji T, Suma K, Togawa T, Nemoto T: Deep body temperature monitoring in cardiac surgery. Jap J Med Biol Engng 14: 220–224, 1976.
33. Tsuji T, Nakajima K, Takeuchi Y, Inoue K, Shiroma K, Yamaguchi T, Koyama Y, Suma K, Togawa T, Nemoto T: Dynamic thermometry by deep body thermometer in man. The Autonomic Nervous System 13: 220–225, 1976.
34. Tsuji T: Circulatory monitoring in cardiac surgery using deep body thermometry. The Autonomic Nervous System 18: 1–11, 1981.
35. Tsuji T, Suma K, Takeuchi Y, Inoue K, Shiroma K, Koyama Y, Narumi J, Yoshikawa T, Ito N, Kobayashi H, Nakajima K, Iwabuchi K: The forehead and sole temperature monitoring with deep body thermometer in cardiac surgery. Nippon Kyobu Geka Gakkai Zasshi 29: 1029–1035, 1981.

36. Tsuji T, Ooe Y, Iwabuchi K, Togawa T, Tamura T, Nemoto T, Toyoshima T, Kaneko H, Suma K: Changes in forehead and sole deep temperature during cardiopulmonary bypass for congenital heart diseases. Masui 33: 532–539, 1984.
37. Yasuura K, Nishiya Y, Hashimoto A, Hayashi H, Konno S: An application of the deep body thermometry to cardiac patients. Bulletin of the Heart Institute, Japan, 1975–1976: 30–36, 1976.
38. Watanabe T, Shimizu T, Abe T, Iyomasa Y: Care of patients during open heart surgery with deep body thermometry – The criteria of poor peripheral circulation. Nippon Kyobu Geka Gakkai Zasshi 29: 1907–1912, 1981.
39. Webb GE: Comparison of esophageal and typanic temperature monitoring during cardiopulmonary bypass. Anesth Analg 52: 729–733, 1973.
40. Whitby LD, Dunkin LJ: Temperature difference in the oesophagus, The effect of intubation and ventilation. Brit J Anesth 41: 615–618, 1969.

Address for offprints:
Takayuki Tsuji
2-3-10 Kanda Surugadai Chiyodaku
Tokyo 101, Japan

Medical Progress through Technology 12 (1987) 39–50

The development of artificial endocrine pancreas

From bedside-, wearable-type to implantable one

Motoaki Shichiri, Ryuzo Kawamori & Yoshimitsu Yamasaki
First Department of Medicine, Osaka University Medical School, 1-1-50 Fukushima, Fukushima-ku, Osaka 553, Japan

Key words: artificial endocrine pancreas; bedside-type artificial endocrine pancreas; wearable-type artificial endocrine pancreas; implantable artificial endocrine pancreas; needle-type glucose sensor; closed-loop control system

Abstract

The artificial endocrine pancreas is a feedback controlled instrument regulating insulin delivery on a minute-by-minute basis according to measured blood glucose levels. It has been proven to be useful not only as the therapeutic tool of diabetes mellitus but also as an elegant research tool for investigating the pathophysiology of the disease.

The wearable type of closed-loop system has been developed recently for the first time by the authors. The breakthrough is the establishment of needle-type glucose sensor.

The trend in development of closed-loop glycemic control system which enables perfectly physiological regulation on long-term basis, is directed to implantable devices. Much efforts have been conducted now to realize these devices.

1. Introduction

The discovery of insulin in 1921 allowed the successful treatment of the acute manifestation of diabetes. But replacement therapy by intermediate-acting insulin injection once a day for diabetics was revealed to be ineffective to normalize the blood glucose concentration, especially in the postprandial period. Thus, high glucose levels in diabetics seem to result in the onset or progress of chronic complications such as retinopathy, nephropathy or neuropathy.

Recently, with introduction of the computer, new techniques for elaborating the measurement, communication and operation to achieve the adaptive blood glucose control have been developed. The earliest external device which achieved this goal was a feedback controlled instrument which regulated insulin on a minute-by-minute basis according to the measured blood glucose levels and their rate of change. This bedside-type of device has been known as the first artificial 'closed-loop' system to function as a living organ [1, 4, 6].

Clinical applications of this bedside-type artificial endocrine pancreas succeeded in normalizing daily glycemic profiles of diabetics. However, to extend the duration of glycemic control with the system, a new approach is required. We have developed a needle-type glucose sensor which is exchangeable and indwellable directly in the subcutaneous tissue. At the present time it works as long as three days. The wearable artificial endocrine pancreas which incorporated a needle-type glucose sensor as a monitoring device could extend the period of glycemic control in diabetics.

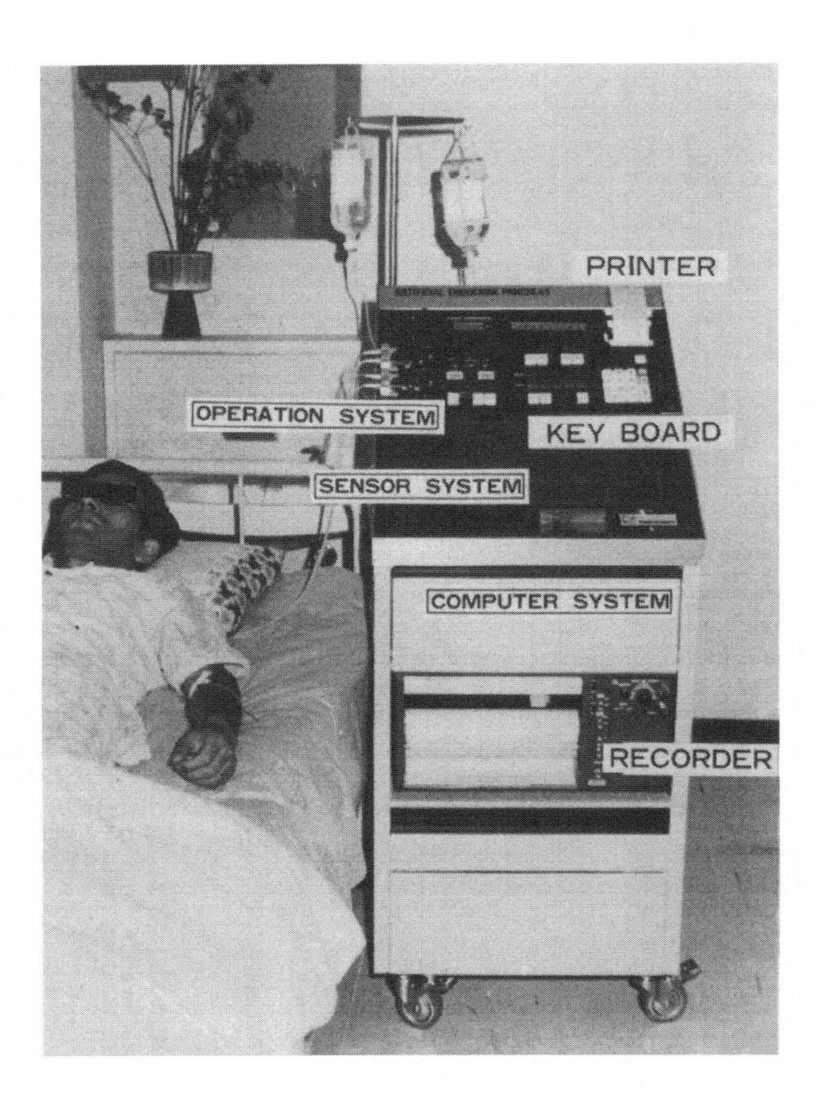

Fig. 1. Bedside-type artificial endocrine pancreas.

2. Bedside-type artificial endocrine pancreas

2.1 Principle of the system

The artificial endocrine pancreas is a device composed of a sensor, a computer and a set of pumps. These components are connected in such a way as to form a closed-loop for the subjects. The system which we have originally developed is shown in Fig. 1. By means of an indwelling dual-lumen catheter, venous blood is drawn into an analyzer modified for continuous blood glucose measurement. The computer receives the electrical signals generated by the glucose analyzer and interprets these in accordance with its internal algorithms which are programmed with specific parameters. In turn the computer instructs one pump to delivery insulin, the amount varying according to the level of the blood glucose and its rate of change. Similarly, glucose or glucagon may be admin-

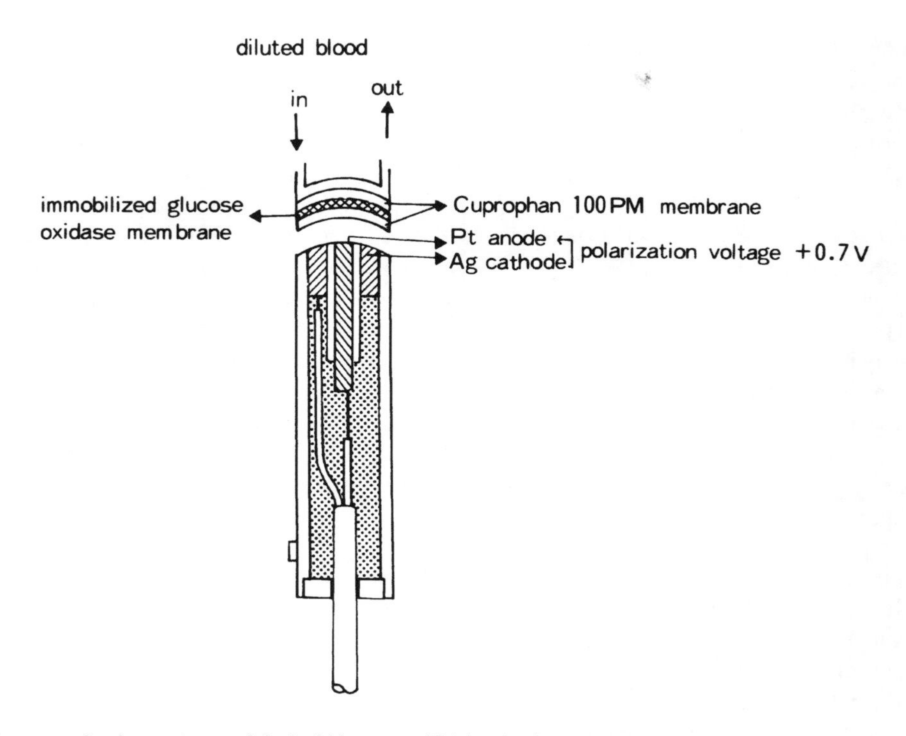

Fig. 2. Structure of a glucose sensor of the bedside-type artificial endocrine pancreas.

istered by another pump in a counter-regulatory manner when hypoglycemia tends to occur.

2.2 Glucose sensor

In our first artificial endocrine pancreas system, continuous glucose measurement had been conducted with a Technicon AutoAnalyzer II using a modification of the glucose oxidase method [4, 9]. But to minimize the blood sampling volume and to make the whole system smaller, a glucose sensor for continuous glucose monitoring in the whole blood has been developed by combining glucose oxidase membrane with an electrode which measures hydrogen peroxide, one of the reaction products, polarographically. Because a key component of a low noise blood glucose sensor with long-term stability is its membrane, hydrophilic Cuprophan 100PM with the pore size of 30 Å, was applied to cover the immobilized glucose oxidase (Fig. 2).

2.3 Computer algorithm for blood glucose control

For the closed-loop regulation of the blood glucose in a diabetic subject a set of relationships is needed to translate information from the glucose sensor into rate of delivery of two agents: insulin if the glycemia is too high and glucose (glucagon) if it is too low.

2.3.1 Insulin infusion algorithm for mimicking insulin secretory dynamics
Mathematical control theory was applied to derive a relationship between glucose levels and insulin secretion. It is well known that biphasic responses of insulin secretion resulted from glucose stimulation was assumed to correspond to the rate of change in glycemia (derivative action), while the second phase or slow rise in insulin secretion was assumed to correspond to the absolute glucose concentration (the proportional action). This relationship could be simulated by using a transfer function with a first order delay in both proportional and

derivative actions. With these considerations, the insulin infusion rates are determined from measured blood glucose concentrations. The details in computer algorithm are described in the previous papers [1,4, 6].

2.3.2 Self-adaptive control algorithm for compensating insulin sensitivity changes

Even though the insulin secretory dynamics of healthy subjects is accomplished in diabetics whose insulin sensitivity is low or super-normal, it is obliged to change the parameters deciding insulin infusion rates for the adaptive control of blood glucose manually. So, a computer algorithm for self-adaptive control is established. Firstly, under the blood glucose regulation with artificial endocrine pancreas, the real rate of change in blood glucose concentration in each subject is calculated and the difference between this and the projected rate of change in blood glucose concentration is assumed to be the index of insulin sensitivity. Secondly, according to the calculated insulin sensitivity, the computer automatically changes the parameters which regulate the insulin infusion rate [7].

2.3.3 Glucose infusion algorithm

A counterregulatory system might be useful and safe for the prevention of hypoglycemia caused by the increased endogenous insulin secretion and the change in insulin sensitivity which are frequently observed during insulin treatment with the artificial endocrine pancreas in diabetics. In glucose infusion algorithm, glucose is infused on the basis of proportional and derivative actions to blood glucose concentration with the time delay constant between blood withdrawal and initiation of glucose infusion [20].

2.4 Clinical results

Normalization of the blood glucose profiles in an insulin-dependent diabetic subject was attempted. The artificial endocrine pancreas enabled the perfect blood glucose and plasma insulin profiles seen in healthy subjects [8, 13]. Two important characteristics of the system recognized in clinical applications are; 1) the rate of insulin infusion is small enough to keep the plasma concentration of insulin physiological; then insulin requirements are reduced compared with those given subcutaneously; ii) glucose or glucagon to rectify hypoglycemia is not essential because the negative derivative mode of blood glucose concentration reduces the insulin infusion rate during the decline of the blood glucose, and hypoglycemia does not result.

The treatments of diabetic coma and ketoacidosis have been explored by the artificial endocrine pancreas with the self-adaptive control algorithm. Return of blood glucose to the normal range had been achieved more rapidly and with smaller quantities of insulin than by the conventional regimens. It is also demonstrated that diabetic ketosis and ketoacidosis are insulin resistant and that serial blood glucose measurements are obligatory to quantify the resistance and to decide treatment regimen.

3. Needle-type glucose sensor

3.1 Principle of the measurement

In the presence of glucose and oxygen, the glucose oxidase used in enzymatic glucose sensors catalyzes the oxidation of glucose and produces gluconic acid and hydrogen peroxide.Because physiological concentration of oxygen in blood or tissue fluid is much lower [2] than the Km values of the enzyme [3], not only glucose concentration but also oxygen tension may regulate the rate of glucose oxidation. Therefore, when a glucose sensor is implanted, output of the sensor might be non-linearly proportional to glucose concentration. In order to solve this problem, a membrane which is more permeable to oxygen than to glucose is useful [5, 21], which limits delivery of glucose to the enzyme layer of the sensor. Thus, output of the sensor with such a membrane shows the linearity on the wide range of glucose concentrations and insensitivity to fluctuation of oxygen tension.

Concerning the host response to a sensor, the size and surface configurations of the intracorporeal device are other important points. Wood-

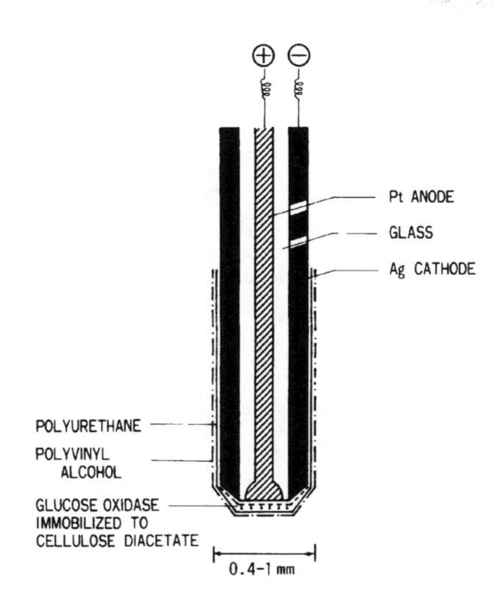

Fig. 3. Structure of a needle-type glucose sensor.

ward [19] suggested that if the sensor could be fabricated in the form of a wire or filament measuring less than about 2 mm in diameter, a minimal host response would be evoked. Therefore, a miniature needle shape is one of the ideal designs for an indwelling glucose sensor rather than a disc shape.

3.2 Preparation of a needle-type glucose sensor

The principle arrangement in a needle-type glucose sensor is shown in Fig. 3. The method for preparing the sensor is mentioned in detail in previous papers [14, 15].

3.3 In vitro characteristics

A needle-type glucose sensor loaded with polarizing voltage of +0.6V is connected to the current-voltage converting amplifier (POG-200A, Unique Medical Co., Ltd., Japan), which amplifies current of one nA to voltage of 100 mV. A pen recorder (VP6621A, Matsushita Communication Industrial Co., Ltd., Japan) is connected to the amplifier to record sensor outputs.

The in vitro characteristics of the sensor are tested in 0.9% NaCl solution containing 7% bovine albumin (Fraction V, Miles, USA) with varying glucose concentrations in a temperature-, flow rate-, and oxygen tension-controllable chamber. The output current of the sensor is calibrated initially after a stabilization period of at least 10 min. Table 1 summarized the in vitro characteristics of the needle-type glucose sensor.

3.4 In vivo characteristics

A glucose sensor is inserted by means of an indwelling needle (gauge #18) into the jugular vein or subcutaneous tissue of healthy and diabetic dogs, or into subcutaneous tissue of the forearm in healthy and diabetic volunteers. The sensor output is compared with blood glucose concentrations si-

Table 1. Characteristics of the needle-type glucose sensor in vitro.

Test	Performance
residual current	1.3 ± 0.6%
baseline drift	0.8%/24hr
noise range	0.3 ± 0.4%
output current generated to 100 mg/100 ml of glucose concentration	1.2 ± 0.4 nA
signal-to-noise ratio	15.8 ± 2.6 decibels
dose-response pattern to glucose concentration (range of a linear function)	0–500 mg/100 ml
T90%	16.2 ± 6.2 sec
temperature coefficient	2.3 ± 1.0%/C
oxygen tension dependency	0.15%/mmHg (25–150 mmHg) 78.0 ± 17.2% (15 mmHg)

Residual current, baseline drift, noise range and temperature coefficient are expressed as percentage of the output current to the solution containing 0.9% NaCl, 7% albumin, 100 mg/100 ml of glucose and 5% oxygen tension (38 mmHg, 37 C).
Residual current denotes the output current of the electrode in the absence of glucose, noise range; the deviation of output current, T90%; the response time to reach 90% of the final plateau value. Output current in response to oxygen tension is expressed as percentage of that of an oxygen tension of 38 mmHg. Results are shown in mean ± SD of 15 sensors examined.

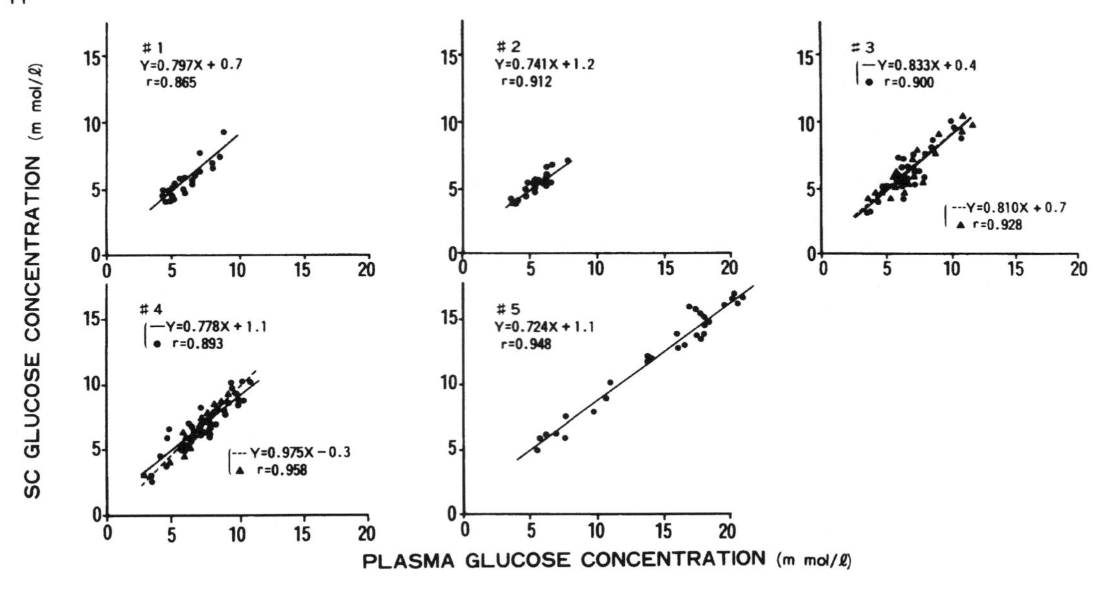

Fig. 4. The relationship between glucose concentration determined by needle-type glucose sensor inserted into subcutaneous tissue and blood glucose concentration determined by a bedside-type artificial endocrine pancreas in five diabetic subjects.

multaneously measured by a bedside–type artificial endocrine pancreas system [8, 13].

The outputs of the sensor when kept in the jugular vein of dogs (Y) was related to the results of intravenous glucose monitoring by the bedside-type of artificial endocrine pancreas system (X) ($Y = 0.98X + 2$, $r = 0.998$, $n = 92$). In each diabetic subject, a high correlation between the glucose concentrations obtained by the needle-type glucose sensors in subcutaneous tissue (Y) and the blood glucose concentrations (X) determined by the bedside-type monitoring system was observed (Fig. 14) [17].

In order to examine changes of the characteristics of sensors inserted into subcutaneous tissue of healthy subjects during continuous monitoring, both relative output current and relative response time of the sensor are determined as follows: Relative output of the sensor kept in subcutaneous tissue for 3 days is calculated by comparing the sensor's outputs with simultaneously measured blood glucose levels. Relative response time of the sensor is calculated from the time lag between the rise in blood glucose and the rise in sensor's output after meal-intake. After three days, the relative sensor output decreased to 73.5% of the initial level and the relative response time increased up to 13.5 min [16]. In vitro characteristics of the sensor determined after removal showed a 23% reduction in output current and a 14 sec delay in response (Table 2).

Scanning electron-microscopic examinations were carried out on glucose sensors kept in subcutaneous tissue of normal dogs for 3, 7, and 14 days. Fig. 5 shows one example of the scanning electron-microscopic examinations on the membrane of the sensor. After a 3-day continuous use in the subcutaneous tissue, a slight fixation of protein was observed but small pits were kept on the surface of the membrane. After seven and fourteen days of continuous use, the membrane was heavily coated with protein and also small pits on the surface were not observed. However, in these situations, fixation of fibroblasts and giant cells was not demonstrated on the surface.

Histologic changes in subcutaneous tissue around the sensor insertion area were examined on normal dogs. After a 3-day application, migration of leukocytes and slight fibrin deposition was recognized in the insertion area.

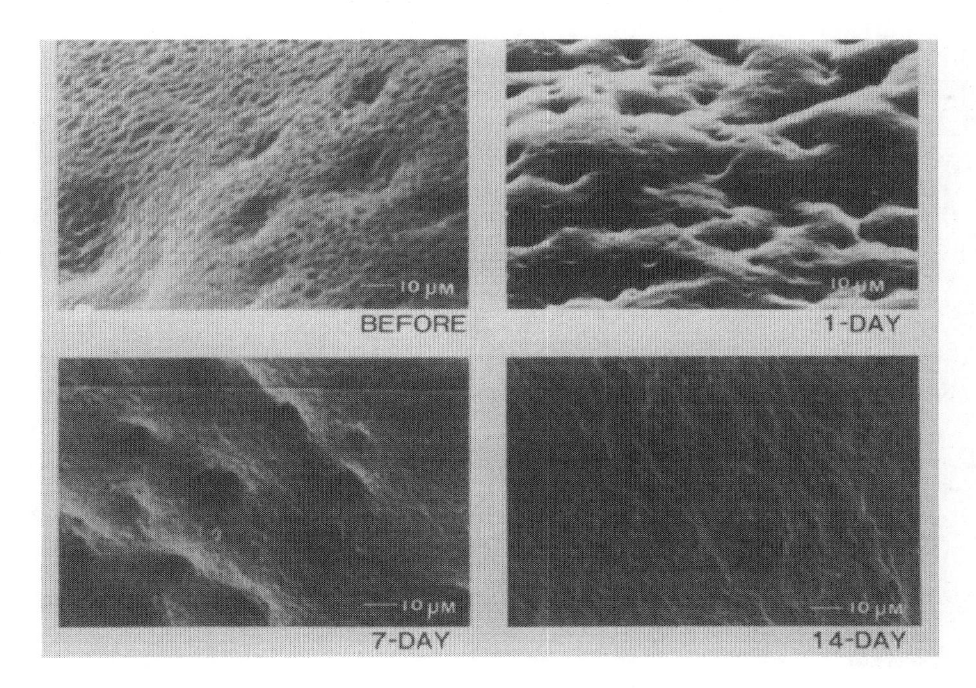

Fig. 5. Scanning electron-mícroscopic examinations on glucose sensors kept in subcutaneous tissue of normal dogs before or after 3, 7, and 14 days of implantation.

4. Wearable artificial endocrine pancreas

4.1 System

A needle-type glucose sensor preserves sensor characteristics suitable to apply in a closed-loop control system and allows wearability at the same time. Thus, the author developed a wearable artificial endocrine pancreas, which consists of a needle-type glucose sensor, a micro-computer system, 2 syringe delivery units for insulin and glucagon infusions, and lithium batteries. Total system was packed into a small unit (12 × 15 × 6 cm) weighing 400 g (Fig. 6) [14, 15].

Table 2. 'Relative' output current and 'relative' response time of sensors inserted into subcutaneous tissue during continuous monitoring.

In vitro characteristics	before application	3-day after
residual current (nA)	1.0 ± 0.4	1.4 ± 1.2
output current generated to 100 mg/100 ml of glucose (nA)	2.2 ± 0.5	1.7 ± 0.1
T90% (sec)	29 ± 6	43 ± 6
In vivo characteristics	**just after application**	**3-day after**
'relative' output current generated to 100 mg/100 ml of glucose (%)	100	74 ± 3
'relative' response time to blood glucose (min)	5.1 ± 2.2	13.5 ± 1.5

Results are shown as mean ± SD (n=5).
'Relative' current output of the sensor kept in subcutaneous tissue for 3 days is calculated by comparing the sensors' outputs against blood glucose concentrations just before application with that after 3-day use.

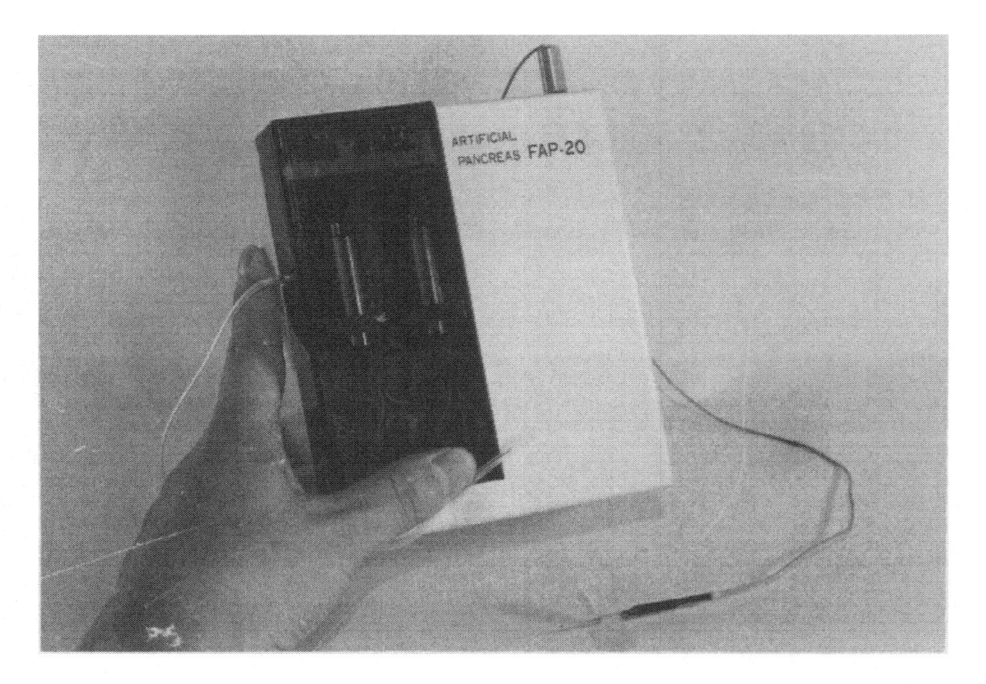

Fig. 6. Wearable artificial endocrine pancreas.

4.2 Computer algorithm for wearable artificial endocrine pancreas

4.2.1 Insulin and glucagon infusion algorithm
Intravenous insulin and glucagon infusion algorithms in this system are the same as those of a bedside-type [8, 13].

4.2.2 Noise reduction filter
Output current generated by a glucose sensor is so small that even tiny noises can disturb the output. Thus, hardware and software noise filters are built in the system. Because the sensor's signal is a direct current, low and high path filters are effective in eliminating noises of low and high frequency waves as a hardware noise filter. As a software noise filter, a computer algorithm has several program steps for noise reduction, such as follows; computer calculates an average of ten samples of output current fetched every ten microseconds and computer rejects new data which has deviation from the 1-min previous one greater than the pre-fixed threshold.

4.3 Closed-loop glycemic control with wearable artificial endocrine pancreas

The glycemic controls in insulin dependent diabetic patients with the wearable artificial endocrine pancreas were attempted. The sensor was replaced with a new one after 3 days' use. Obtained glycemic controls were compared in each patient with those by intensified multiple insulin injection regimens and continuous subcutaneous insulin infusion therapy. The typical glycemic controls for six days in an insulin dependent diabetic patient is depicted in Fig. 7. In all patients studied, physiological glycemic regulations were established [16]. Indices of daily glycemic excursions such as MBG (mean blood glucose), M-value [10], and MAGE [11] were improved significantly in diabetics controlled by the wearable artificial endocrine pancreas, compared with the patients treated with the conventional insulin therapy, multiple insulin injections therapy, and continuous subcutaneous insulin infusion therapy.

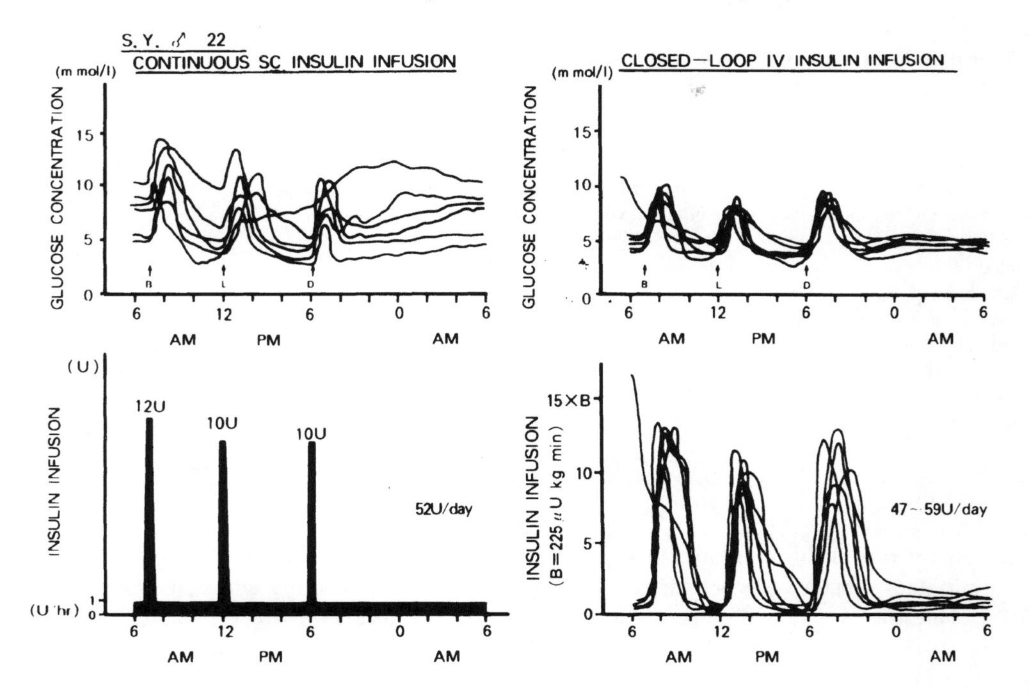

Fig. 7. A 6-day continuous glycemic control in an insulin-dependent diabetic patient with a wearable artificial endocrine pancreas and with continuous subcutaneous insulin infusion.

5. Toward implantable artificial endocrine pancreas

The trend in development of an artificial endocrine pancreas is now from bedside-type to wearable and even implantable ones. However, there still remain many problems to be solved in each part of the device. Technologies derived in the process of the development of various implantable artificial organs will be very beneficial for the accomplishment of long-term clinical applications of the device.

Problems awaiting solution in glucose sensor, processor and effector are listed in Table 3, 4, 5, respectively.

5.1 Problems awaiting solution in long-term clinical application of glucose sensor (Table 3)

It is of no doubt that the most crucial point regulating the system on a long-term basis is the stability of sensor characteristics. So far, many enzyme sensors measure hydrogen peroxide produced in the enzymatic reaction with a platinum electrode. Since these electrodes consume oxygen for enzymatic reaction, low oxygen tension in sensor-inserted area affects sensor outputs. In order to solve this problem, Williams et al. [18] used quinone in place of oxygen as an electron mediator. Using glucose oxidase trapped in a porous or jelled layer and covered with a dialysis membrane over a platinum electrode, glucose could be determined by monitoring the electrode oxidation of quinone. Unfortunately, about 3–10 min was required to obtain a steady state current so far.

The other factor affecting the sensor output is temperature. In order to compensate the dependency of the sensor outputs on the temperature, the addition of a micro-thermistor will be beneficial.

Since glucose sensor detects ultra-small amounts in current change, noises generated from the wire or electricity may interfere with the measurement.

Table 3. Long-term clinical application of glucose sensor: Problems awaiting solution.

1. maintenance of excellent sensor characteristics
   dependency on oxygen tension – application of electron-mediator
   dependency on temperature – development of self-calibration system for temperature change
2. noise elimination – development of noise filter system
3. longevity
   selection of biomaterials – membrane design
   development of automatic internal calibration system
4. interface between the living organism and sensor preservation of natural environment
   safety of immobilized enzyme
   immunological response to biomaterials
5. light and small system – development of FET enzyme sensor
6. noninvasiveness for measurement
7. low-cost

To reduce these noises, a membrane is applied which permits the transfer of hydrogen peroxide and at the same time restricts the penetration of other charged substances. The shortage or elimination of wired electric circuits may be effective in reducing the current induction by electric charges.

More intensive investigations would be necessary on membrane design for glucose sensors. The sensor detects the substance in the tissue which has a narrow range of its concentration. And the tissue fluid contains some substances which interfere the sensors' outputs. Therefore, a membrane which shows semipermeability against various substances should be sought for the specifiity in measurement.

Most electrochemical sensors for glucose are amperometric, which means that the electrical signals are derived from a Faradayic reaction. On the other hand, a chemically sensitive field effect transistor (FET) is a potentiometric device. If this mismatch could be solved then the benefit would be a device simultaneously sensor and amplifier. Small size, sterilizability, and high signal-to-noise ratio make FET attractive for those applications. The main problems that remain to be solved are biocompatibility, long-term stability, and electrical safety. For in vivo glucose sensing, an ion-selective FET employing glucose dehydrogenase and pH sensing would have a higher probability of success than other devices.

5.2 Problems awaiting solution in processor (Table 4)

In case of implantation of a closed-loop device, insulin infusion route is one of the subjects of controversy. To investigate the glycemic regulating property of intraportally-infused insulin, we exam-

Table 4. Implantation of processor: Problems awaiting solution.

1. Substantiality in soft-ware
   1) analysis in controllability of portally-infused insulin
   2) monitoring of individuals' glycemic regulatory ability and its adaptive control – development of self-adaptive control algorithm
   3) safety of the system
      fool-proof, fail-safe system
      noise elimination – noise filter system

2. Substantiality in hard-ware
   1) small-size – application of one-chip microcomputer
   2) improvement in system design for preservation of natural environment

ined the effects of portal and peripheral venous administration of insulin on glycemic responses as well as glucose fluxes during iv glucose loads in depancreatized dogs. As a result, with intraportal insulin infusion, the smaller gain in glucose regulation was observed. In other words, to establish physiological glycemic responses the range in insulin doses required was a twice large as peripheral insulin infusion. In addition, the role of the liver in glucose handling was also revealed to be more dominant. Thus, the clinical significance of intraportal insulin delivery on glucose regulation was demonstrated.

As described previously, during glycemic regulations in diabetics by closed-loop control system, sensitivity of subject to exogenous insulin varied on moment-to-moment basis. Therefore, if the parameters for insulin infusion algorithms are fixed, unexpected hypo- and hyper-glycemias may happen due to the mismatch of insulin delivery to its demand. The self-adaptive control algorithm which contains glucose-insulin regulatory mechanism for evaluating the suitable parameters for hormone infusion on moment-to-moment basis should be developed.

Since during the application of closed-loop regulatory system false glycemic changes induced by the sensor's noises modifies insulin infusion rates, it is obligatory to eliminate noises by both hard- and soft-ware basis. A hard-ware noise filter is effective in reducing the electrical noises and soft-ware one reduces the noises passed through the hard-ware noise filter and noise-drift. Band path filter which is designed to cut-off the excessive change of glycemia is one of the candidates of such soft-ware noise filter system.

5.3 Problems awaiting solutions – implantation of effector (Table 5)

For implantation of the whole system a small but powerful, long-life battery is required. A transcutaneous energy transmission (TET) system which inductively couples energy between a superficial primary coil of wire and an implanted secondary coil of wire separated by an unbroken layer of skin [12], would be one of the candidates of those attempts.

Since highly concentrated insulin solutions (100–500 U/ml) have to be used in the small insulin reservoir, insulin aggregation forming an insulin plug in the pump system should be avoided. Stable and biologically active insulin solutions are now under investigation.

Obviously, the nearest future will require concentration on continuous improvement of the presently available technologies, and a totally implantable artificial endocrine pancreas will be realized. At this time point, it should not be necessary to transplant all these parts of the apparatus intracorporeally. It would be adequate to implant the computer and infusion pumps, and the glucose sensor extracorporeally would regulate insulin infusion rates by telemetric means.

6. Conclusion

The successful glycemic control in human diabetics with the artificial pancreas underlined the importance of continuous glycemic monitoring on strict glycemic control. However, the major obstacle for extending the term of glycemic control on human

Table 5. Implantation of effector: Problems awaiting solution.

1. maintenance of excellent operation ability and endurance	
2. security control	– introduction of fool-proof, fail-safe system
3. light-weight, small-size	
4. long-life battery	– application of transcutaneous energy transmission to recharge battery
5. interface between the living organism and the artificial system, preservation of the natural environment	
	system design
	the selection of biocompatible
	biomaterials
6. insulin solution	– development of nonaggregatable highly concentrated insulin solution

diabetics is the development of an implantable glucose sensor with high precision in tissue glucose determination.

A needle-type glucose sensor, which is a miniature hydrogen peroxide electrode covered by membrane with biological activities, can be easily implanted and exchangeable. The sensor has the in vitro and in vivo characteristics suitable for continuous tissue glucose monitoring.

Wearable artificial endocrine pancreas, which incorporates a needle-type glucose sensor, has been devised and has regulated glycemia physiologically in human diabetics for more than six days.

Further improvements in sensor design especially in membranes with biocompatibility might reduce the host reactions to the sensor implanted in tissue and thus extend its biological long-life.

References

1. Albisser AM, Leibel BS, Ewart TG, Davidovac Z, Botz CK, Zingg W, Schipper H, Gander R: Clinical control of diabetes by the artificial pancreas. Diabetes 23: 397–404, 1974.
2. Bartlett D Jr, Tenney SM: Tissue gas tensions in experimental anemia. J Appl Physiol 18: 734–8, 1963.
3. Gibson QH, Swoboda BEP, Massey V: Kinetics and mechanism of action of glucose oxidase. J Biol Chem 239: 3927–34, 1964.
4. Goriya Y, Kawamori R, Shichiri M, Abe H: The development of an artificial beta cell system and its validation in depancreatized dogs: The physiological restoration of blood glucose homeostasis. Med Prog Technol 6: 99–108, 1979.
5. Ikeda S, Sawafa Y, Mino K, Ishida M, Ito K, Ichikawa K, Yukawa M, Ichihashi H, Kondo T: Improvement of membranes for glucose sensor. Jpn J Artif Organ 11: 992–5, 1982.
6. Kawamori R, Shichiri M, Goriya Y, Yamasaki Y, Shigeta Y, Abe H: Importance of insulin secretion based on the rate of change in blood glucose concentration in glucose tolerance, assessed by the artificial beta cell. Acta Endocrinol 87: 339–51, 1978.
7. Kawamori R, Shichiri M, Kikuchi M, Yamasaki Y, Abe H: Perfect normalization of excessive glucagon responses to intravenous arginine in human diabetes mellitus with the artificial beta cell. Diabetes 29: 762–765, 1980.
8. Kawamori R, Yamasaki Y, Murata T, Morishima T, Yagi T, Goriya Y, Shichiri M, Abe H: Validation of self-adaptive control algorithm for blood glucose concentration in artificial beta cell. Automedica 3: 183–9, 1980.
9. Pfeiffer EF, Thum Ch, Clemens AH: The artificial beta-cell: A continuous control of blood sugar by external regulation of insulin infusion (glucose controlled insulin infusion system). Horm Metab Res 6: 339–42, 1974.
10. Schlichtkrull J, Munk O, Jersild M: The M-value, an index of blood-sugar control in diabetes. Acta Med Scand 177: 95–102, 1965.
11. Service FJ, Molnar GD, Rosevear JW, Ackerman E, Gatewood LC, Taylor WF: Mean amplitude of glycemic excursions, a measure of diabetic instability. Diabetes 19: 644–755, 1970.
12. Sherman C, Delay BDT, Clay W, Desse K: In vivo evaluations of transcutaneous energy transmission (TET) system. Trans Am Soc Artif Intern Organs 30: 143–50, 1984.
13. Shichiri M, Kawamori R, Abe H: Normalization of paradoxic secretion of glucagon in diabetics who were controlled by the artificial beta cell. Diabetes 28: 272–5, 1979.
14. Shichiri M, Kawamori R, Yamasaki Y, Hakui N, Abe H: Wearable-type artificial endocrine pancreas with needle-type glucose sensor. Lancet 2: 1129–31, 1982.
15. Shichiri M, Kawamori R, Goriya Y, Yamasaki Y, Hakui N, Asakawa N, Abe H: Glycaemic control in pancreatectomized dogs with a wearable artificial endocrine pancreas. Diabetologia 24: 179–84, 1983.
16. Shichiri M, Kawamori R, Hakui N, Yamasaki Y, Abe H: Closed-loop glycemic control with a wearable artificial endocrine pancreas – Validations in daily insulin requirements to glycemic response. Diabetes 33: 1200–1202, 1984.
17. Shichiri M, Asakawa N, Yamasaki Y, Kawamori R, Abe H: Telemetry Glucose monitoring device with needle-type glucose sensor: A useful tool for blood glucose monitoring in diabetic individuals. Diabetes Care 9: 298–301, 1986.
18. Williams D, Doig A, Korosi A: Electrochemical enzymatic analysis of blood glucose and lactate. Anal Chem 42: 118–21, 1970.
19. Woodward SC: How fibroblasts and giant cells encapsulate implants: Considerations in design of glucose sensors. Diabetes Care 5: 278–281, 1982.
20. Yamasaki Y, Shichiri M, Kawamori R, Goriya Y, Sasai T, Morishima T, Nomura M, Tohdo R, Abe H: Counter-regulatory system in an artificial endocrine pancreas – Glucose infusion algorithm. Artif Organs 3: 265–70, 1979.
21. Yamasaki Y: The development of a needle-type glucose sensor for wearable artificial endocrine pancreas. Med J Osaka Univ 35: 25–34, 1984.

Address for offprints:
Dr. M. Shichiri
First Department of Medicine
Osaka University Medical School
1-1-50 Fukushima, Fukushima-ku
Osaka 553, Japan

Medical Progress through Technology 12 (1987) 51–63

Functional electrical stimulation for the control of the upper extremities

Yasunobu Handa[1] & Nozomu Hoshimiya[2]
[1] *Dept. of Anatomy, Shinshu University School of Medicine, Matsumoto 390;* [2] *Research Institute of Applied Electricity, Hokkaido University, Sapporo 060, Japan*

Key words: functional electrical stimulation, upper extremity, quadriplegia, microcomputer, percutaneous electrode

Abstract

A multi-channel functional electrical stimulation (FES) system for the restoration of hand function of the quadriplegic is described. The system is composed of a personal computer NEC PC-8801mkII, peripheral electronic circuits and two kinds of sensors, i.e. an analog displacement sensor for volitional control (channel 1) and a logical sensor (high pitch sound or head switch, channel 2). Combination of the two channel signals allow three major function: 1) designation of the desired prehension pattern among cylindrical grasp, key grip and parallel extension grip; 2) selection of the operation status – 'start', 'proportional control', 'hold', 'stop' – and, 3) volitional control which can be controlled by the shoulder movement. In the clinical application, Caldwell-Reswick type multistrand stainless steel percutaneous electrodes were used. In this FES system, standard multi-channel stimulation patterns were obtained from electromyographical analysis of joint movement of the upper extremities in normal subjects which gave us precise information about a role of each muscle during various kinds of motion. Such stimulation patterns have enabled us to restore motor function of the paralyzed upper extremities for activities of daily living (ADL).

Abbreviations: ECRB: Extensor carpi radialis brevis; FPL: Flexor pollicis longus; FCU: Flexor carpi ulnaris; FDP: Flexor digitorum profundus; FDS: Flexor digitorum superficialis; ED: Extensor digitorum; 1DI: 1st dorsal interosseus; AdD: Adductor pollicis; OpP: Opponens pollicis; AbPB: Abductor pollicis brevis; FPB: Flexor pollicis brevis; EPB: Extensor pollicis brevis; Med: Median nerve; PQ: Pronator quadratus.

1. Introduction

Functional electrical stimulation (FES) to the paralyzed extemities caused by spinal cord injury or cerebrovascular disorders has been investigated to restore their motor function. Especially, FES systems for gait assistance of the stroke patient have already been commercially available. Much work has also been carried out on electrically-induced locomotion in paraplegic patients [2, 4, 5, 13, 19–22, 24]. As compared with the lower extremity FES, studies on restoration of upper extremity function by FES remained less advanced because of functional complexity of the upper extremities and of limitation of residual function as sources for control commands in the quadriplegic. However, recent advances in computer technology as well as in biomedical research have enabled us to overcome such difficulty. A multi-channel FES computer system can simultaneously control many muscles of the hand and arm with a greater degree of freedom. Peckham and his associates have been developing FES system for the paralyzed hand in C5 or C6 quadriplegics [1, 16–18]. They succeeded to restore functional prehension and release for practical usage by using intramuscular electrodes which were percutaneously implanted to the intrinsic and extrinsic hand muscles. Volitional control of the paralyzed hand was obtained by two dimensional movements of the shoulder. Nathan has proposed a closed loop FES computer system controlled by voice commands. Activation of hand muscles was provided by surface electrode arrays arranged in the vicinity of the motor points of these muscles [15].

Our research group has also been working on a FES system for the paralyzed upper extremities in the quadriplegic [6–10, 12, 14, 15]. In our computerized FES system, standard multi-channel stimulation patterns were obtained from electromyographical analysis of joint movements of the upper extremities in normal subjects which gave us precise information about role of each muscle during various kinds of motion. Stimulating data obtained by adding threshold and maximum stimulating voltages to the standard stimulation patterns have provided the patient to execute precise, reliable and well-coordinated movements of the paralyzed upper extremities. This allowed us to fabricate a versatile and sophisticated FES system for the patient with impaired upper motorneurons.

2. Principle of the functional electrical stimulation (FES).

2.1 Electrode

In general, following three types of electrodes have been utilized in the FES application: 1) surface electrode; 2) percutaneous wire electrode; 3) implanted cuff or wire electrode [5, 23, 24]. For the restoration of hand function, Caldwell-Reswick type multistrand percutaneous wire electrodes have been used [1, 6–10, 12, 14, 16, 17] in order to realize fine control of the individual muscles. An example of the electrode which we have utilized is shown in Fig. 1. The electrode was a helical coil wound from a teflon-insulated seven strand stainless steel wire (type 316, A-M Systems Co.). The outermost diameter of the coil was about 0.7 mm,

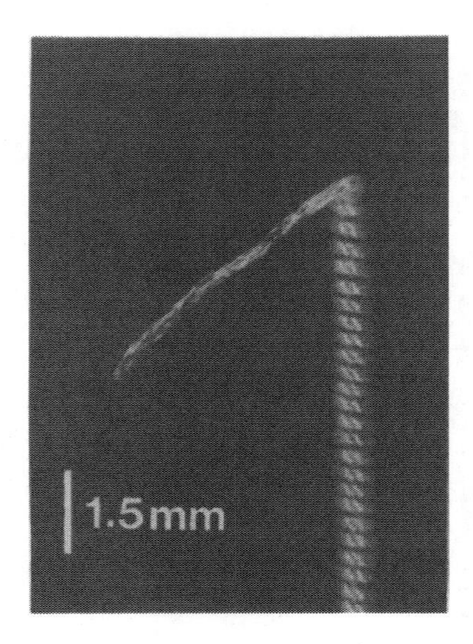

Fig. 1. Multistrand stainless steel percutaneous electrode.

and the tip of the electrode was deinsulated for applying the stimulus to the neuromuscular systems. There has been no serious problem during long term implantation in the forearm of the quadriplegics (more than 4 years).

2.2 Stimulation method

Basic design principle of our FES system is illustrated in Fig. 2. As shown here, this system itself is an open-loop system. As a total system including a user (a patient), however, auditory and/or visual information is utilized for feedback control.

For the stimulation to the neuromuscular system, the voltage pulse train has been utilized. Methods for controlling force of electrically-induced muscle contraction are categorized into AM (amplitude modulation), PWM (pulse width modulation) and FM (frequency modulation). In the case of AM or PWM, an increase in amplitude or pulse width increases the number of the excited motor units (the recruitment characteristics), thus resulting in an increase in muscle force. Fig. 3 (a) shows the relationship between pulse width and amplitude for stimulation and resulting contractile force of the extensor digitorum in a C5 quadriplegic. The contractile force increased non-lin-

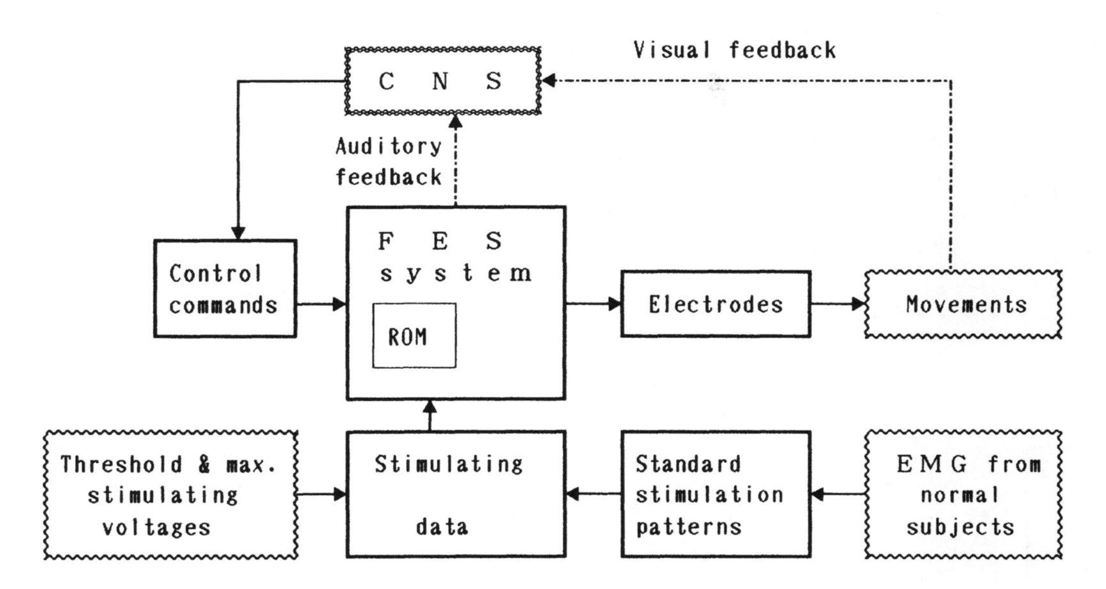

Fig. 2. Principle of our FES system.

early with an increase in stimulus pulse width or amplitude, and reached plateau when the pulse width or amplitude exceeded more than 0.06 ms or 2 volts, respectively. Fig. 3 (b) shows the relationship between stimulus frequency and resulting contractile force when the stimulus pulse width was fixed at 0.2 ms. Although an increase in the frequency caused an increase in the contractile force, it resulted in a time-dependent decrease in the contractile force. In addition, vibratory contraction appeared at lower frequencies of stimulation below 15 Hz. For these reasons, FM method has not been used for the control of the paralyzed upper extremities in our FES system.

The authors, therefore, have utilized AM pulse trains with the following parameters: pulse duration = 0.2 ms, pulse frequency = 20 Hz. Although stimulus amplitude depended on the distance between an active eletrode and a nerve to be stimulated, the maximum output voltage was set at −15 volts. The load impedance of this stimulator system ranged from 0.8 to 1.2 kohms.

In the AM method, it is very important to realize the smooth recruitment characteristics for practical use of FES, so that the non-linearity mentioned above is disadvantageous to proportional control of the movements by the patient. Crago et al. have proposed to include the inverse function of the non-linear curve as an element of the modulator [3]. It has been known that closed loop feedback can also improve the non-linearity. In addition, authors reported that coactivation of the antagonistic muscles linearized the non-linear curve of agonists [10]. Electromyographical analysis in normal subjects revealed that not only synergists but also antagonists cocontracted with agonists during motion of the upper extremities. For this reason, we have adopted standard stimulation patterns determined from the EMG analysis in our open loop FES system. This method has enabled the patient to realize the proportional control more easily.

One important factor is that the average current of the stimulation should be nearly zero to guarantee the charge equality for the stimulation waveforms. Otherwise, irreversible electrochemical changes are produced at the electrode-tissue interface, which vary the electro-physiological excitability of the neuromuscular system. A coupling capacitor or isolation transformer is introduced in the circuit for this purpose.

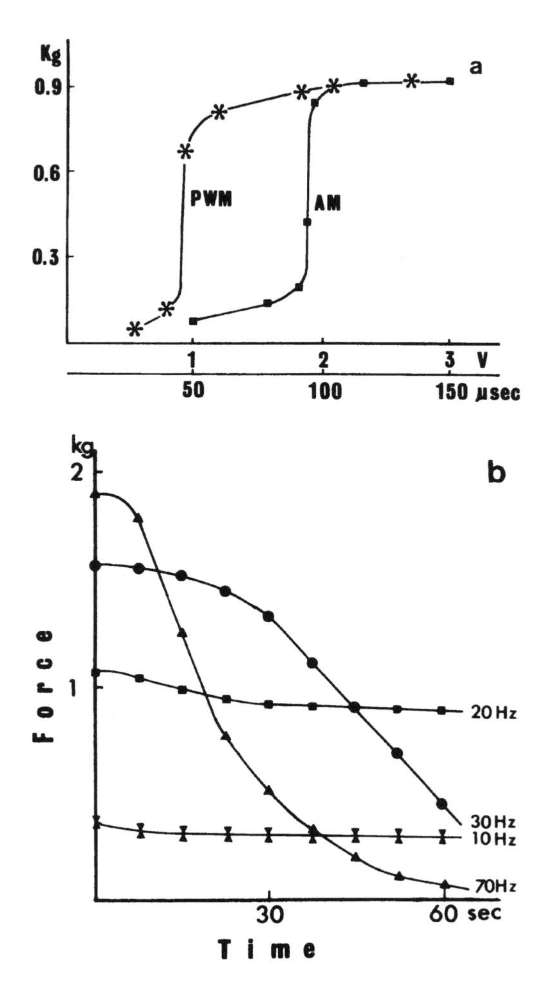

Fig. 3. Characteristics of muscle contraction of the extensor digitorum in a C5 quadriplegic by electrical stimulation. (a) Changes of muscle force by amplitude modulation (AM) and pulse width modulation (PWM). In AM, pulse width was 0.2 ms. Pulse amplitude in PWM was set to −4 volts. Frequency of the pulse trains in AM and PWM was 20 Hz. (b) Time-dependent changes of muscle force in various stimulation frequencies. Pulse width and amplitude were 0.2 ms and −4 volts, respectively.

3. Multi-channel FES system

3.1 Structure of a FES system

Fig. 4 shows a block diagram of a multi-channel FES system which we developed. A commercially available personal computer (NEC PC-8801 mkII) is used for a central processing unit for the FES system. Peripheral devices of the system are composed of dual floppy drives, a CRT display, 3 channels of A/D converters and 16 channels of D/A converters. In addition, the computer system is connected to analog circuits for controlling manually the stimulus amplitude of individual output channels. Final stage of this output circuit consists of 16 channels of transformers. A major role of these transformers is to eliminate DC component of the stimulus for preventing electrode breakage and electrochemically induced tissue reaction.

Several kinds of standard stimulation patterns for executing desired movements of the limbs and other parts of the body are stored on floppy disks through a key board. Stimulating data for each patient were automatically created by inputting threshold and maximum stimulating voltages of muscles to the standard stimulation patterns. Commands for selection of a file of the stimulating data registered and for execution of control of the movement selected are generated by the patient, and the command signals are fed to the central processing unit through A/D converters. According to a proportional control command, amplitude-modulated rectangular pulses with the pulse width of 0.2 ms and the frequency of 20 Hz are produced through D/A converters and the analog circuits mentioned above, and fed to the percutaneous electrodes.

3.2 System program

System program of our FES system consists of the job control program and the key command control program as shown in Fig. 5. The key command control program was written by BASIC while the job control program was written by Z-80 assembler for real-time processing. The job control program controls the following subroutines:

1. Input subroutine: for the control of command input.
2. Function subroutine: for the selection of a data file (transaction file) from the master file according to a selection command and for the readout of the data of stimulating amplitude from the

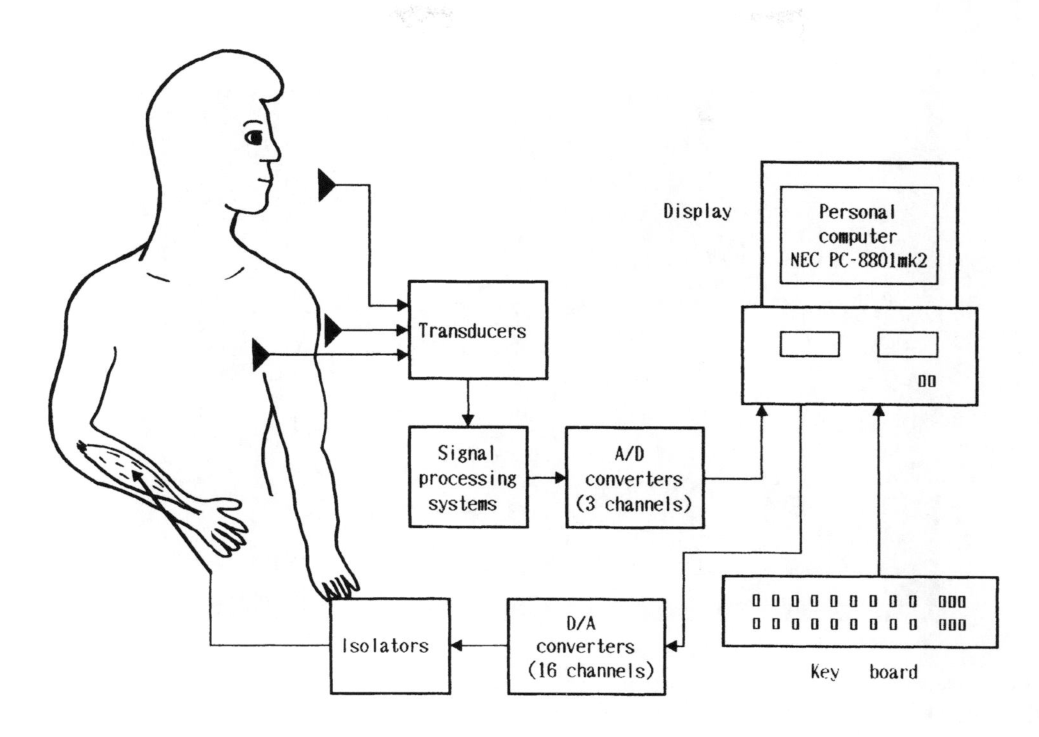

Fig. 4. A block diagram of a microcomputer based multi-channel FES system.

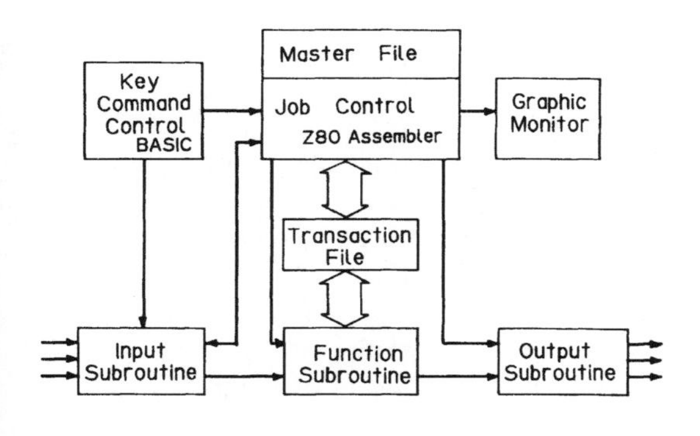

Fig. 5. System program organization.

transaction file by excution and proportional commands.

3. Output subroutine: for the control of stimulating output.

These jobs are displayed on a graphic monitor during the execution. One phase of the CRT display is shown in Fig. 6. At the left hand side, present status is shown. Multichannel stimulation patterns are also displayed at the right hand side.

The system program is processed sequencially as shown in Fig. 7. One phase of 100 ms is one unit of this sequence of time sharing and the phase is divided into two frames. The duration of each frame is 50 ms. The output of stimulating pulses is performed every 50 ms (20 Hz) and its processing time is 10 ms. The input and function jobs are also processed every one frame. Display processing for the graphic monitor requires 20 ms and is performed every one phase. The rest of the processing time is used for the key control job. This system program is activated by interruption of every 50 ms provided by a timer on the A/D converter board.

3.3 Creation of stimulating data for each patient

In order to execute the desired movements of the limbs and other parts of the body, the temporal and spatial sequence of stimulation are required. For this purpose, kinematic and electromyographic

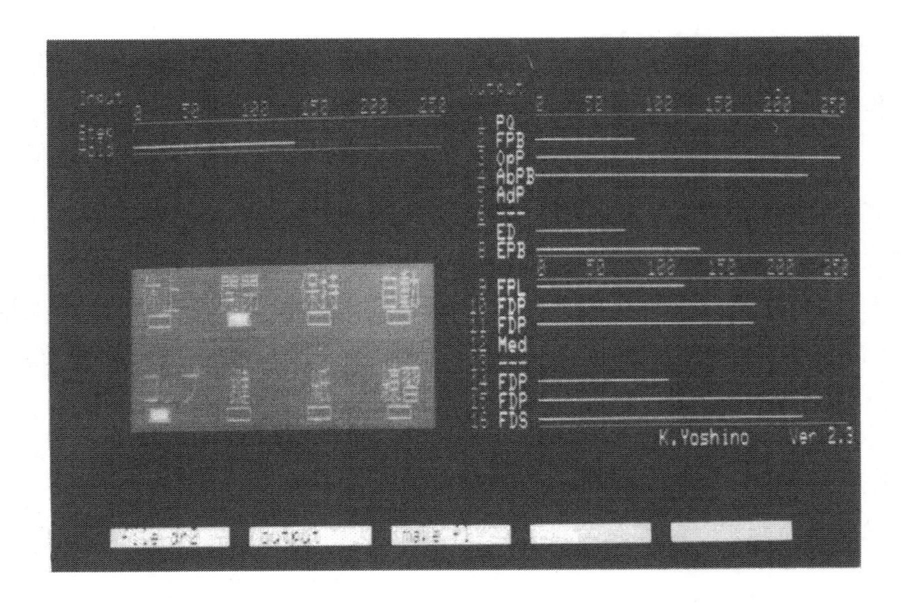

Fig. 6. An example of the CRT display. In this display, 'Input' indicates the level of proportional control commands, while a bar graph in 'Output' shows stimulating intensities applied to the hand muscles. Japanese words show the present status of the FES control as follows;

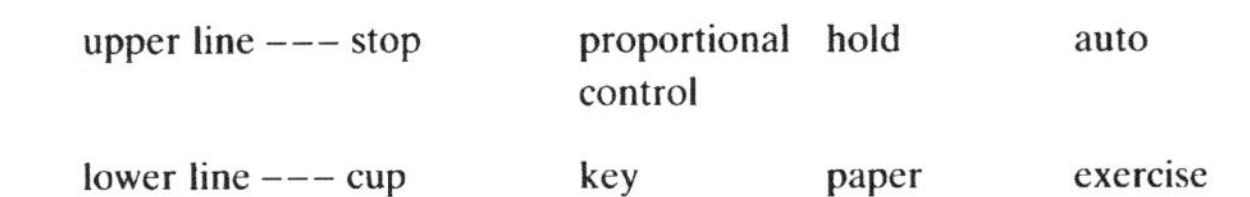

upper line --- stop	proportional control	hold	auto
lower line --- cup	key	paper	exercise

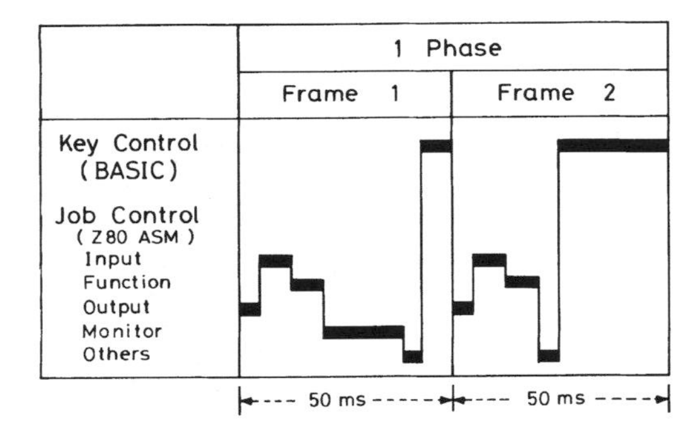

Fig. 7. Sequential scheduling on the program execution.

analyses of the movements have been achieved in normal subjects and utilized for the creation of standard stimulation patterns [7–9, 12, 14]. Especially, determination of stimulation patterns taking account for coordinated activities of the agonists, synergists, stabilizers and antagonists during movements, seems to be essential for the control of reliable and well-coordinated movements of the paralyzed body. Actually, programmed coactivation of nine thumb muscles based upon the EMG analysis resulted in fine gradation of movements and joint stability of the thumb [12]. This is partly explained from our result that non-linearity of the recruitment characteristics of electrically-induced muscle contraction [3] is improved by simultaneous stimulation of the antagonist with an agonist [10]. Fig. 8 shows an example of EMG activities of extrinsic and intrinsic hand muscles during grasp motion. A schemetic representation in Fig. 9 indicates a standard stimulation pattern created from these activities. Stimulating intensities for a patient are automatically determined by inputting the threshold and maximum stimulating voltages of the paralyzed muscles of the patient through a key board. Fig. 10 shows an example of stimulating data for providing cylindrical grasp for a C5 quadriplegic. These data are read out by pointing the memory

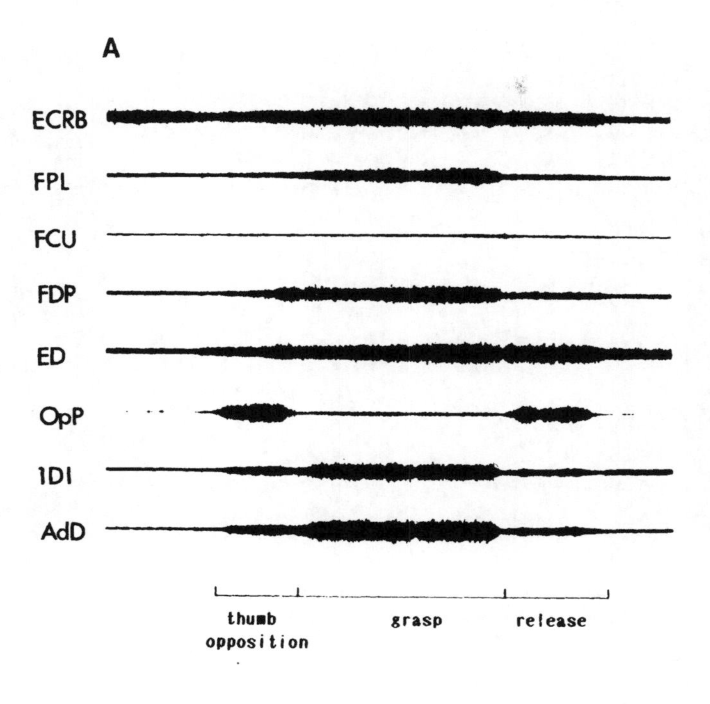

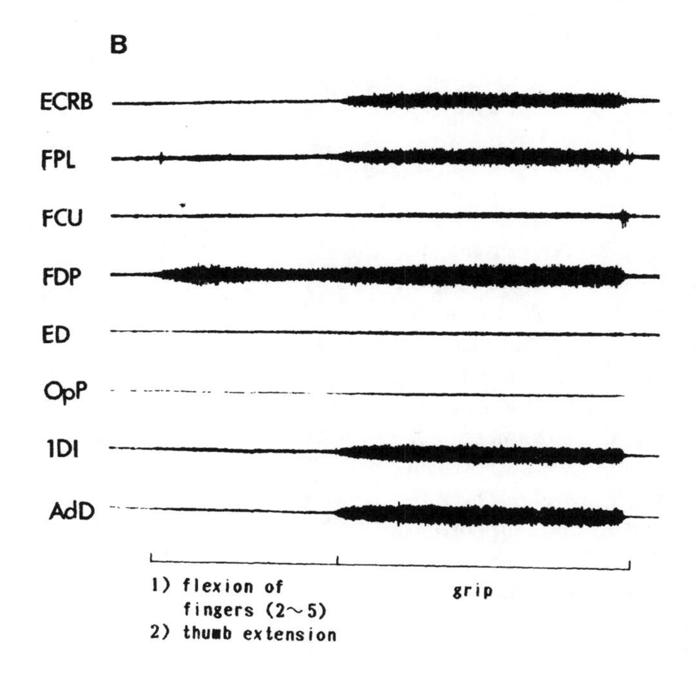

Fig. 8. EMG activities of the hand muscles during grasp motion.
(A) cylindrical grasp, and (B) key grip.

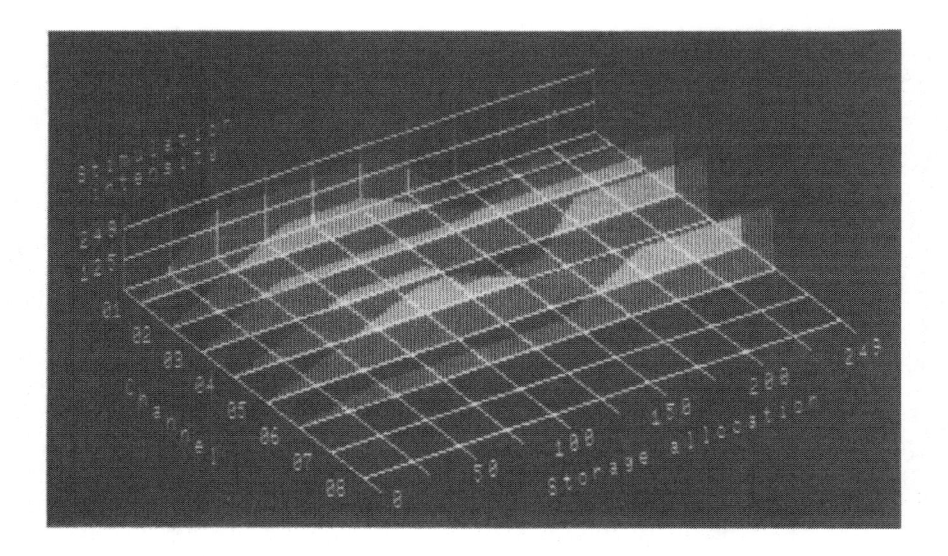

Fig. 9. Three dimensional representation of the standard stimulation patterns created from multi-channel EMG activities.

allocations corresponding to the level of the proportional control commands generated by the patients.

3.4 Control commands

Various kinds of transducers have been tried for providing control commands. At present, two kinds of transducers were used for C5 and C6 quadriplegics. One was a silastic tube filled with conductive fluid. One end of the tube was placed on the anterior chest wall just above the sternum, and the other was on the shoulder. Expansion and contraction caused by the shoulder movement on the coronal plane (vertical axis) resulted in resistance change between both ends of the tube. This transducer was mainly used for detecting a proportional analog signal which reflected the patient's volitional activities. The other was a small electric capacitor microphone (WM-063Y, Matsushita Tsushin Co., 5 mm diameter) for picking up high pitch humming sound (falsetto) of the patient. This microphone was attached to an anterior portion of the patient's chest. In order to eliminate usual speech input, a CR high-pass filter was introduced

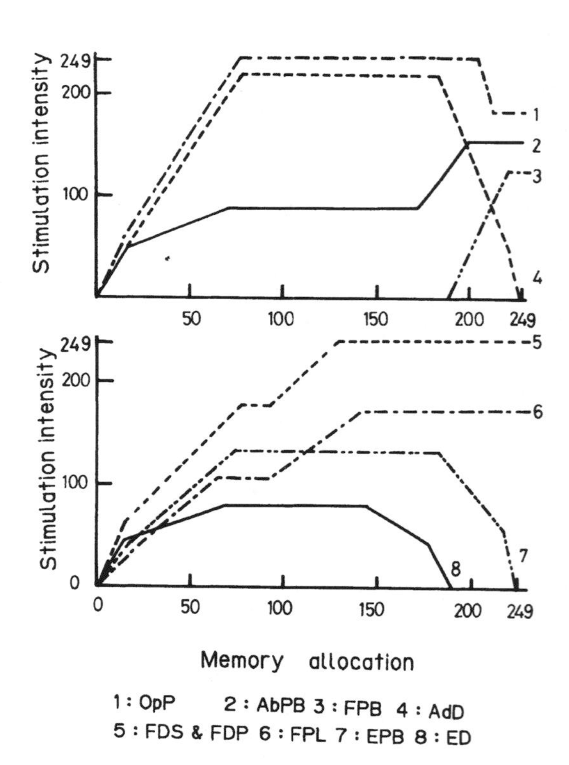

Fig. 10. Stimulating data for cylindrical grasp in a C5 quadriplegic.

Present Status	Input 1 / Input 2: 0 / 0	0 / 1	1 / 0	1 / 1
(A) Initial Status		*	To(B)	
(B) Start			To(C)	To(E)
(C) Prop. Cont.		To(D)		
(D) Hold		To(C)		To(E)
(E) Stop	To(A)			

* Selection of grasping pattern

Table 1. Command table.

Input 1: Shoulder movement
('1'): maximum elevation of the shoulder)
Input 2: Logical input (falsetto or head movement)

to a preamplifier. Frequency of the patient's sound was converted to DC voltages by an F/V converter. Only the sound with higher frequency than a certain threshold was utilized as a logical command for the control. When a patient was not willing to use falsetto, a simple on/off signal produced by the head movement was used instead.

Control commands consist of a selection command for desired movements registered, execution command for the selected movement and the proportional control command. The proportional control parameters were obtained only from the shoulder positions on a vertical axis (channel 1). On the other hand, certain degrees of shoulder elevation and depression were also logically used as 1 and 0, respectively. The control logic for the selection and execution commands is shown in Table 1. At the beginning, patient specifies his maximum position of the shoulder elevation together with a logical input (channel 2, falsetto or head) '1'. This initiates the system operation and also allows the patient to compensate his postural changes. After this, logical input command can sequentially call a file of desired grasping pattern from three types of hand tasks (cylindrical grasp, key grip and parallel extension grip), and the system is ready to accept an execution command 'start'. The start command is obtained by shoulder depression to a resting position (zero position) after maximum shoulder elevation. Thus the system begins 'proportional control' of a desired task selected. The 'hold' command is accepted by a logical input command when the patient intends to maintain the presently obtained task by the proportional control regardless of the subsequent shoulder movements. Stimulating data stored in a specified allocation is continuously readout and sent to D/A converters. Versatile controllabilities have been realized by introducing a new data allocation method [7–9], i.e. allocation address can be directly assigned by the analog voltage of the proportional input (channel 1). Restart of the proportional contol is performed by giving a logical command '0(ch.1),1(ch.2)' and subsequent shoulder position adjustment to the previously held position. A logical input '1,1' causes 'stop' operation. A sequence of the operation is schematically illustrated in Fig. 11.

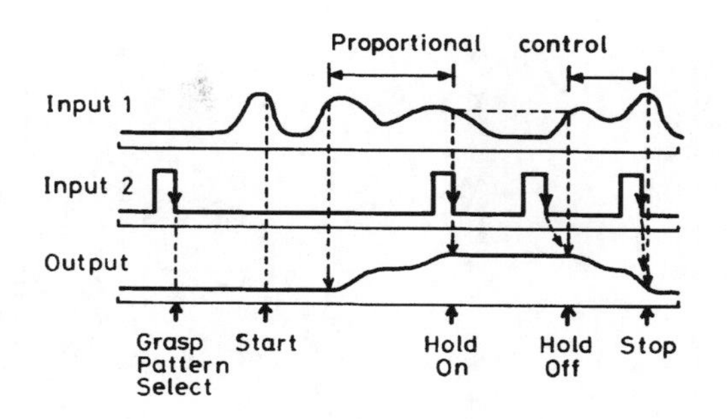

Fig. 11. Control sequence in the FES system.

4. Example of the clinical application

In C5-6 quadriplegics, musculatures of distally located joints of the upper extremities such as the joints of the hand are mainly paralyzed. Therefore, volitional conrol of the paralyzed hand may restore function of the upper extremities for daily use. For this purpose, the FES system which we developed has been applied to the paralyzed hand of C5 and C6 quadriplegic patients.

In order to utilize electrically-induced hand movements to activities of daily living (ADL), three kinds of stimulating data files for cylindrical grasp, key grip and parallel extension grip were stored into the master file [6, 7]. Giving a command by a falsetto or head movement, the patient could

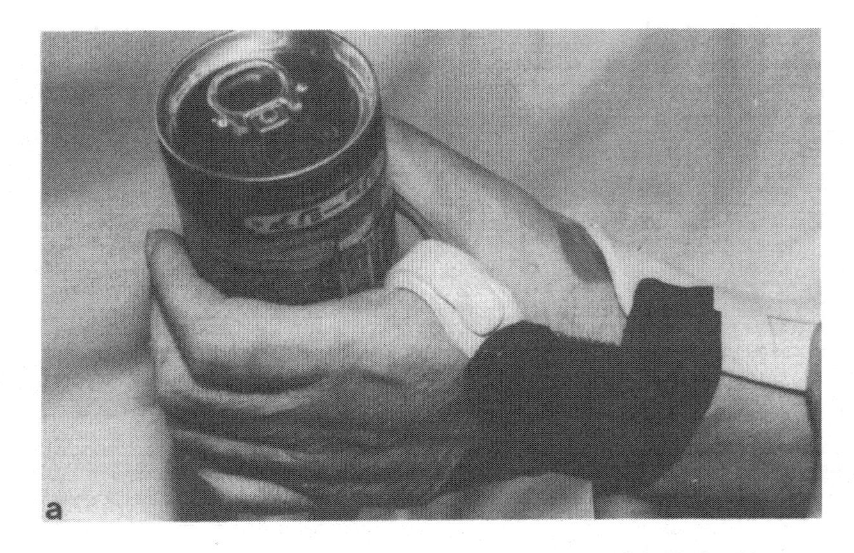

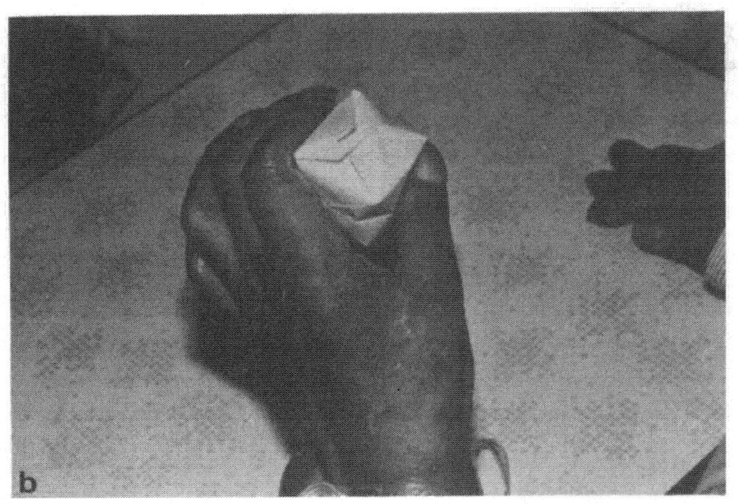

Fig. 12. Examples of FES-induced hand tasks in quadriplegics. (a) cylindrical grasp for a heavy object; (b) cylindrical grasp for a soft paper baloon; (c) key grip for holding a pen; and (d) parallel extension grip for tooth brushing.

select one grasping pattern from these three patterns.

Almost complete recognition of control commands was obtained in this system. Usual speech, a sneeze and a cough were not misread as a sound command. After selecting one grasping pattern, the maximum elevation of the shoulder gave a 'start' command to the system and successively provided acceptance of the proportional control command by shoulder elevation and depression for the selected hand task. By this proportional control command, the patient could voluntarily open and close his paralyzed hand in a highly coordinated manner. The 'hold' command provided by a falsetto or head movement could maintain the position of the thumb and fingers when the command

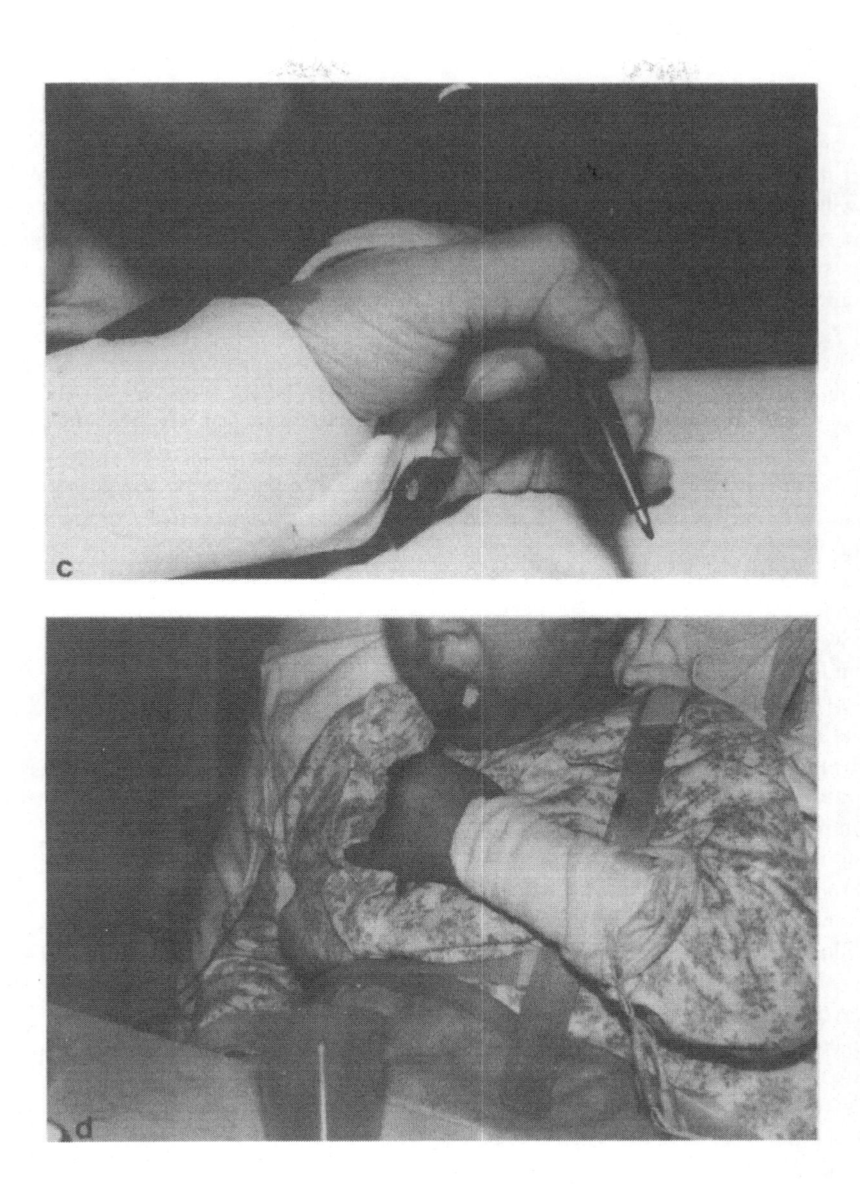

was just applied. Joint stability during 'hold' state was reliable and reproducible, and thus the patient could perform a constant tonic task without paying attention to the shoulder position. As shown in Fig. 12(a)–(d), C5 quadriplegics could keep holding a soft object such as a paper baloon as well as a hard and heavy object such as a full can of juice. Consequently, the patient whose peripheral motor function of the shoulder, elbow and wrist was almost intact could perform eating, drinking, writing, shaving, brushing the teeth and other ADL by use of these three grasping tasks induced by FES.

5. Discussion

In order to control the paralyzed extremities or other parts of the body by FES, versatility of the FES system will be needed because of differences in the part and types of paralysis, i.e. causes, levels, complications such as contracture of muscles or joints, shortening or spasticity of muscles and degeneration due to damage of the peripheral nervous system. The complexity of muscle coactivation for well-coordinated control of electrically-induced movements will also necessitate the system versatility. The FES system developed by us could partly satisfy such needs. The standard stimulation patterns obtained from the EMG analysis of the movements of the thumb and fingers of the hand in normal subjects could be basically applied to those of the paralyzed hand of C5 and C6 quadriplegics. In addition, we could also control the paralyzed wrist and hand of C4 quadriplegic by using the same methods [14]. These results suggest that creation of standard stimulation patterns for restoring function of the paralyzed part of the body is one of the most important factors to fabricate a multipurpose FES computer system.

In high cervical cord injury, almost all of the extremities are paralyzed while residual voluntary function of the patient for control commands of FES is quite limited. Movement of the head [8, 17], shoulder [7–9, 16–18] and the upper arm [6], voice [8, 15] and myoelectric signals [17] have been utilized as the control commands. However, such commands are not enough to control the paralyzed extremities with a multidegree of freedom. The patient requires the FES systems which operate with easiest and simplest control commands and perform dexterous and reliable movements in the paralyzed extremities. From this point of view, investigations of control commands including the way for picking up the command and its signal processing are also required.

By the way, quadriplegic patients are deprived of not only motor function but also sensory function. To restore the sensation relating to the hand movements produced by FES, efficient sensory feedback capabilities should be introduced into the total FES system [11].

Acknowledgement

Authors wish to thank to Prof. Y. Shimizu and Prof. K. Terayama of Shinshu University and Dr. T. Ikeda of Okukakeyu Onsen Rehabilitation Center for their constant interest and guidance in this investigation. Thanks are also due to members of our FES research group for their cooperation. This work was greatly indebted Mr. K. Yoshino and Miss M. Suejima. This work was supported by the Ministry of Education, Science & Culture of Japan under a Grant-in-Aid for Developmental Scientific Research No. 60850073 (1985–1986) and No. 61890007 (1986–1987), and Japan Research & Development Cooperation (1985).

References

1. Buckett JR, Braswell SD, Peckham PH, Thrope GB, Keith MW: A portable functional stimulation system. IEEE/7th Ann Conf Eng 314–317, 1985.
2. Chizeck HL: Helping paraplegic walk: Looking beyond the Media Blitz. Technol Rev 88: 55–63, 1985.
3. Crago PE, Peckham PH, Thrope GB: Modulation of muscle force by recruitment during intramuscular stimulation. IEEE Trans Biomed Eng BME-27: 679–684, 1980.
4. Cybulski GR, Pen RD, Jaeger RJ: Lower extremity functional neuromuscular stimulation in case of spinal cord injury. Neurosurg 15: 132–146, 1984.
5. Hambrecht FT, Reswick JB (eds): Functional electrical stimulation. Application in neural prosthesis. Marcel Dekker, New York, 1977.
6. Handa Y, Shimada Y, Komatsu S, Naito A, Ichie M, Nakatsuchi Y, Yagi R, Sugimoto Y, Iijima K, Futami R, Hoshimiya N: Electrically induced hand movements and their application for daily living. Proc 8th Int Symp ECHE (Dubrovnik): 169–180, 1984.
7. Handa Y, Ichie M, Handa T, Yagi R, Hoshimiya N: Control of the paralyzed hand by a computer-controlled FES system. IEEE/7th Ann Conf Eng Med & Biol Soc (Chicago), 322–326, 1985.
8. Handa Y, Handa T, Nakatsuchi Y, Hoshimiya N: A voice-controlled functional electrical stimulation system. Japan J Med Electron & Biol Eng 23: 292–298, 1985.
9. Handa Y, Handa T, Hoshimiya N: A portable FNS system for the paralyzed upper extremities. IEEE/8th Ann Conf Eng Med &Biol Soc (Dallas), 658–660, 1986.
10. Hoshimiya N, Iijima K, Futami R, Handa Y, Ichie M: A new FES system for the paralyzed upper extremities. IEEE/7th Ann Conf Eng Med & Biol Soc (Chicago), 327–330, 1985.

11. Hoshimiya N, Izumi T, Fujii A, Futami R, Ifukube T, Handa Y: Sensory feedback for the 'FNS' system. IEEE/8th Ann Conf Eng Med & Biol Soc (Dallas), 661–663, 1986.
12. Ichie M, Handa Y, Naito A, Handa T, Matsushita N, Hoshimiya N: EMG analysis of the thumb and its application to FNS. IEEE/8th Ann Conf Eng Med & Biol Soc (Dallas), 538–590, 1986.
13. Kobetic R , Marsolais EB: Automated electrically induced paraplegic gait. Proc 38th Ann Conf EMB 293, 1985.
14. Matsushita N, Handa Y, Ichie M, Naito A, Handa T, Hoshimiya N: Analysis of wrist movements and its application to FNS. IEEE/8th Ann Conf Eng Med &'Biol Soc (Dallas), 618–619, 1986.
15. Nathan RH: The development of a computerized upper limb electrical stimulation system. Orthop 7: 1170–1180, 1984.
16. Peckham PH, Mortimer JT: Restoration of hand function in the quadriplegic through electrical stimulation. In: Hambrecht FT, Reswick JB (eds) Functional electrical stimulation: Applications in neural prostheses. Marcel Dekker, New York, 1977, pp 83–95.
17. Peckham PH, Mortimer JT, Marsolais EB: Controlled prehension and release in the C5 quadriplegic elicited by functional electrical stimulation of the paralyzed forearm musculature. Ann Biomed Eng 8: 369–388, 1980.
18. Peckham PH, Poon CW, Ko WH, Marsolais EB, Rosen JJ: Multichannel implantable stimulator for control of paralyzed muscle. IEEE Trans Biomed Eng BME-28: 530–536, 1981.
19. Petrofsky JS, Phillips CA: Computer controlled walking in the neurological paralyzed individual. J Neurol Orthop Surg 4: 153–164, 1983.
20. Petrofsky JS, Phillips CA, Heaton HH: Feedback control systems for walking in man. Comput Biol Med 14: 135–149, 1984.
21. Schwanda G, Freg M, Holle J, Kern H, Mayr W, Stöhr H, Thoma H: 18-month experience in clinical application of implantable mutichannel devices for paraplegic patients. Proc 8th Int Symp ECHE (Dubrovnik), 79–88, 1984.
22. Schwanda G, Mayr W, Stöhr H, Thoma H: Analysis of FES treated paraplegic patients with implants. Proc 38th Ann Conf EMB, 294, 1985.
23. Special issue on the 'Applied neural control'. IEEE Eng Med & Biol Eng Magazine 2–2: 11–36, 1983.
24. Special issue on the 'Applied neural control'. IEEE Eng Med & Biol Eng Magazine 2–3: 29–49, 1983.

Address for offprints:
Dr. Yasunobu Handa
Dept. of Anatomy
Shinshu University School of Medicine
Matsumoto 390, Japan

Medical Progress through Technology 12 (1987) 65–76

Blood flow in the heart and large vessels

Motoaki Sugawara
The Heart Institute of Japan, Tokyo Women's Medical College

Key words: blood flow, aorta, left ventricle, pulmonary artery, carotid artery

1. Introduction

The rapid progress in haemodynamics over the last twenty years has depended greatly on the development of instrumentation. The quantities necessary for the description of blood flow are the pressure and velocity (or flow-rate) of the blood. Since the blood flow in large arteries has periodic, transient, and sometimes random characteristics, a system for measuring pressure or velocity must have a sufficiently large frequency response to cover the spectrum associated with the pressure or velocity waveform. The practical application of the catheter-tip transducer led to the improvement of the quality of blood pressure data even in terms of fluid dynamics. Various systems for measuring the blood velocity, each having its merits and faults, have been developed, and a considerable amount of experimental and clinical data are now available. The present stage of research in cardiovascular fluid dynamics is described here in relation to several methods of measurement.

2. Blood flow in the aorta

The electromagnetic flowmeter, which is currently regarded as the standard method for the measurement of blood flow in the aorta, measures the volumetric flow rate with a sensitivity that is independent of the velocity profile, and with an accuracy of ± 5% [4]. The introduction of the hot-film anemometer with its high spatial resolution and frequency response to the measurement of blood flow has greatly extended our knowledge of the development and distribution of the velocity of blood in the aorta [22].

2.1 Development of flow and transition to turbulence

Blood flow in the ascending aorta pulsates periodically, but its velocity (or flow-rate) waveform is not like that of an oscillating flow superposed on a steady flow (Fig. 1). The velocity rises rapidly to a peak, and promptly, but more slowly, falls again. Then the blood comes almost to rest for the remainder of the cardiac cycle. At resting heart-rates, the period of forward flow occupies only about a quarter to a third of the cardiac cycle. In a sense, therefore, the blood flow in the ascending aorta can be regarded as a combination of starting flow and stopping flow [28, 30].

Fig. 2 shows the velocity recording of a stopping and starting flow from a large reservoir through a tube with a well-rounded entrance [27]. The flow was started and stopped repeatedly by actuating a solenoid valve placed at a point far from the entrance of the tube. The hot-film anemometer was set near the entrance. The ordinate of Fig. 2 shows the Reynolds number calculated from the velocity. Prominent fluctuations were seen during the first steady flow. When the flow was stopped suddenly, fluctuations remained until the Reynolds number became as low as 1000. On the other hand, during the first few seconds after the flow was restarted, no irregular changes in velocity were seen and the Reynolds number reached a value higher than 15000. Then it decreased, and a steady turbulent

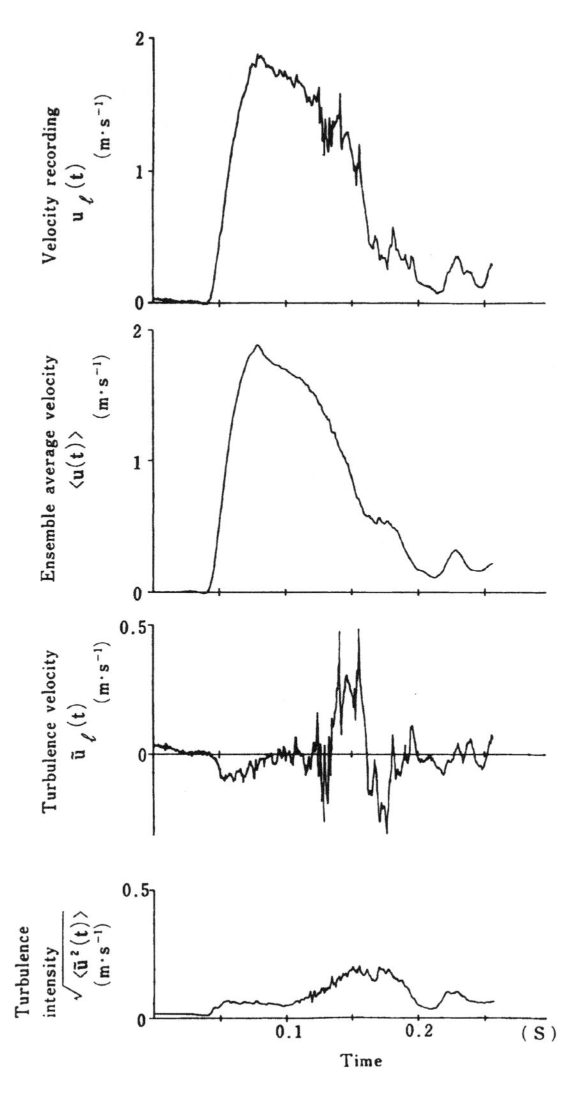

Fig. 1. Turbulence in the aorta of a dog. The first panel shows a recording of blood velocity history. The second panel gives an ensemble average of many beats. The third panel is a sample of turbulence velocity history. The fourth panel gives the turbulence intensity. (From Yamaguchi T et al.: J Biomech Eng 105: 183, 1983 [31].)

flow began suddenly. Bearing in mind these features of the starting and stopping flow, now look again at Fig. 1. No irregular changes in velocity are seen during the acceleration phase. However, prominent fluctuations suddenly appear near the peak of the velocity (Reynolds number ≒ 10000)

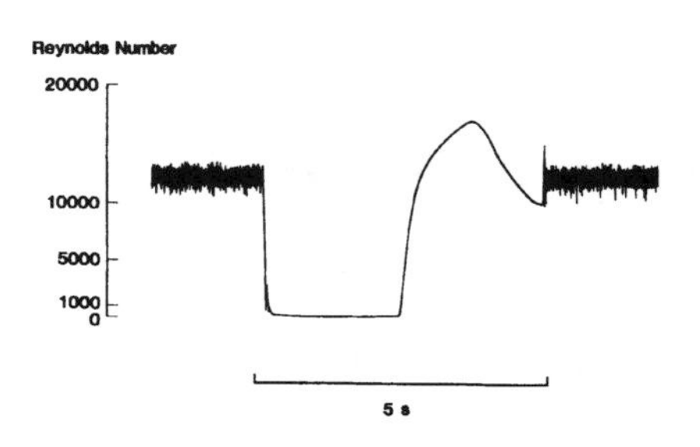

Fig. 2. Velocity record of stopping and starting flow in a straight tube made with a hot-film anemometer. (From Sugawara M and Yamaguchi T: In: Okino H et al. (eds) Shinzokekkankei No Rikigaku To Kisokeisoku. Kodansha, Tokyo, p 185, 1980 [27].)

and persist all the way through the deceleration phase. The turbulence intensity reaches a maximum value during the later half of the deceleration phase [31].

Fig. 3 shows the development of the average-velocity profile across the diameter of the ascending aorta in the plane of the main curvature of the aortic arch [34].The profiles are more or less blunt, but the flow close to the outer wall of the arch, i.e., the anterior wall, is a little more accelerated, which skews slightly the velocity profiles at peak systolic velocity. However, there are variations in the profile from dog to dog. One dog shows symmetrical profiles, but another dog shows skewing with higher velocities towards the inside wall, i.e., the posterior wall [5, 6]. The reasons for these variations are as yet not understood. Fig. 4 shows the time-varying turbulence intensity profile corresponding to the velocity profile in Fig. 3. The profile is reasonably symmetrical and two peaks appear near the anterior and posterior wall as the intensity increases. There are also variations in the turbulence intensity profile from dog to dog. Some dogs show rather flat profiles [32].

Turbulence in blood flow has been of interest not only from a phenomenological but also from a pathological viewpoint. It has often been assumed that turbulence may be a cause of a variety of pathophysiological changes [24]. Nothing has been made clear in this respect, although the knowledge of the characteristics of turbulence in the aorta has been greatly extended by the use of the hot-film anemometer [5, 6, 18, 19, 22, 23, 31–34].

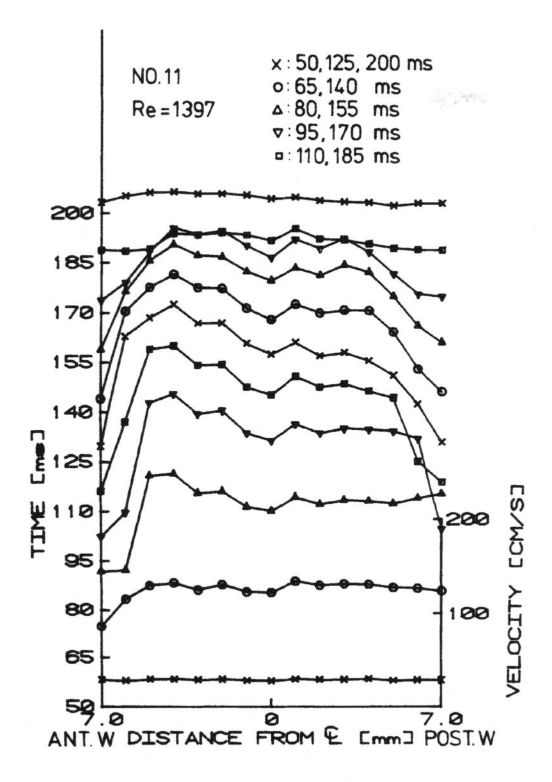

Fig. 3. Time-varying velocity profile in the ascending aorta of a dog. The ensemble-averaged velocity at a phase of the cardiac cycle at each site on the vessel diameter is expressed at an interval of 15 ms. The left end of the abscissa corresponds to the anterior wall of the ascending aorta and the right end corresponds to the posterior wall of the ascending aorta. Re = mean Reynolds number during one cardiac cycle. (From Yano et al.: Proc Jpn Soc Biorheol 9: 317, 1986 [34].)

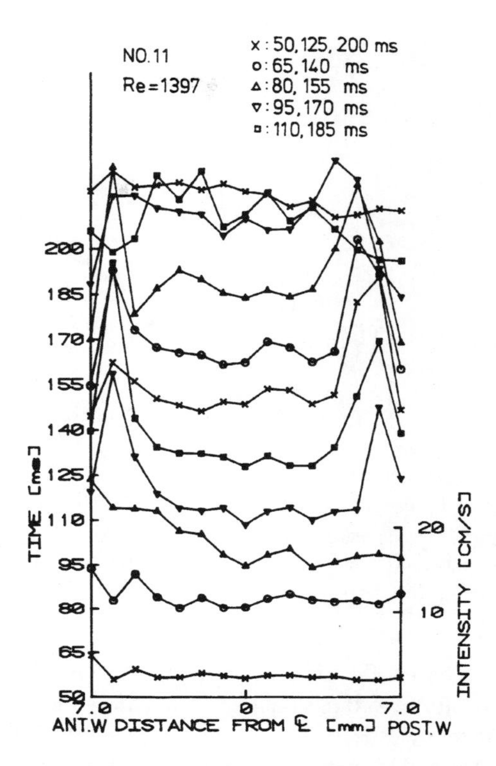

Fig. 4. Time-varying turbulence intensity profile corresponding to the velocity profile in Fig. 3. Different symbols correspond to those in Fig. 3. (From Yano et al.: Proc Jpn Soc Biorheol 9: 317, 1986 [34].)

2.2 *Clinical measurements of turbulence*

The hot-film anemometer is usually used in animal experiments, but turbulence in the cardiovascular system can also be detected with clinically used devices, such as the catheter-tip pressure transducer. Records of blood velocity and pressure measured with a multi-sensor catheter (a catheter with pressure and velocity transducers) in the aorta in a 4-year-old boy with congenital aortic stenosis are shown in Fig. 5. The so-called 'anacrotic notch' is seen in the pressure wave, which is shown by an arrow. Immediately after the anacrotic notch, fluctuations appear in the pressure recording, which are turbulent signals detected by the pressure transducer. Fluctuations are also seen in the velocity recording. However, because the frequency response of the velocity measuring system is limited to 30 Hz, it cannot follow the turbulent velocity fluctuation precisely. It does, however, sense the existence of fluctuations.

Sabbah et al. [21] pointed out that the transition from laminar to turbulent flow plays a significant role in the development of anacrotic notch. They tried to explain the pressure drop in an anacrotic notch by the transformation of pressure energy into kinetic energy of turbulence [12]. The pressure drop caused by this mechanism is reversible (recoverable) and cannot exceed the mean amplitude

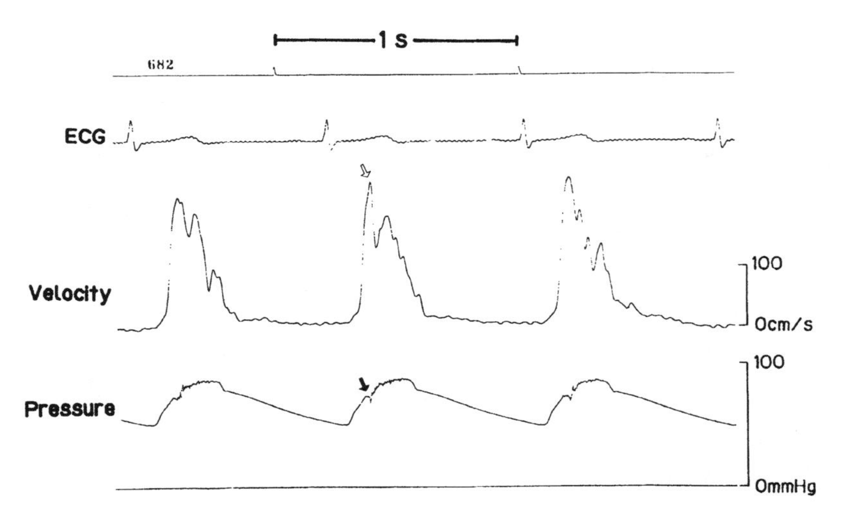

Fig. 5. Velocity and pressure recordings made with catheter-tip velocity/pressure transducers in the aorta of a 4-year-old boy with congenital aortic stenosis. (Panels by courtesy of Dr. S. Hanya, Dept. of Thoracic & Cardiovascular Surgery, School of Med., Kitasato Univ.).

of turbulent fluctuations of pressure. So far as the pressure recordings Sabbah et al. showed in their paper and the pressure recording in Fig. 5 are concerned, it seems that the reversible pressure drop accounts for the development of an anacrotic notch. However, in the case of severe aortic stenosis, the reversible pressure drop fails to explain the development of an anacrotic notch. Fig. 6 shows blood velocity and pressure recordings from the aorta in a 43-year-old man with severe aortic stenosis [10]. The anacrotic notch is initiated first by a sudden pressure drop shown by an arrow, which is succeeded by pressure fluctuations. These fluctuations persist until the downstroke of the systolic pressure wave. The amplitude of the pressure fluctuations first increases until the mean pressure

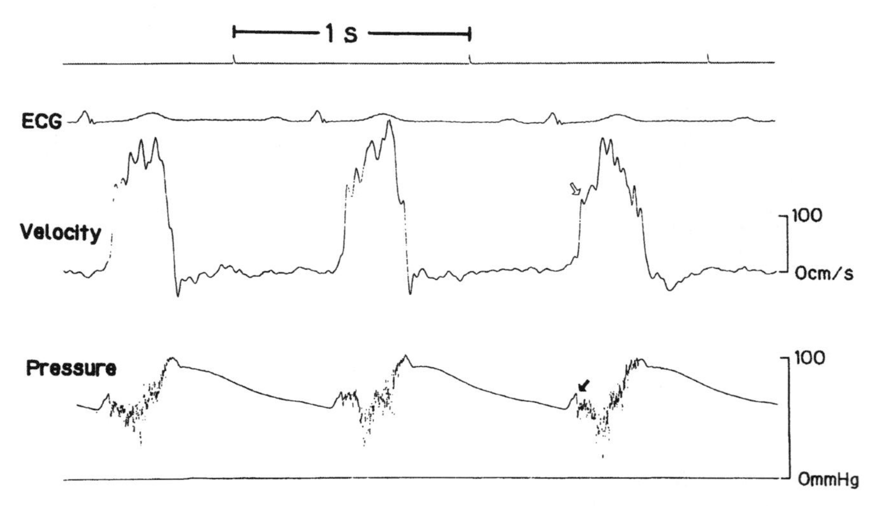

Fig. 6. Velocity and pressure recordings made with catheter-tip velocity/pressure transducers in the aorta of a 43-year-old man with severe aortic stenosis. (From Hanya S et al.: Kokyu To Junkan 33: 553, 1985 [10].)

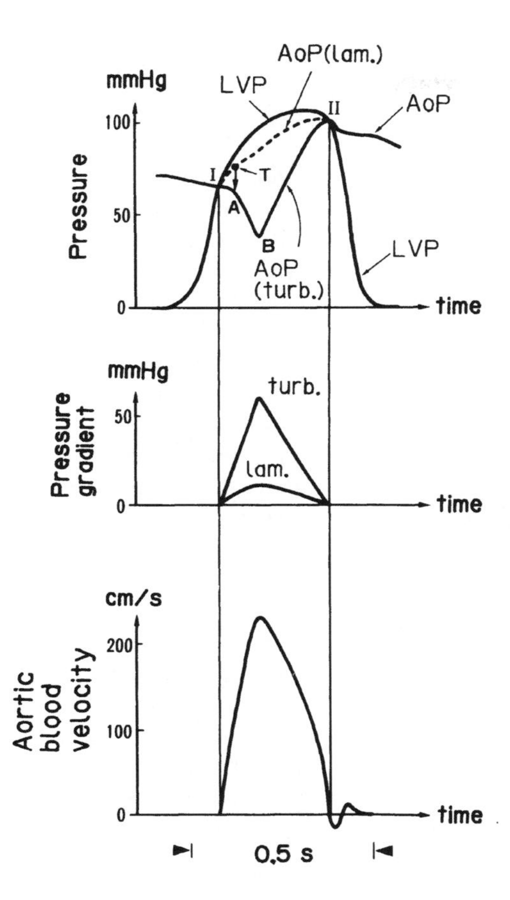

Fig. 7. Schematic waveforms in a patient with severe aortic stenosis. In calculating the pressure losses from the velocity in the aorta, the proportional constants were chosen in order to make the results realistic. The aortic pressure was obtained by subtracting the pressure loss (gradient) from the left ventricular pressure. AoP = aortic pressure, LVP = left ventricular pressure, lam. = laminar, turb. = turbulent. (From Hanya S et al.: Kokyu To Junkan 33: 556, 1985 [10].)

reaches its minimum and then begins to decrease or disappears when the systolic pressure wave reaches its peak. The sudden pressure drop is always coincident with sudden changes in the contour of the velocity curve. The fluctuations in the velocity wave always appear at the same time and are of the same duration as the pressure fluctuations. According to the characteristics of the pressure and velocity recordings, it seems clear that the transition from laminar to turbulent flow plays the main role in the development of an anacrotic notch. However, the initial and succeeding pressure drop is much larger than the mean amplitude of the pressure fluctuations. Therefore, the reversible transformation of pressure energy to turbulent kinetic energy cannot account for this large pressure drop. It is necessary to take into account the pressure drop caused by irreversible energy dissipation.

The pressure drop due to irreversible energy dissipations, such as the frictional loss in a straight tube and the loss caused by flow separation in a stenosed tube, is proportional to the velocity when the flow is laminar, and proportional to the square of the velocity when the flow is turbulent [3, 37]. At the bottom of Fig. 7, a typical waveform of the velocity in the aorta in a patient with aortic stenosis is shown. Fluctuations are superposed on this waveform when the flow is turbulent. Using this velocity wave, we can calculate the pressure loss across the stenosis for both laminar and turbulent flows [10]. The results are shown in the middle of Fig. 7. The lower curve is the pressure loss (gradient) obtained when assuming that the flow is laminar. The upper curve is that obtained when assuming that the flow is turbulent. Subtracting the pressure loss from the left ventricular pressure, we obtain the aortic pressure. Here, we neglect the pressure gradient due to inertia. At the top of Fig. 7, the left ventricular pressure curve and two calculated aortic pressure curves are shown. The dashed curve I-T-II is the aortic pressure obtained on the assumption that the flow is laminar. The curve I-A-B-II is the aortic pressure obtained on the assumption that the flow is turbulent. In the early accelerating period, the aortic flow is laminar. Therefore, the aortic pressure varies along the dashed line at first. But, when the transition occurs, the aortic pressure curve changes from the laminar to the turbulent curve, which is shown by the change from T to A. After the transition, the aortic pressure varies along the curve A-B-II. Therefore, the overall aortic pressure curve is the curve I-T-A-B-II. In real recordings, the fluctuations due to turbulence are superposed on this curve (see Fig. 6).

The anacrotic notch is also seen in the pressure contour in the left pulmonary artery downstream of the stenosis [10]. Whether in the aorta or pulmo-

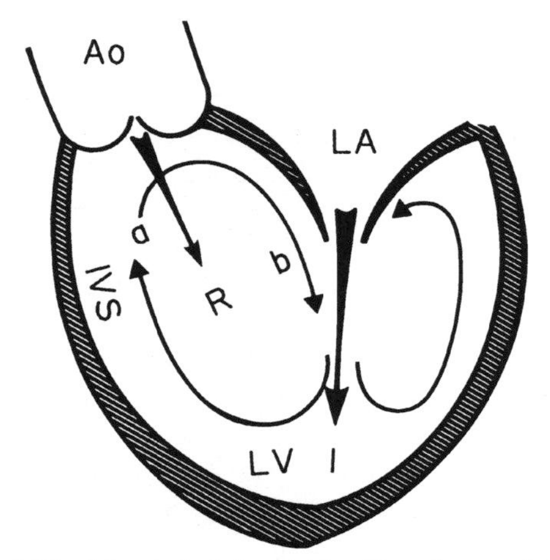

Fig. 8. Blood flow in the left ventricle with aortic regurgitation. R = regurgitant flow, I = inflow, Ao = aorta, LA = left atrium, LV = left ventricle, IVS = interventricular septum.

nary artery, turbulent flow initiates a pressure drop followed by pressure fluctuations. Furthermore it should be emphasized that the anacrotic notch is not only characteristic of patients with semilunar valve stenosis or any other type of obstruction to flow but it is also seen in normal subjects in whom high peak velocity exceeding the critical Reynolds number would result in the development of turbulence [10].

3. Blood flow in the left ventricle

The swirling motion of the blood in the left ventricle during diastole was first suggested by Bellhouse and Bellhouse [1] in relation to the closing mechanism of the mitral valve. When analyzing the results of flow measurements in the left ventricle, we always have to keep this swirling motion in mind.

Fig. 8 shows schematically the blood flow pattern in the left ventricle during diastole in a patient with aortic regurgitation. The swirling motion generated by the inflow from the atrium is considered to be superposed on the aortic regurgitation flow. If a blood velocity measurement is made at a site near the interventricular septum (a in Fig. 8), the measured regurgitant velocity will be relatively low, and a velocity toward the aortic valve may be detected in late diastole when the swirling motion becomes fully developed. On the other hand, if a measurement is made at a site near the anterior cusp of the mitral valve (b in Fig. 8), the regurgitant velocity will be relatively high, and it will become higher in late diastole with the development of swirling motion [8, 9]. Keeping these in mind, let us see the results of actual clinical measurement. Fig. 9 shows the pressure and blood velocity recordings from the outflow tract of the left ventricle in a patient with isolated aortic regurgitation [8, 9]. It shows the variations of the pressure and velocity waveforms according to the sites of measurement in the outflow tract of the left ventricle. By gradual counterclockwise rotation of the catheter, its tip, namely, the measuring site, was moved from a point near the interventricular septum to one near the anterior cusp of the mitral valve. The variations of the waveforms caused by the repositioning of the catheter tip were similar to those speculated in the previous considertion. In the pressure recording, fluctuations were observed, which increased in intensity with the increase of regurgitant flow velocity. When the catheter-tip was near the interventricular sepum, it detected a flow toward the cardiac base in late diastole. On the other hand, when the catheter-tip was near the anterior cusp, it detected greater regurgitant velocity in late diastole.

3.2 Flow in systole

Compared with the diastolic flow pattern, the systolic flow pattern in the left ventricle is rather simple. However, prior to the major ejection wave of the blood velocity and posterior to the P wave of the ECG, there is a spiky velocity wave. An example is seen in the velocity recording at the bottom of Fig. 10, which was obtained with a hot-film anemometer from the outflow tract of the left ventricle of a dog [33]. Fig. 11 shows recordings taken with a multisensor catheter from the left ventricular outflow tract of a human [8]. The velocity wave is in the middle, which has the spiky wave, indicated by A, prior to the systolic ejection wave, indicated by B. The similar spiky wave is often detected with the pulsed Doppler velocity meter, too [14]. We speculated that this spike is caused by the closing motion

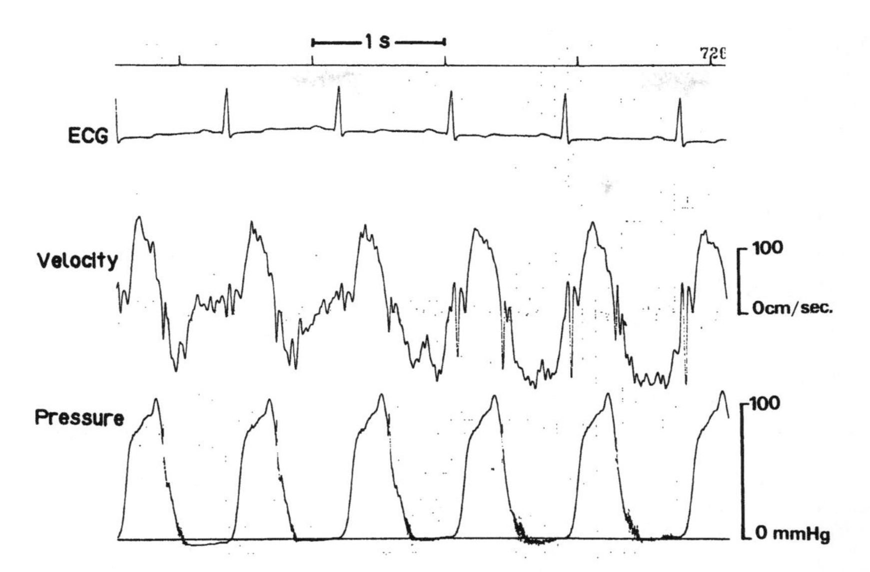

Fig. 9. Velocity and pressure records made with catheter-tip velocity/pressure transducers in a 45-year-old man with aortic regurgitation. The waveforms change as the site of measurement is moved in the outflow tract of the left ventricle from a point near the septum to one near the anterior cusp of the mitral valve. (From Hanya S et al.: Kokyu To Junkan 30: 415, 1982 [9].)

of mitral leaflets [25]. Later, Mizushige et al. [17] made a close investigation of this wave using a pulsed Doppler velocity meter. They detected the spiky wave in healthy subjects, subjects with atrial fibrillation and those with Wenckebach A-V block. The amplitude of the spiky velocity wave varied according to the sites of measurement. When the sampling site was moved from a level near the cardiac base to one near the tip of anterior mitral

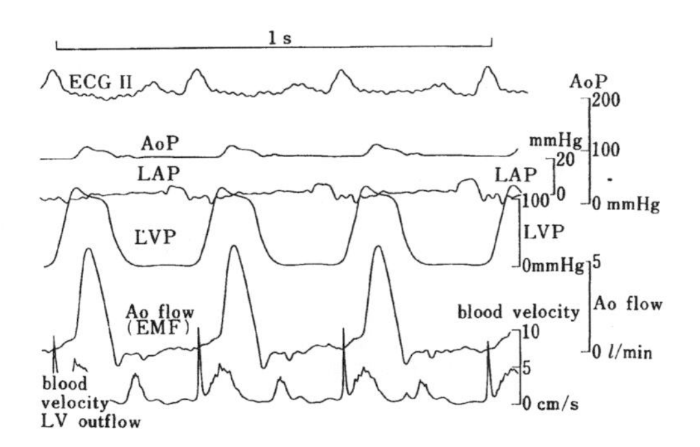

Fig. 10. Blood flow velocity pattern in the outflow tract of the left ventricle of a dog measured with a hot-film anemometer. A spiky wave is seen in the velocity recording at the bottom. (From Yamaguchi T et al.: Iyodenshi To Seitai Kogaku 16: 132, 1978 [33].)

cusp, the amplitude increased. And the amplitude was larger when the sampling site was closer to the mitral cusp. The fact that this wave was detected also in subjects with atrial fibrillation suggests that it may be caused by ventricular contraction. However, in subjects with Wenckebach A-V block, the wave was also detected during the cardiac cycle without ventricular contraction. And in the cardiac cycle with prolonged P-Q interval the wave showed two peaks. Therefore, they concluded that this wave is related to both the atrial contraction and the ventricular contraction during the pre-isometric contraction period, and may be caused by deceleration of the left ventricular inflow after the atrial contraction and the succeeding left ventricular contraction which brings about the mitral valve closure.

4. Blood flow in the pulmonary artery

4.1 Characteristics of the flow

There have been few reports on the velocity profile in the pulmonary artery. Reuben et al. [20] mea-

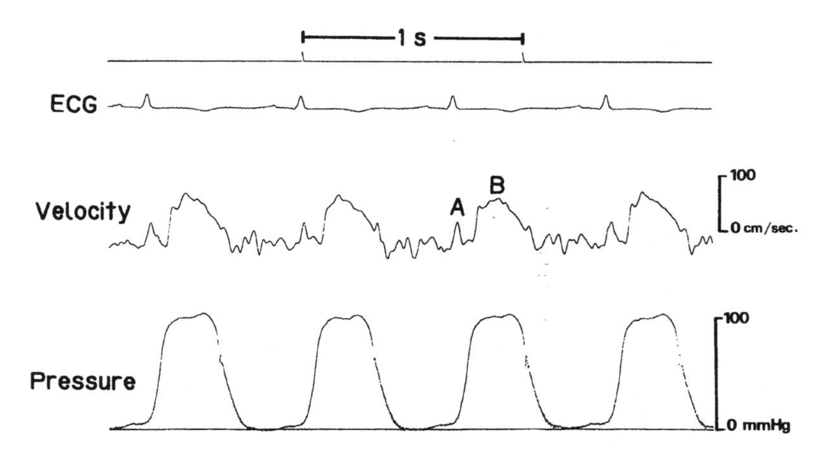

Fig. 11. Blood flow velocity pattern measured with catheter-tip velocity/pressure transducers in the outflow tract of the left ventricle of a 46-year-old man without heart disease. A spiky wave is seen in the velocity recording in the middle. (From Hanya S et al.: Proc 3rd Inter Conf Mech Med Biol: 106, 1982 [8].)

sured velocity profiles in the main pulmonary artery of dogs and man with the hot-film anemometer. The results were that the velocity profile was approximately flat both in dogs and in man. This suggests that blood velocity measured at any point in a cross-section of the main pulmonary artery is representative of the blood velocity at all other points in that cross-section. Whether the transition from laminar to turbulent flow can occur in the normal pulmonary artery has not yet been clarified.

Fig. 12 shows pressure and flow waves measured in the pulmonary artery (top) and the ascending aorta (bottom) under control conditions [29]. In the pulmonary artery, pressure and flow waves look alike, but this is not so in the aorta. The differences between aortic and pulmonary pressure and flow waves can be explained by pulse wave reflection. General theories of pulse wave in an elastic tube assert that when the effects of wave reflection are negligible, the following equation holds [2, 13, 16]:

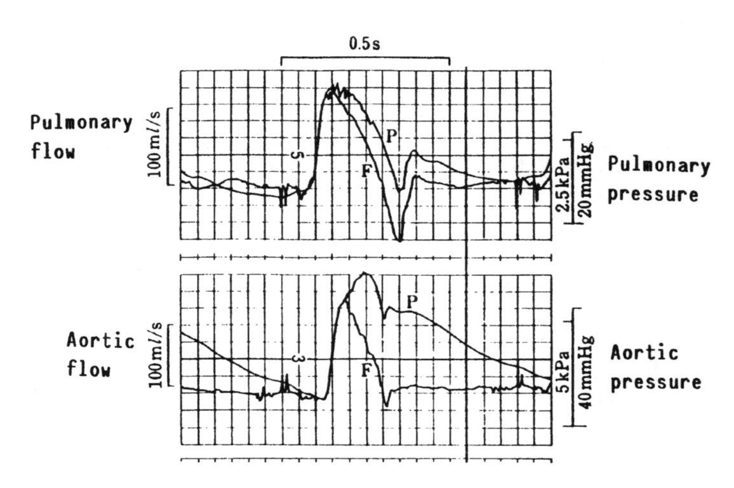

Fig. 12. Blood flow-rate and pressure waveforms in the pulmonary artery and the aorta. P = pressure, F = flow-rate. (From van den Bos GC et al.: Circ Res 51: 480, 1982, by permission of American Heart Association, Inc. [29].)

$$P - P_O = \varrho c u, \qquad (1)$$

where P is the instantaneous pressure at time t at a point in the artery, P_O is the pressure at the same point at the end-diastole, ϱ the density of blood, c the velocity of the pulse wave, and u the velocity of blood at time t at the same point in the artery (when $P=P_O$, $u=O$). In Eq. (1), there is no phase difference between P and u. When the effects of wave reflection become significant, the phase difference between P and u appears. In the circulatory system, the major sources of reflection are the peripheral vessels, which furnish most of the total resistance to flow. The pulmonary circuit under control conditions offers a resistance which produces a pressure loss of about 20 mm Hg, while the systemic circuit offers a resistance which produces a pressure loss of about 100 mm Hg. Therefore, the effects of wave reflection are much smaller in the pulmonary artery than in the aorta. This explains the difference in the resemblance of pressure and flow waves between the pulmonary artery and the aorta. In clinical situations, however, this normally existing resemblance of pressure and flow waves is often lost in the pulmonary artery when the pulmonary vascular bed is diseased, as in pulmonary hypertension.

4.2 Clinical measurements: Application of the pressure loss coefficient

The severity of aortic or pulmonary stenosis is conventionally evaluated by the pressure difference across the stenosis. However, the pressure difference depends strongly on the blood velocity, and consequently changes with the change in cardiac output. In the field of fluid dynamics, the commonly used index indicating the degree of resistance to flow is the pressure-loss coefficient, which is nearly independent of the fluid velocity when the Reynolds number of the flow is sufficiently high or the flow is highly disturbed. It is well known that the presence of a stenosis within a large artery gives rise to a region of turbulent flow downstream of the obstruction. In the cardiovascular system, the pressure loss coefficient λ can be defined by the following equation:

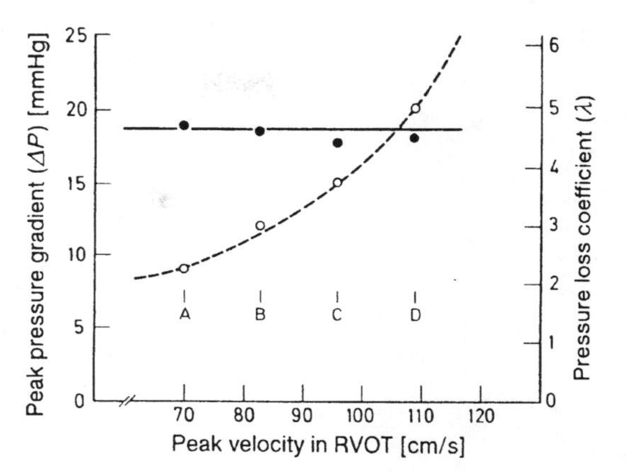

Fig. 13. Peak pressure gradient and pressure loss coefficient plotted against peak blood velocity in the right ventricular outflow tract (RVOT) in a 6-year-old boy with pulmonary valvular stenosis during pharmacological loading. Open circles denote the peak pressure gradient and the pressure-loss coefficient is represented by closed circles. (From Hanya S et al.: Heart Vessels 1: 38, 1985, by permission of Springer-Verlag [11].)

$$\lambda = \Delta P / \{(1/2)\,\varrho U^2\}, \qquad (2)$$

where ΔP is the peak systolic pressure gradient between pre- and poststenotic sites, ϱ is the density of blood, and U is the peak blood velocity. To apply the pressure loss coefficient to the evaluation of cardiovascular stenosis, it is necessary to measure both the pressure gradient and the blood velocity. Using the multisensor catheter, Hanya et al. [11] measured simultaneously the pressure in the pulmonary artery and the right ventricular outflow tract and the velocity in the right ventricular outflow tract in patients with pulmonary stenosis, and calculated the pressure loss coefficient. Fig. 13 shows the λ and the peak pressure gradient across the stenosis plotted against the peak blood velocity in the right ventricular outflow tract obtained from a patient during pharmacological loading (0.02 mg/kg orciprenaline sulfate) [11]. The pressure gradient changed parabolically with the blood velocity, but λ was almost constant during the pharmacological loading. This confirmed that λ is more appropriate for evaluating the severity of stenosis than the pressure gradient which depends on the blood velocity.

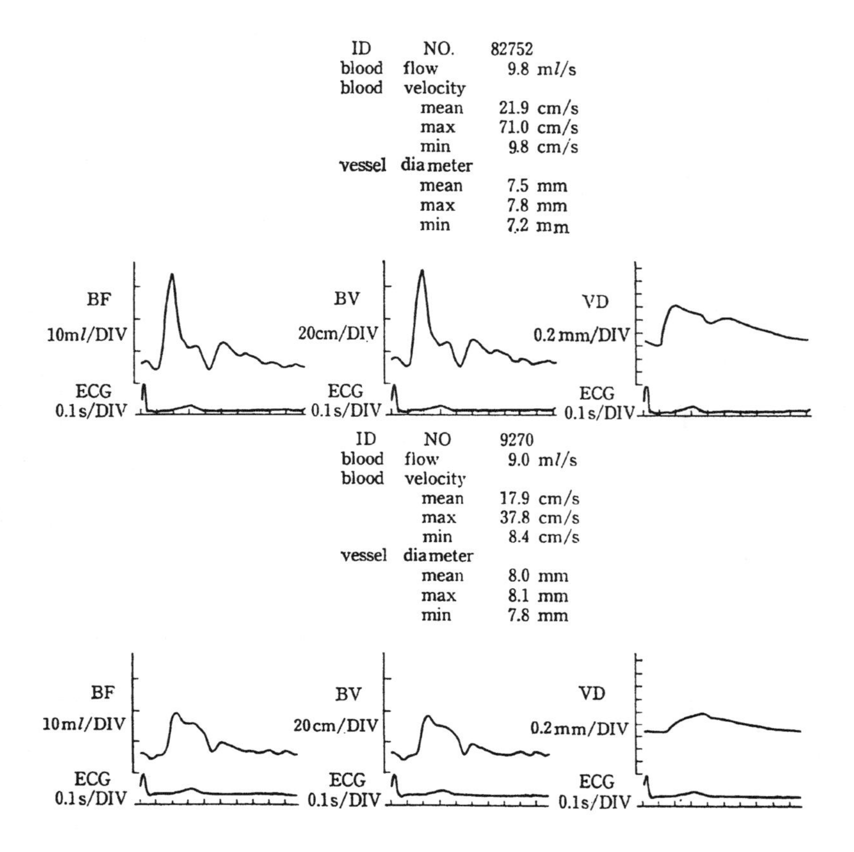

Fig. 14. Typical records of blood flow-rate, blood velocity and vessel diameter change made with QFM system in the carotid artery of a young (top panel) and an old (bottom panel) subject. BF = blood flow-rate, BV = blood velocity, VD = vessel diameter change. (From Yoshimura S et al.: In: Sugawara M et al. (eds) Ketsuryu. Kodansha, Tokyo, 1985, p 264, by permission of Kodansha [35].)

5. Blood flow in the carotid artery

Yoshimura and Furuhata et al. [7, 35, 36] developed a new system named QFM for measuring the carotid arterial blood flow using ultrasound wave. Four transducers are assembled in the probe of the QFM; one for pulsed echo to measure the diameter of the vessel, and the other three are for continuous Doppler ultrasound. One is the transmitter and the other two are the receivers. In the calculation of the absolute blood velocity, the use of the output from two receivers cancels the error due to the uncertainty in determining the angle between the directions of ultrasound beam and the blood flow. Fig. 14 shows the print-outs of the QFM system [35]. Typical waveforms obtained from the carotid artery of a young subject are in the top row. Those of an old subject are in the bottom row. The differences in the waveforms of the blood velocity and the vessel wall motion between the two subjects are obvious.

We proposed an idea for measuring the blood pressure waveform using this system [26]. We performed simultaneous measurements of the diameter of the left common carotid artery with the QFM system and the pressure in the left common carotid artery with a catheter-tip transducer inserted through the femoral artery. On the left of Fig. 15, simultaneous recordings of the pressure and the diameter for a single cardiac cycle are shown. On the right, instantaneous relationship of the pressure to the diameter is shown [26]. There is a good

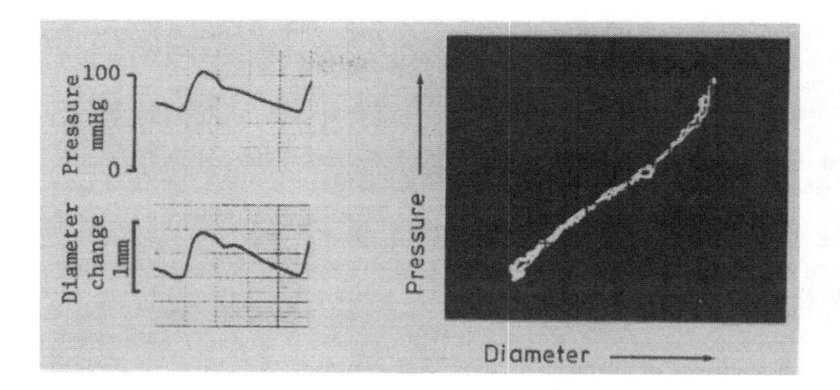

Fig. 15. Left: simultaneous records of pressure and diameter from the left common carotid artery in a 31-year-old woman after open mitral commissurotomy. Right: instantaneous relationship of pressure to diameter for this same cycle. Pressure was measured with a catheter-tip micromanometer, and vessel diameter change was measured with the QFM system. (From Sugawara M et al.: Iyodenshi To Seitai Kogaku 21 (Suppl): 429, 1983 [26].)

similarity between the pressure and the diameter curves, on the basis of which the diameter change waveform can be regarded as the pressure waveform. The peak and bottom values of the pressure pulse can be calibrated by other non-invasive methods, such as Riva-Rocci's sphygmomanometer.

Thus, the blood flow and pressure waveforms in the carotid artery can be obtained simultaneously by the QFM system. The measured flow and pressure waveforms give the input impedance of the cerebrovascular system, which is used for an index of the severity of cerebral arteriosclerosis [35].

References

1. Bellhouse BJ, Bellhouse FH: Fluid mechanics of the mitral valve. Nature 224: 615–616, 1969.
2. Caro CG, Pedley TJ, Schroter RC, Seed WA: The mechanics of the circulation. Oxford University Press, Oxford, 1978, pp 282–283.
3. Clark C: The fluid mechanics of aortic stenosis: I. Theory and steady flow experiments. J Biomech 9: 521–528, 1976.
4. Cobbold RSC: Transducers for biomedical measurements: Principles and applications. John Wiley & Sons, New York, 1974.
5. Falsetti HL, Carroll RJ, Swope RD, Chen CJ, Cramer JA, Length RA, Laughlin DE: Turbulent blood flow in the ascending aorta of dogs. Cardiovasc Res 17: 427–436, 1983.
6. Falsetti HL, Kiser KM, Francis GP, Belmore ER: Sequential velocity development in the ascending and descending aorta of the dog. Circ Res 31: 328–338, 1972.
7. Furuhata H, Kanno R, Kodaira K, Aoyagi T, Matsumoto H, Hayashi J, Yoshimura S: Ultrasonic Doppler method aimed at the absolute measurement of blood velocity. Iyodenshi To Seitai Kogaku (Jpn J Med Elec Biol Eng) 16: 264–268, 1978 (in Japanese).
8. Hanya S, Sugawara M, Ishihara A: Blood flow velocity patterns in the left ventricular outflow tract studied with a catheter-tip velocity/pressure transducer system (Abstract). Proc 3rd Inter Conf Mech Med Biol: 105–106, 1982.
9. Hanya S, Sugawara M, Ishihara A: Studies on flow velocity patterns in the left ventricular outflow tract using catheter-tip velocity/pressure transducers. Kokyo To Junkan (Respiration and Circulation) 30: 411–418, 1982 (in Japanese).
10. Hanya S, Sugawara M, Ishihara A: A fluid dynamical analysis of the development of anacrotic notch in the pressure wave in patients with semilunar valve stenosis. Kokyu To Junkan (Respiration and Circulation) 33: 553–558, 1985 (in Japanese).
11. Hanya S, Sugawara M, Inage H, Ishihara A: A new method of evaluating the degree of stenosis using a multisensor catheter: Application of the pressure loss coefficient. Heart Vessels 1: 36–42, 1985.
12. Hinze JO: Turbulence. McGraw-Hill, New York, 1975, pp 305–310.
13. Jones RT: Fluid dynamics of heart assist devices. In: Fung YC, Perrone N, Anliker M (eds) Biomechanics: Its foundations and objectives. Prentice-Hall, Englewood Cliffs, 1972, pp 549–565.
14. Kitabatake A, Inoue M, Asao M, Mishima M, Tanouchi J, Morita H, Masuyama T, Hori M, Abe H, Chihara K, Sakurai Y, Senda S, Matsuo H: Non-invasive visualization of intracardiac blood flow in human heart using computer-aided pulsed Doppler technique. Clin Hemorheol 2: 85–91, 1982.
15. Maruyama T, Kato Y, Mizushina T: Transition to tur-

bulence in starting pipe flows. J Chem Eng Jpn 11: 346–353, 1978.
16. McDonald DA: Blood flow in arteries. Edward Arnold, London, 1974, p 284.
17. Mizushige K, Matsuo H: Spike in the velocity wave in the outflow tract of the left ventricle. In: Sugawara M, Matsuo H, Kajiya F, Kitabatake A (eds) Ketsuryu (Blood flow). Kodansha, Tokyo, 1985, pp 42–50 (in Japanese).
18. Nerem RM, Seed WA, Wood NB: An experimental study of the velocity distribution and transition to turbulence in the aorta. J Fluid Mech 52: 137–160, 1972.
19. Paulsen PK, Hasenkam JM: Three-dimensional visualization of velocity profiles in the ascending aorta in dogs, measured with a hot-film anemometer. J Biomech 16: 201–210, 1983.
20. Reuben SR, Swadling JP, Lee G de J: Velocity profiles in the main pulmonary artery of dogs and man, measured with a thin-film resistance anemometer. Circ Res 27: 995–1001, 1970.
21. Sabbah HN, Blick EF, Anbe DT, Stein PD: Effect of turbulent blood flow on systolic pressure contour in the ventricles and great vessels: Significance related to anacrotic and bisferious pulses. Am J Cardiol 45: 1139–1147, 1980.
22. Schultz DL: Pressure and flow in large arteries. In: Bergel DH (ed) Cardiovascular fluid dynamics, 1. Academic Press, London, 1972, pp 287–314.
23. Stein PD, Sabbah HN: Turbulent blood flow in the ascending aorta of humans with normal and diseased aortic valve. Circ Res 39: 58–65, 1976.
24. Stein PD, Sabbah HN: Hemorheology of turbulence. Biorheology 17: 301–319, 1980.
25. Sugawara M: Biofluid mechanics: Fluid mechanics of the heart and large vessels. Iyodenshi To Seitai Kogaku (Jpn J Med Elec Biol Eng) 19: 511–517, 1981 (in Japanese).
26. Sugawara M, Furuhata H, Kikkawa S, Suzuki S, Ohnishi S, Takabayashi W, Suzuki N, Kurokawa T, Yoshimura S, Caro CG: Development of a non-invasive method of measuring blood pressure wave (Abstract). Iyodenshi To Seitai Kogaku (Jpn J Med Elec Biol Eng) 21 (Suppl): 429, 1983 (in Japanese).
27. Sugawara M, Yamaguchi T: Basic ideas in fluid dynamics. In: Okino H, Sugawara M, Matsuo H (eds) Shinzokekkankei No Rikigaku To Kisokeisoku (Cardiovascular mechanics and fundamental measurements). Kodansha, Tokyo, 1980, pp 156–186 (in Japanese).
28. Szymański P: Sur l'écoulement non permanent du fluide visqueux dans le tuyau. Proc Inter Cong Appl Mech Stockholm 1: 249–254, 1930.
29. van den Bos GC, Westerhof N, Randall OS: Pulse wave reflection: Can it explain the differences between systemic and pulmonary pressure and flow waves? A study in dogs. Circ Res 51: 479–485, 1982.
30. Weinbaum S, Parker KH: The laminar decay of suddenly blocked channel and pipe flows. J Fluid Mech 69: 729–752, 1975.
31. Yamaguchi T, Kikkawa S, Yoshikawa T, Tanishita K, Sugawara M: Measurement of turbulence intensity in the center of the canine ascending aorta with a hot-film anemometer. J Biomech Eng 105: 177–187, 1983.
32. Yamaguchi T, Sugawara M: Turbulence in the aorta. In: Okino H, Sugawara M, Matsuo H (eds) Shinzokekkankei No Rikigaku To Kisokeisoku (Cardiovascular mechanics and fundamental measurements). Kodansha, Tokyo, 1980, pp 199–216 (in Japanese).
33. Yamaguchi T, Sugawara M, Sakurai Y: The application of hot-film anemometer to blood flow velocity measurements. Iyodenshi To Seitai Kogaku (Jpn J Med Elec Biol Eng) 16: 130–133, 1978 (in Japanese).
34. Yano T, Sawaguchi H, Tsuchihashi K, Kikkawa S, Yamaguchi T, Sugawara M: Time-space distribution of some statistical parameters of aortic turbulence. Proc Jpn Soc Biorheol 9: 315–318, 1986 (in Japanese).
35. Yoshimura S, Furuhata H, Kodaira K: Cerebral arteriosclerosis. In: Sugawara M, Matsuo H, Kajiya F, Kitabatake A (eds) Ketsuryu (Blood flow). Kodansha, Tokyo, 1985, pp 260–301 (in Japanese).
36. Yoshimura S, Kodaira K, Fujishiro K, Furuhata H: A newly developed non-invasive technique for quantative measurement of blood flow: With special reference to the measurement of carotid arterial blood flow. Jikei Med J 28: 241–246, 1981.
37. Young DF: Fluid mechanics of arterial stenoses. J Biomech Eng 101: 157–175, 1979.

Address for offprints:
Motoaki Sugawara
Department of Surgical Science
The Heart Institute of Japan
Tokyo Women's Medical College
8-1 Kawada-cho, Shinjuku-ku
Tokyo 162, Japan

Medical Progress through Technology 12 (1987) 77–85

An optical-fiber laser Doppler velocimeter and its application to measurements of coronary blood flow velocities

Fumihiko Kajiya, Osamu Hiramatsu, Keiichiro Mito, Yasuo Ogasawara & Katsuhiko Tsujioka
Dept. of Medical Engineering and Systems Cardiology, Kawasaki Medical School, Matsushima 577, Kurashiki, 701–01, Japan

Key words: laser Doppler velocimeter, optical fiber, coronary blood flow velocity

Abstract

In this paper we describe a laser Doppler velocimeter (LDV) with an optical fiber that measures blood flow velocities accurately in a small sample volume. The principle, optical arrangement, spatial and the temporal resolutions and accuracy for blood flow measurements are delineated, followed by a report of the results of measurements of coronary artery and vein blood flow velocities in dogs. Finally, we touch upon some recent progress made in the LDV with an optical fiber pickup.

1. Introduction

Laser Doppler velocimetry has been considered to be a promising new technique capable of measuring blood flow velocity accurately in a small sample volume [6, 13]. Riva et al. [12] first applied a laser Doppler velocimeter (LDV) to measurement of the blood flow velocity in a 200-μm-diameter tube. Blood velocity measurements by LDV subsequently were made in the retinal and skin vessels as well as in the small vessels of frog webs and the rat renal cortex [2, 14, 15, 16].

The application of this method, however, had been restricted to measurement of the blood flow velocity in superficial fine vessels with a thin wall because of the relatively low transparency of blood and the vessel wall to laser light.

Tanaka and Benedek [17] were the first to use a thick fiber-optical catheter (500 μm o.d.) to introduce laser light into a blood vessel. They measured the average blood flow velocity in the rabbit femoral vein by taking an auto-correlation of scattered light. Their method, however, was unable to detect instantaneous changes in pulsatile blood flow and to differentiate reverse from forward flow.

In order to apply LDV to real time observation of phasic arterial and venous blood flow velocity, one should be able to measure the blood flow velocity with a high temporal resolution and also to discriminate the reverse from the forward component. In this study, we developed a high-resolution LDV using an optical fiber to assess local, detailed characteristics of pulsatile blood flow. Kilpatrick also developed an LDV with an optical fiber and demonstrated its utility for blood velocity measurements in the coronary vein [10]. We particularly intended to apply our method to an analysis of the blood flow velocity in the coronary vascular system. Our LDV with an optical fiber has the following advantages: 1) high spatial resolution (~100 μm); 2) high temporal resolution (~8 ms); and 3) excellent accessibility with a flexible thin fiber sensor [3, 4, 5, 19]. This enabled us to measure local blood flow velocities point by point in a coronary artery and blood flow velocities in the small epicardial arteries and veins. We are also trying to measure blood velocities in intramyocardial arteries and veins.

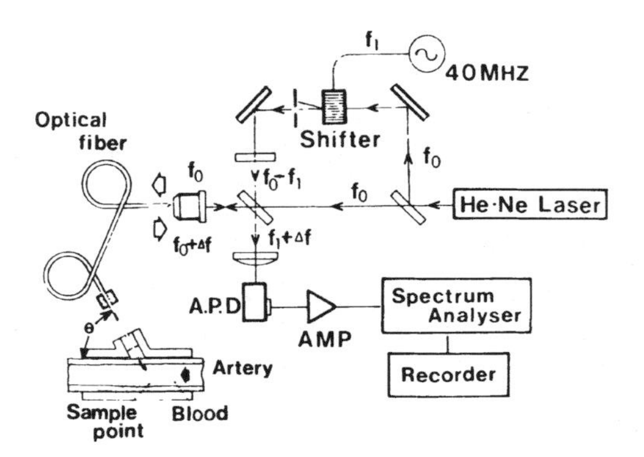

Fig. 1. Schematic diagram of our LDV with an optical fiber system.

2. System of LDV with an optical fiber

2.1 Arrangement of our LDV and measuring principle

A schematic diagram of our LDV and a photograph of the complete system are shown in Figs 1 and 2.

A linearly polarized He-Ne laser beam (frequency of f_O) was divided into incident and reference beams by a polarization beam splitter. The incident beam was focused onto the entrance of an optical fiber using a microscope objective and was guided into the blood stream through the fiber. A portion of the back-scattered light from flowing erythrocytes with diameters of approximately 7 μm is collected by the same fiber and the signal is transmitted back to its entrance.

The back-scattered light signal has a Doppler shift frequency (Δf) given by,

$$\Delta f = 2nV\cos\theta/\lambda \quad (1)$$

where V is the blood flow velocity; n is the refractive index of blood, approximately 1.33; θ is the angle between the fiber axis and the axis of the blood vessel and λ is the laser wave-length of 632.8 nm in a free space. When θ is 60° and λ is 632.8 nm, a Doppler shift frequency of 1 MHz corresponds approximately to blood velocity of 48 cm/sec.

The other beam divided by the beam splitter is used as a reference beam. A frequency shifter, which is a Bragg cell of the driving frequency f_1 (40 MHz), is interposed in the path of the reference beam to distinguish the forward blood flow from the reverse flow. Thus the reference beam is frequency shifted, the resulting frequency being $f_0 + f_1$, where f_O is the original laser frequency. Optical heterodyne detection is done by mixing this reference beam with the Doppler shifted signal of the frequency $f_O + \Delta f$. An avalanche photodiode (APD) was employed as a photodetector since a high signal to noise ratio was predicted. The photocurrent from the APD is fed into a spectrum analyzer to analyse the Doppler shift frequency $f_1 + \Delta f$. Accordingly, the signal spectrum appears to the right of the shifter frequency f_1 for forward blood flow and to the left for reverse blood flow.

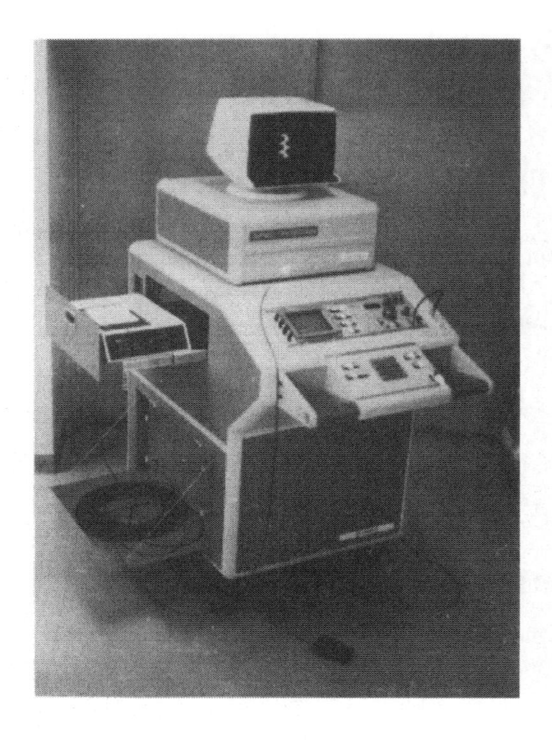

Fig. 2. Photograph of our LDV with an optical fiber.

2.2 Laser and fibers

The laser used is a 5 mW He-Ne (Hughes 3224 H-

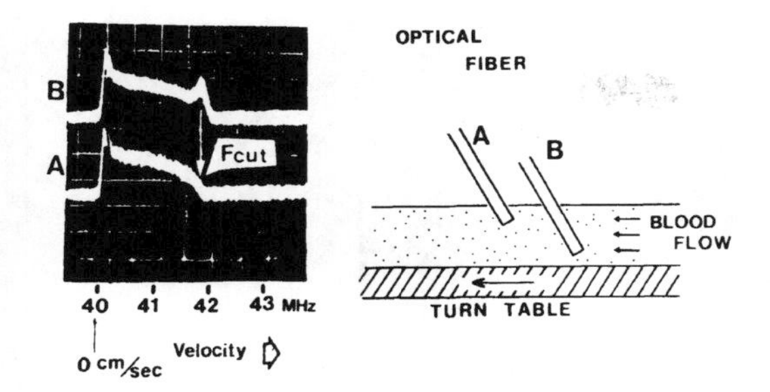

Fig. 3. Doppler signals obtained through an optical fiber from blood flow in the groove on the rotating turntable.

PC), which provides linearly polarized radiation at a wavelength of 632.8 nm. Three types of fibers, step-index multimode fibers, graded-index multimode fibers and step-index single mode fibers, were examined. Multimode fibers have higher efficiency for laser coupling, but lower heterodyne efficiency for the photodetector. Single mode fibers show the reverse characteristics. As a result of several experiments, a multimode graded-index fiber of 125 μm outer diameter and 50 μm core diameter was chosen as a compromise. The excitation was adjusted in such a manner that the number of modes excited was small; i.e., two or three. The total length of the fiber has been optimized to achieve maximum heterodyne efficiency.

2.3 Doppler signal and accuracy of measurement

To evaluate the accuracy of the present method, known blood flow velocities in the circular groove on the rotating turntable were measured at various revolution speeds. The fiber was inserted into the blood flow at an angle of 60°. The typical spectrums of the Doppler signal patterns are shown in Fig. 3. In case A, the power spectrum of the Doppler signal was almost flat from 40 MHz to higher frequencies and then fell to the shot noise level. The spectrum is broadened because the shape contains information about the flow variation of velocities of erythrocytes in the vicinity of the fiber tip. When the fiber tip was moved very close to the bottom of the groove of the rotating turntable as in case B, a Gaussian type sub-peak appeared on the slope of the spectrum (arrow). This sub-peak is due to the Doppler signal from the bottom of the groove, which indicated the actual blood flow velocity. Then we designated the frequency corresponding to the sub-peak as the F-cut and detected this as the measure of the blood velocity. Practically, the frequency interval from 40 MHz to the F-cut was read by keeping the cursor level at an appropriate position.

To evaluate the accuracy of the present measurement, known blood flow velocities in a circular groove on a rotating turntable were measured at various rotational speeds. The frequency interval Δf from 40 MHz to the F-cut was plotted against the known blood flow velocities (Fig. 4). An excellent linear relationship ($r=0.998$) was obtained between the two not only for the forward flow but also for the reverse flow, indicating the high accuracy of our system for measuring blood flow velocities.

2.4 Spatial and temporal resolution

The cross sectional area of the sample volume can be considered to be nearly equal to that of the incident beam ($\pi \times 0.0025\ mm^2$), since the angle of incidence of the laser into blood is small, i.e., about 5 degrees. Then the maximum detectable length for the back-scattered light in the blood was examined repeatedly in the rotating turntable. The maximum distance was found to be around 300 μm in most experiments. However, the actual axial length of the sample volume will be much smaller than 300 μm, because we delete the flow information of regions with lower velocities by taking the F-cut. We estimated that the actual axial length of the sample volume had an order of 100 μm. The frequency response of our system is almost compatible with the sampling rate, i.e., 8 msec.

3. Blood flow velocity measurements in the proximal and distal epicardial coronary arteries [7, 8]

Eleven mongrel dogs were anesthetized with sodium pentobarbital (30 mg/kg) and ventilated with

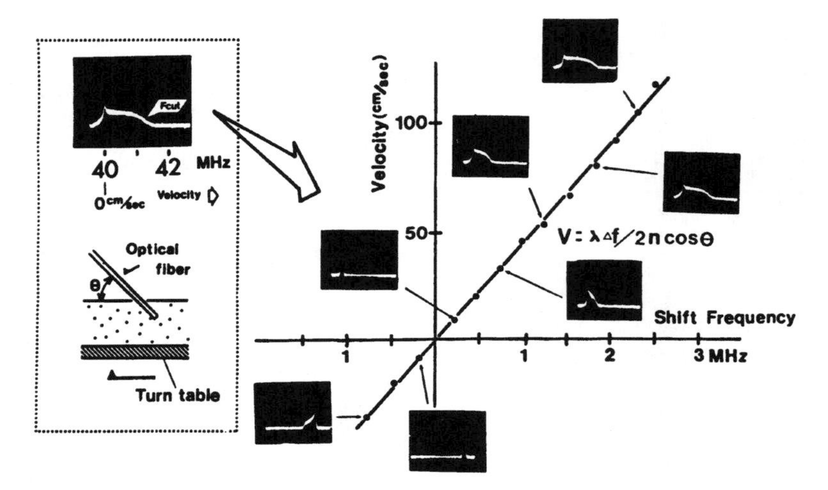

Fig. 4. Relationship between the known blood velocities and the Doppler shift frequency.

room air by a Harvard respirator pump. A thoracotomy in the left intercostal space was performed, the pericardium was opened, and a cradle was formed. The left circumflex coronary artery (LCX) was isolated at its proximal and distal portions. The fiber tip was inserted into vascular lumen at an angle of 60° with the aid of a small plastic cuff, selected out of several types of different diameters (1.0–3.6 mm) to fit the vessel snugly (Fig. 5). The fiber tip was traversed stepwise from the near to the far wall to measure local blood velocity at each sampling point. The position of the fiber tip on the vessel wall was determined by the position where the Doppler signals disappeared. Coronary blood velocity was recorded on a tape recorder (TEAC, R-210) simultaneously with other tracings including pressure and electrocardiography (ECG) [4, 8]. Direct paper recordings were also made on an 8 channel mingograph (NIHON-KODEN, RIJ-2108). By keying on the R wave in the ECG, the velocity profile in the proximal portion of the left circumflex coronary artery was reconstructed during one cardiac cycle.

A representative velocity profile in the proximal

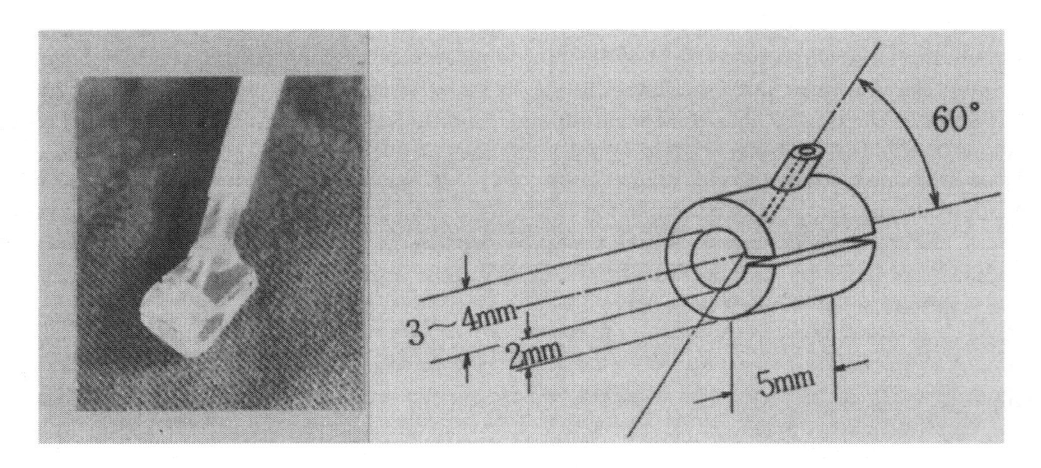

Fig. 5. The plastic cuff to assist fiber insertion into a vessel.

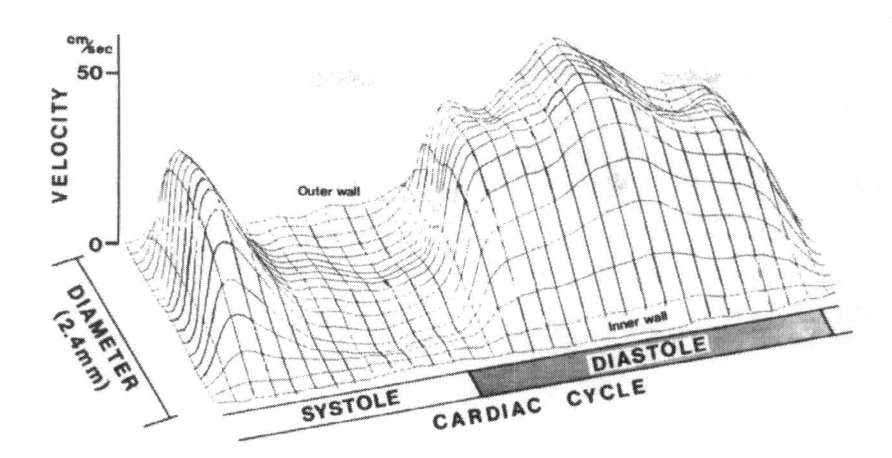

Fig. 6. Three dimensional display of the blood velocity profiles in the coronary artery of a mongrel dog. This is reconstructed from the velocity wave-forms at more than 20 sampling points across the vessel by keying on the R wave in ECG.

LCX is shown in Fig. 6. The characteristics of coronary arterial velocity profiles are readily comprehensible using the three dimensional display.

The velocity waveform showed a diastole predominant pattern which is a characteristic of the coronary arterial flow. The velocity profile across the vascular lumen was flat near the central region and declined abruptly at the vicinity of the vessel wall. The profiles were not symmetric in many cases and, in this case, skewing towards the outer walls was observed.

Fig. 7 shows an example of the blood flow velocity profile in the distal portion of the left circumflex coronary artery. Compared with the velocity profile in the proximal portion, the magnitude of blood velocity was smaller in the distal portion throughout the cardiac cycle. A small reverse flow was observed in some other cases during early systole. The velocity profile across the vascular lumen was developed in the distal portion.

Isoproterenol administration enhanced the difference between the proximal and distal velocity waveforms. Fig. 8 shows an example of the flow velocities. In the proximal portion, the early systolic flow component increased (white arrow) and the reverse flow appeared in mid-systole (black

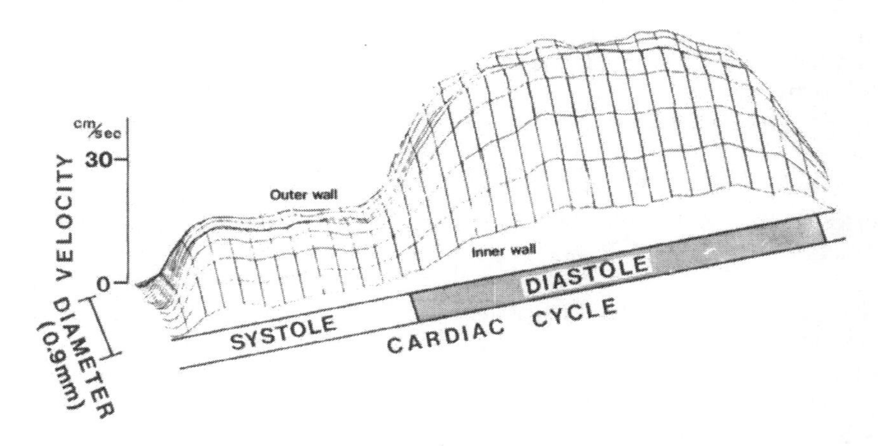

Fig. 7. Three dimensional display of the blood velocity profiles in the distal left circumflex artery.

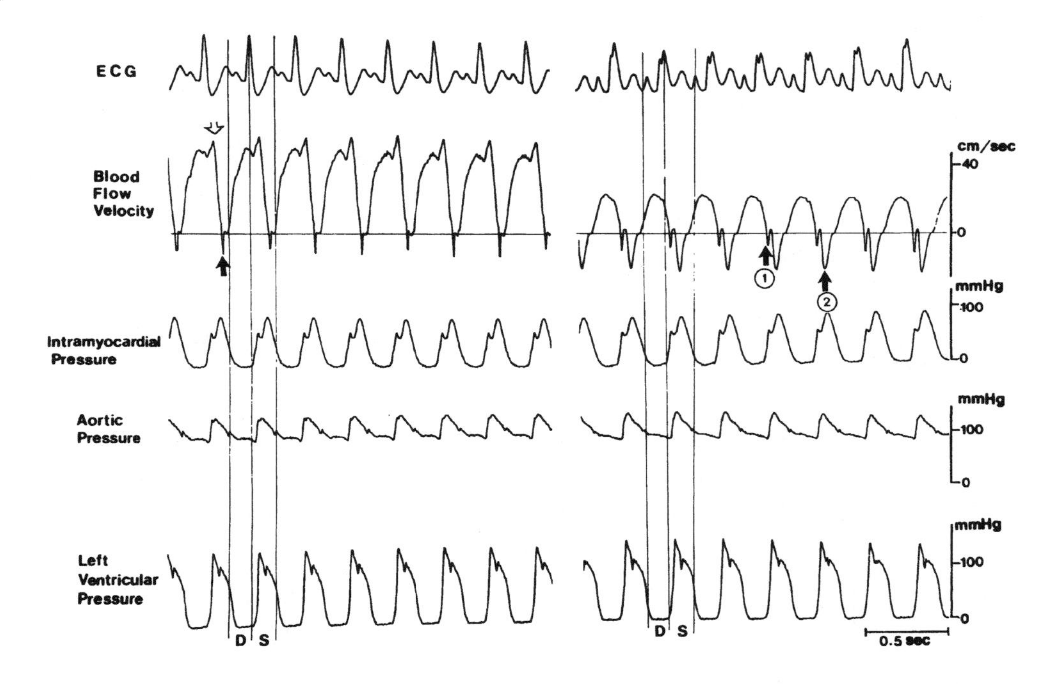

Fig. 8. Effect of isoproterenol on blood velocity in the proximal and distal coronary arteries.

arrow), whereas in the distal portion, the systolic forward flow component became smaller and the reverse flow was divided into two components, i.e., the early and mid-systolic components (arrow 1, 2). The difference in the blood velocity waveforms between the proximal and distal portions probably is mainly caused by the compliance of the epicardial artery, as indicated by Chilian et al. [1]. Therefore, it is necessary to measure the blood flow velocity in the distal portion to evaluate the blood inflow into myocardium.

4. Velocity waveform of blood flow in the great cardiac vein and in an intramyocardial small vein [9]

The optical fiber probe was inserted into the vascular lumen of the great cardiac vein (GCV) with the aid of a cuff in a similar manner to the procedure for coronary artery flow measurements. The tip of the fiber probe was fixed at an optimal position to measure the central maximum velocity after briefly traversing this position from the near to the far wall of the vessel.

The blood velocity wave-form obtained in the great cardiac vein was always characterized by a prominent systolic flow wave in contrast to the coronary artery flow (see Figs 6 and 7). As shown in the representative tracing of blood flow velocity in Fig. 9, the blood velocity increased around the onset of left ventricular ejection and decreased gradually after the peak formation at midsystole. Besides this systolic forward flow, two small backflow components were found in the phase of atrial contraction and during the isovolumic contraction phase of the left ventricle in this particular case.

Recently we have attempted to measure the intramyocardial venous flow velocity in a distal branch of the anterior interventricular vein in the dog. Fig. 10 shows a typical recording of the intramyocardial venous flow velocity. In contrast to coronary arterial flow, coronary venous flow is always characterized by a prominent systolic flow wave. The vein flow appeared at the onset of left ventricular isovolumic contraction. After peak for-

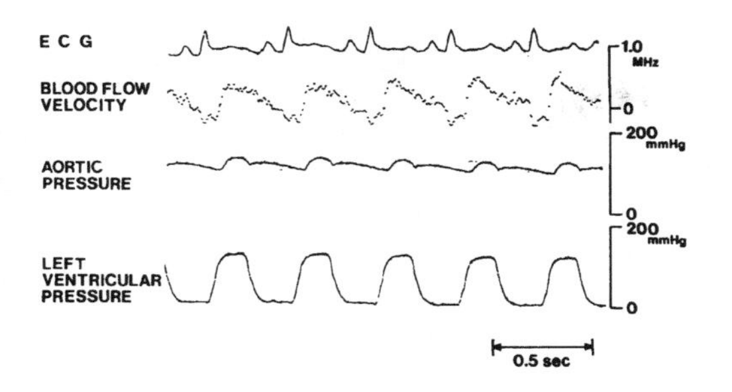

Fig. 9. Velocity wave-form of blood flow in the central axial portion of the great cardiac vein.

mation, the flow velocity decreased with ventricular relaxation. It should be noted that the phase of the velocity pattern in an intramyocardial vein is faster than that in the great cardiac vein or in the coronary sinus.

5. Recent progress on the LDV with an optical fiber pickup

As explained so far, our LDV with an optical fiber is promising for making detailed measurements of arterial and vein flow velocities. Several attempts are being made to improve this velocimeter. Below, we describe two of these.

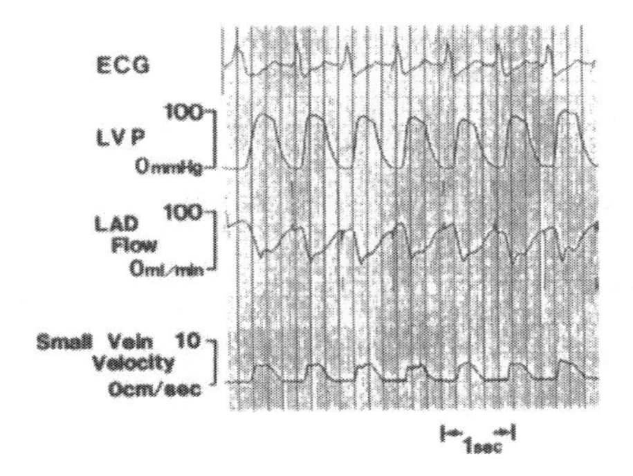

Fig. 10. Velocity wave-form in an intramyocardial coronary vein distal to the anterior interventricular vein measured by our laser Doppler velocimeter.

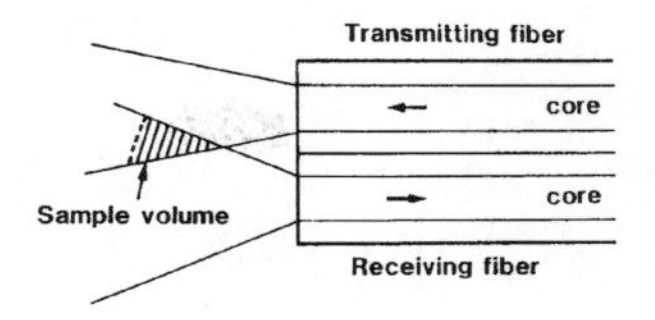

Fig. 11. Schematic drawing of the laser Doppler velocimeter with a two fiber pickup.

5.1 LDV with an optical dual fiber

First, we developed an LDV with a single fiber and succeeded in measuring coronary blood velocities. However, the one fiber system suffers from a broad Doppler spectrum due to flow disturbance in the vicinity of the fiber tip.

To improve the Doppler shift spectrum we tested an LDV with two fibers, which extends the sensing field away from the fiber tip (Fig. 11). The two fibers were placed side by side as proposed by Ohba et al. [11]. The He-Ne laser beam was focused on the entrance of a graded-index multimode fiber (clad diameter: 0.0625 mm, core diameter: 0.05 mm). The light was emitted into a blood flow field with a spreading angle of 5°. The back-scattered light was collected by another fiber with a receiving angle of 17.3°. Doppler signals were analyzed by a spectrum analyser. Evaluation of the Doppler signal was performed using an annular open channel blood flow on a rotating turntable. The spectrum pattern of the Doppler shift frequency showed a peaked pattern (Fig. 12, left). Compared with the original pattern, the spectrum pattern was improved and it became easier to detect the Doppler shift frequency using the two fiber pickup. The accuracy of blood flow velocity measurements was satisfactory, since the Doppler shift frequency showed an excellent linearity with the known blood velocities (Fig. 12, right).

5.2 Integrated-optic fiber laser Doppler velocimeter

The LDV with an optical fiber used until now has been rather bulky and a careful optical alignment has been required. Recently, our collaborators

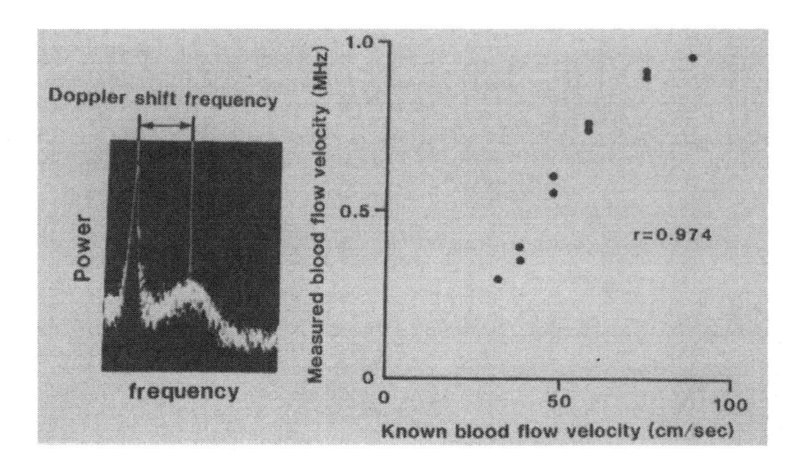

Fig. 12. Doppler signal obtained by the two fiber pickup system (left). Relationship between the known-blood velocities and the Doppler shift frequency.

Nishihara et al. [18] introduced integrated optical technology into the LDV with an optical fiber (Fig. 13). The optical arrangement has now become very compact. A Z-propagation $LiNbO_3$ is used as the substrate and a 4-μm wide Ti-diffused $LiNbO_3$ is employed as the waveguide. The incident TE guided mode is divided into two parts at the Y-junction. The light propagating along the upper arm is fed into a polarization maintaining optical fiber through the TE/TM mode splitter. The output light is transmitted to moving particles through the quarter-wave plate. The reflected light with Doppler signals is received by the same fiber and transmitted back to the entrance. Half of the incident TE mode is converted to the TM mode by the mode converter so that the polarization state coincides with that of the signal light. The light reflected by an aluminum-film mirror is used as a reference light after shifting the frequency with a serrodyne SSB modulator. The reference and signal lights are heterodyne-detected by an avalanche photodiode.

Although the principle is the same as that of our earlier LDV, the optical IC LDV is promising because of the ease of handling.

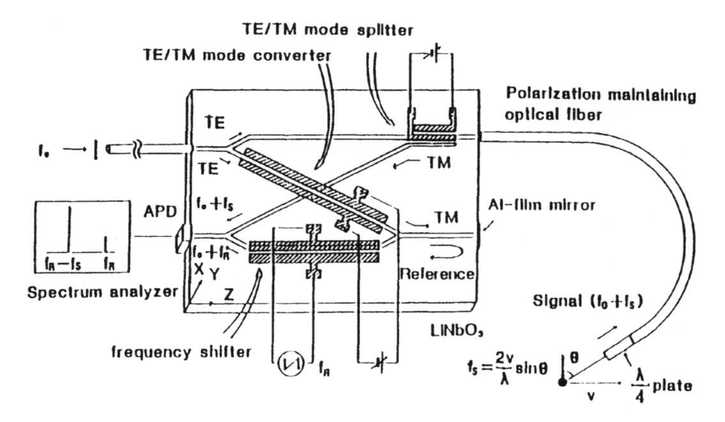

Fig. 13. Configuration of an integrated circuit of a laser Doppler velocimeter with an optical fiber. The circuit consists of a waveguide interferometer and key waveguide components such as a frequency shifter, a TE-TM mode converter and a mode splitter in a Z-propagation $LiNbO_3$ substrate (courtesy of Prof. H. Nisihara and Dr. M. Haruna).

Acknowledgment

We are grateful to the SPIE, ASME, and Springer-Verlag for permission to partly reproduce our papers published in Proceedings of SPIE 494: 25–31 (1984), J. Biomech. Eng 107: 10–15 (1985), and Heart and Vessels 1: 16–23 (1985).

References

1. Chilian WM, Marcus ML: Coronary venous outflow persists after cessation of coronary arterial inflow. Am J Physiol 247: H984–H990, 1984.
2. Horimoto M, Koyama T, Mishina H, Asakura T: Pulsatile blood flow in arteriole of frog web. Biorheology 16: 163–170, 1979.
3. Kajiya F: Laser Doppler blood velocimetry with optical fiber. Digest of 2nd International Conference on Mechanics in Medicine and Biology 16–17, 1980.
4. Kajiya F, Hoki N, Tomonaga G: Evaluation of blood velocity profile in dog coronary artery by laser Doppler method. Circulation (Abstract) 64: IV–40, 1981.
5. Kajiya F, Hoki N, Tomonaga G, Nishihara H: A laser-Doppler-velocimeter using an optical fiber and its application to local velocity measurement in the coronary artery. Experientia 37: 1171–1173, 1981.
6. Kajiya F, Hoki N, Tomonaga G, Saito M: Engineering approaches to the evaluation of cardiac function in future. Med Prog Technol 9: 57–65, 1982.
7. Kajiya F, Mito K, Ogasawara Y, Tsujioka K, Tomonaga G: Laser Doppler blood flow velocimeter with an optical fiber and its applications to detailed measurements of the coronary blood flow velocities. Proceedings of SPIE 494: 25–31, 1984.
8. Kajiya F, Tomonaga G, Tsujioka K, Ogasawara Y, Nishihara H: Evaluation of Local Blood Flow Velocity in Proximal and Distal Coronary Arteries by Laser Doppler Method. Trans ASME J Biochem Eng 107: 10–15, 1985.
9. Kajiya F, Tsujioka K, Goto M, Wada Y, Tadaoka S, Nakai M, Hiramatsu O, Ogasawara Y, Mito K, Hoki N, Tomonaga G: Evaluation of phasic blood flow velocity in the great cardiac vein by a laser Doppler method. Heart and Vessels 1: 16–23, 1985.
10. Kilpatrick D, Linderer T, Sievers RE, Tyberg JV: Measurement of coronary sinus blood flow by fiber-optic laser Doppler anemometry. Am J Physiol 242: H1114, 1982.
11. Ohba K, Matsuno T: Local velocity measurement of opaque Fluid Flow using laser Doppler velocimeter with optical dual fiber pickup. In: Coleman HW, Pfund PA (eds) Engineering applications of laser velocimetry (Book No. H00230). ASME, New York, NY, 1982, pp 145–152.
12. Riva C, Ross B, Benedek GB: Laser-Doppler measurements of blood flow in capillary tubes and retinal arteries. Invest Ophthalmol 11: 936–944, 1972.
13. Roach MR: Biophysical analyses of blood vessel walls and blood flow. Annu Rev Physiol 39: 51–71, 1977.
14. Stern M: In vivo evaluation of microcirculation by coherent light scattering. Nature 254: 56–58, 1975.
15. Stern M, Lappe DL, Bowen PD, Chimosky JE, Holloway GA, Keiser HR, Bowman RL: Continuous measurement of tissue blood flow by laser-Doppler spectroscopy. Am J Physiol 232: H441–448, 1977.
16. Tanaka T, Riva C, Ben-Sira I: Blood velocity measurements in human retinal vessels. Science 186: 830–831, 1974.
17. Tanaka T, Benedek GB: Measurement of the velocity of blood flow (in vivo) using a fiber optic catheter and optical mixing spectroscopy. Appl Optics 14: 189–196, 1975.
18. Toda H, Haruna M, Nishihara H: Integrated-optic fiber laser Doppler velocimeter: Proposal and first demonstration. Fourth International Conference on Optical Fiber Sensors (Technical Digest) 97–100, 1986.
19. Tomonaga G, Mitake H, Hoki N, Kajiya F: Measurement of point velocity in the canine coronary artery by laser Doppler velocimeter with optical fiber. Jpn J Surg 11: 226–231, 1981.

Address for reprints:
Dr. Fumihiko Kajiya
Dept of Medical Engineering and Systems Cardiology
Kawasaki Medical School
Matsushima 577
Kurashiki 701-01, Japan

Medical Progress through Technology 12 (1987) 87–99

Current development in Doppler echocardiography

The real-time two-dimensional Doppler flow imaging system

Akira Kitabatake, Hiroshi Ito & Michitoshi Inoue
The First Department of Medicine, Osaka University School of Medicine, 1-1-50 Fukushima, Fukushima-ku, Osaka 553, Japan

Key words: real-time two-dimensional Doppler flow imaging system, valvular regurgitation, congenital heart disease, flow distribution map

Summary

Recent advances in ultrasound instrumentations have provided a new Doppler modality capable of displaying the spatial distribution of blood flow velocities by colors on the monochromatic echo image on the real time basis, called the real-time two-dimensional Doppler flow imaging system. With this new Doppler technique, we can noninvasively relate the dynamic flow pattern to the anatomy and the motion of the cardiac structures and can further our understandings of flow dynamics in the circulatory system in health and disease. In clinical cardiology, the Doppler flow imaging technique offeres a quite sensitive approach to the detection of flow abnormalities caused by valvular insufficiency or stenosis and congenital shunt diseases. The spatial distribution of the regurgitant jet flow visualized by the Doppler flow imaging technique provides a semiquantitative approach to the evaluation of the severity of the valvular insufficiency. Furthermore, we can appreciate the spatial and angular orientation of the stenotic or regurgitant jet flow, which allows us to measure the velocity of the jet flow with the optimal beam direction. Though there are some limitations and pitfalls in the Doppler flow imaging system at present, it has provided the mapping of the dynamic distribution of flow velocities, which has never been available with the conventional Doppler technique, and has expanded Doppler capabilities and utilities in clinical cardiology. The Doppler flow imaging system is now widely used as a routine part of noninvasive cardiac examination and is improving its clinical significance.

1. Introduction

Since the initial ultrasonic Doppler device was developed and applied to the measurement of blood flow velocity in peripheral artery by Satomura et al. [15] in Japan in 1960, the ultrasonic Doppler instruments have been technically advanced and are now being widely used as a routine part of noninvasive cardiac axamination. The Doppler echocardiography provides direct data on blood flow velocities in the heart and vessels, which are complementary to the structural information obtained by M mode or two-dimensional echocardiography, and has enhanced our understandings of the blood flow dynamics in the cardiovascular system in health and disease. In clinical cardiology, the Doppler echocardiography provides a sensitive approach to detecting flow abnormalities generated by valve stenosis or regurgitation, and by congenital heart disease. It also offers quantitative methods to measure cardiac output as a product of flow area and the time integral of flow velocity [6, 7], and to estimate the pressure drop across the valve stenosis using the maximal jet flow velocity according to the simplified Bernoulli equation [1, 2].

In the conventional Doppler echocardiography, the sample volume (target of the measurement) for Doppler flow signals is only a single point in the cardiac chamber, and it is difficult to determine the spatial distribution of blood flow velocities. In order to establish the distribution map of the flow, the point by point Doppler searching should be performed, which is quite troublesome. Recent advances in ultrasound instrumentations have provided a new Doppler modality capable of displaying the spatial distribution of blood flow velocities by colors on the echo image on the real time basis, called the real-time two-dimensional Doppler flow imaging system or color flow mapping [10, 11]. This Doppler flow imaging technique has extended Doppler capabilities and provides a number of utilities in clinical cardiology [8, 12, 14].

The purpose of this article is firstly to describe the principles and instrumentations of the new Doppler flow imaging technique and, then, to demonstrate the clinical significance of the Doppler flow imaging technique in the diagnosis and evaluation of valvular lesions and congenital heart diseases.

2. Principles and instrumentations

2.1 Principles of the Doppler flow imaging system

The basic concept of the real-time Doppler flow imaging technique stems from our previous works with a computer-aided multigated pulsed Doppler technique combined with two-dimensional echocardiography. In the multigated Doppler technique, color-coded flow velocity data were plotted on the echo image for the establishment of the distribution map of blood flow velocities at any desired period during a cardiac cycle [4]. The Doppler flow imaging system also uses a pulsed Doppler technique to serially build a number of sampling gates along any particular ultrasound beam within the sector image.

Emitted ultrasound pulses are reflected from either cardiac structures or moving red cells. The reflected ultrasound pulses are devided into two electric circuits: one is used for the two-dimensional echo imaging based on the amplitude analysis, and the other is used for Doppler velocity analysis. Doppler signals are assembled from any and all of sampling gates of each beam within the sector image and processed by a digital autocorrelator to establish a dynamic distribution map of blood flow on the two-dimensional echo image (Fig. 1). In the digital autocorrelator, the emitted and received ultrasound waveforms are compared with each other on the time domain, and the time difference between the two ultrasound waveforms is computed. The time difference is theoretically related to the phase difference between the two waveforms, according to the principle of Wiener-Khinchine. Since the magnitude of the phase difference is proportional to the blood flow velocity, the blood flow velocity at any depth of the beam of sight within the sector image is separetely and quickly calculated in the autocorrelator. The Doppler velocity data within any particular location are sent to a digital scan converter where they are read out into a color converter and are displayed in the corresponding portions by colors on the monochromatic echo image.

During processing of Doppler signals in the digital autocorrelator the signals derived from cardiac structures are effectively canceled out because slowly moving cardiac structures yield little or no detectable time shift in the reflected ultrasound as compared with rapidly moving red cells and the detected time shift is eliminated by the digital filter. Thus, the autocorrelator technique is advantageous for detecting and processing weak Doppler signals generated by red cells.

The output of the Doppler flow imaging technique include mean flow velocity and the variance of velocity components around the mean velocity. The variance is interpreted to represent the degree of flow disturbances. In commercially available instruments, the flow toward the transducer is coded in red and that away from the transducer, in blue. The magnitude of the flow velocity is expressed by increasing the brightness of the color. The degree of the flow disturbances is represented by mixing green to the color.

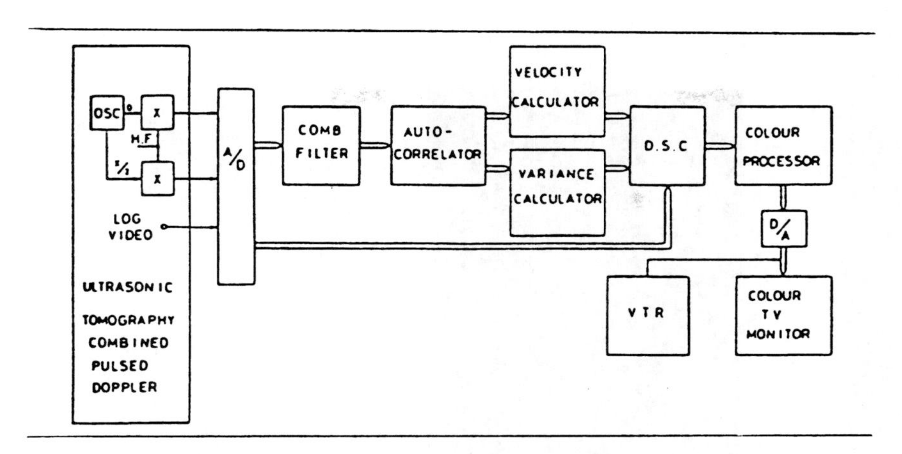

Fig. 1. Blockdiagram of the real-time two-dimensional Doppler flow imaging system. The received ultrasound pulses are analysed by the digital autocorrelator to calculate the mean flow velocity and the variance of the velocity components around the mean flow velocity, which are sent to the digital scan converter (DSC). The Doppler velocity information is read out in the colour processor and displayed by colours on the screen together with the monochromatic echo image.

2.2 Instrumentations

In commercially available Doppler flow imaging systems, the color flow imaging unit is incorporated in the real-time two-dimensional echocardiograph. The carrier frequency we are employing is 2.5 to 5.0 MHz, and the pulse repetition frequency is variable; i.e., 4, 6 or 8 kHz. Two-dimensional echocardiogram and color-coded Doppler velocity imaging are simultaneously obtained from a phased-array transducer composed of 48 or 64 piezoelectric elements. In the Doppler flow imaging system, besides performing 90 degree anatomic sector scanning, the dynamic color flow imaging can also be obtained within 30, 45 or 60 degree sector image. When 45 degree sector scan is applied to the color flow imaging, the sector image is composed of 30 or 32 lines of the sight in commercially available devices. Each line displays the flow and structural data obtained from the 8 successively transmitted ultrasound pulses. It takes 66 or 77 msec to establish one sector image, and the rate of sector scanning is 13 or 15 frames/sec.

2.3 Limitations and pitfalls

The real time display of the Doppler flow imaging system is obviously dynamic and furthers our understandings of flow patterns in the circulatory system in health and disease. However, we should take possible limitations and pitfalls of this Doppler system into account in the interpretation of the flow patterns. The limitations are mostly related to the frequency aliasing, signal-to-noise problems of Doppler signals originating from the deep portion, angular dependency of Doppler velocity signals and Doppler gain setting.

Frequency aliasing. Since the sampling of Doppler signals is intermittent due to the finite transit time of the pulsed signals, the Doppler frequency shifts corresponding to flow velocity can be assessed without ambiguity only if its magnitude is less than one half of the pulse repetition frequency (Nyquist frequency (limit)) according to the 'sampling theory'. If the flow velocity exceeds the Nyquist limit, the Doppler flow imaging system provides a unique display of high velocity flow. Velocity components that exceed the Nyquist limit wrap around to the reverse color as if it goes to the opposite direction to the expected one. Color reversal is often encountered when we record the stenotic or regurgitant jet flow.

Signal-to-noise problem. Signal-to-noise problems

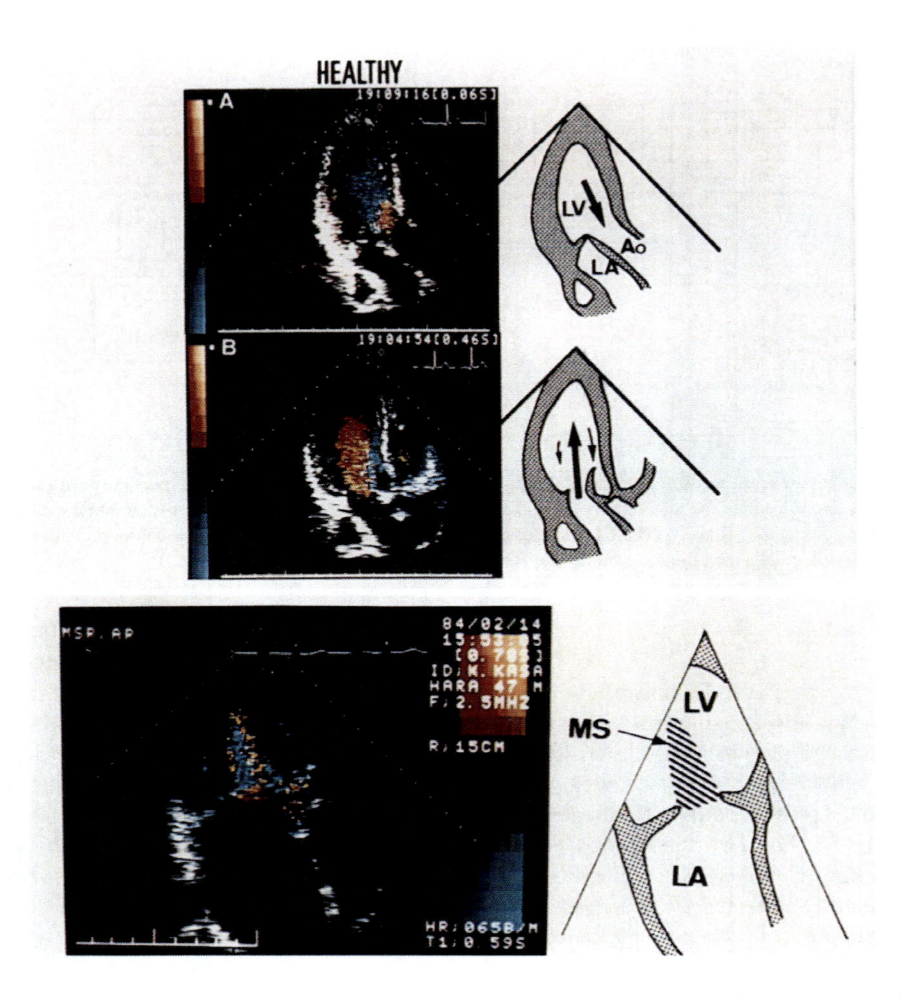

Figs 2A & B. Normal distribution map of flow velocities in the left ventricle observed from the cardiac apex in systole (A) and in diastole (B). In systole (A), the left ventricular cavity is filled with the bluish color representing the flow velocity components away from the transducer. The ejection flow is spatially accelerated from the apex toward the outflow tract as represented by increasing the brightness of the color. The color reversal is observed just below the aotic valve in the outflow tract. In diastole (B), in turn, the transmitral flow is expressed by the reddish color going toward the cardiac apex. In the apical region, the part of the transmitral flux turns its direction to go down along the interventricular septum or along the free wall toward the body of the left ventricle, representing the eddy current formation. Abbrevations: Ao = aorta, LA = left atrium, LV = left ventricle.

Fig. 3. Mitral stenosis (apical view). In the patient with mitral stenosis, the transmitral flow is expressed by a reddish hue band with the bluish central area representing the color reversal. It spurts from the mitral orifice into the central portion of the left ventricle.

should be taken into account in interpreting the color-coded Doppler velocity data obtained at the deep portion of the heart; for example, in the detection of mitral insufficiency. Poor signal-to noise ratio often makes the true Doppler flow signals illegible.

Angular dependency. It should be emphasized that color-coded velocity display of the Doppler flow imaging system represents not a distribution map of actual velocities but that of the velocity components on the direction of the interrogation beam.

Therefore, the color-coded velocity is the cosine function of the angle between the direction of the blood stream and the interrogation beam. If the direction of the blood stream is perpendicular to that of the interrogation beam, the velocity information is not displayed on the screen. The maximal flow velocity is measured only when the interrogation beam is aimed parallel to the direction of the blood stream.

Gain setting. The color-coded display of Doppler velocity data is much influenced by the Doppler gain setting, and the appropriate gain setting for Doppler flow imaging is important to obtain correct flow information. Where Doppler flow gain is insufficient, the blood flow with low velocity cannot be displayed on the screen. If it is too high, the background of color-coded flow image comes to be so noisy and blurred that the identification of true flow signals may be difficult. Optimal gain setting is usually accomplished by increasing the Doppler flow gain just before the background noise appears.

In spite of these limitations and pitfalls, the Doppler flow imaging technique provides dynamic display of the spatial distribution of blood flow velocities, which is not available from the conventional wave-form display of the pulsed Doppler technique, and has extended Doppler capabilities. It is now expanding its applications and usefulness in clinical cardiology. We will introduce its clinical significance in the following chapters.

3. Clinical applications

3.1 Normal flow pattern in the left ventricle

Figs 2 A and B represent displays of color-coded flow velocity in the normal left ventricle, in which ultrasound beam is interrogated from the cardiac apex.

In systole (Fig. 2A), the ejection flow displayed by the bluish color runs down through the body toward the outflow tract of the left ventricle. As the ejection flow approaches to the outflow tract, the ejection flow velocity is spatially accelerated, which is represented by increasing the brightness of the bluish color, and the color reversal showing the frequency aliasing is observed just below the aortic valve in the outflow tract. No green hue is observed, and the ejection flow is considered to be relatively laminar.

In diastole (Fig. 2B), the transmitral flow, in turn, appears with reddish color. The transmitral flow firstly goes toward the cardiac apex and, then, turns its course in the apical region to run down along the ventricular free wall and interventricular septum toward the base of the left ventricle. This phenomenon is refered to as eddy current associated with the interruption of the transmitral flow at the cardiac apex. This eddy current flow is considered to play a significant role in the closing of the mitral valve. No orange hue is found during diastole, so that the transmitral flow as well as the ejection flow seem not to be turbulent in normal subjects.

3.2 Mitral stenosis

In patients with mitral stenosis, Doppler flow imaging system shows the transmitral jet flow spurting from the stenotic mitral orifice into the left ventricle during diastole (Fig. 3). The width of the transmitral flux in the patients with mitral stenosis is narrow compared with that in normal subjects, representing the stenosis of the mitral orifice. The stenotic jet flow usually represents a layered appearance like a candle flame [8. 14]. The center area of the highest velocity which exceeds the Nyquist limit aliases into the bluish color surrounded by the reddish color, though the center area shows velocity components going toward the transducer. In some cases, the mitral stenotic jet flow goes toward the interventricular septum, and in another cases it spurts toward the central portion of the left ventricular cavity. The direction of the jet flow may vary even in one cardiac cycle. We can easily observe the spatial distribution and the dynamic motion of the mitral stenotic jet flow by the Doppler flow imaging system.

The layered appearance is helpful to recognize the angular orientation of the stenotic jet flow.

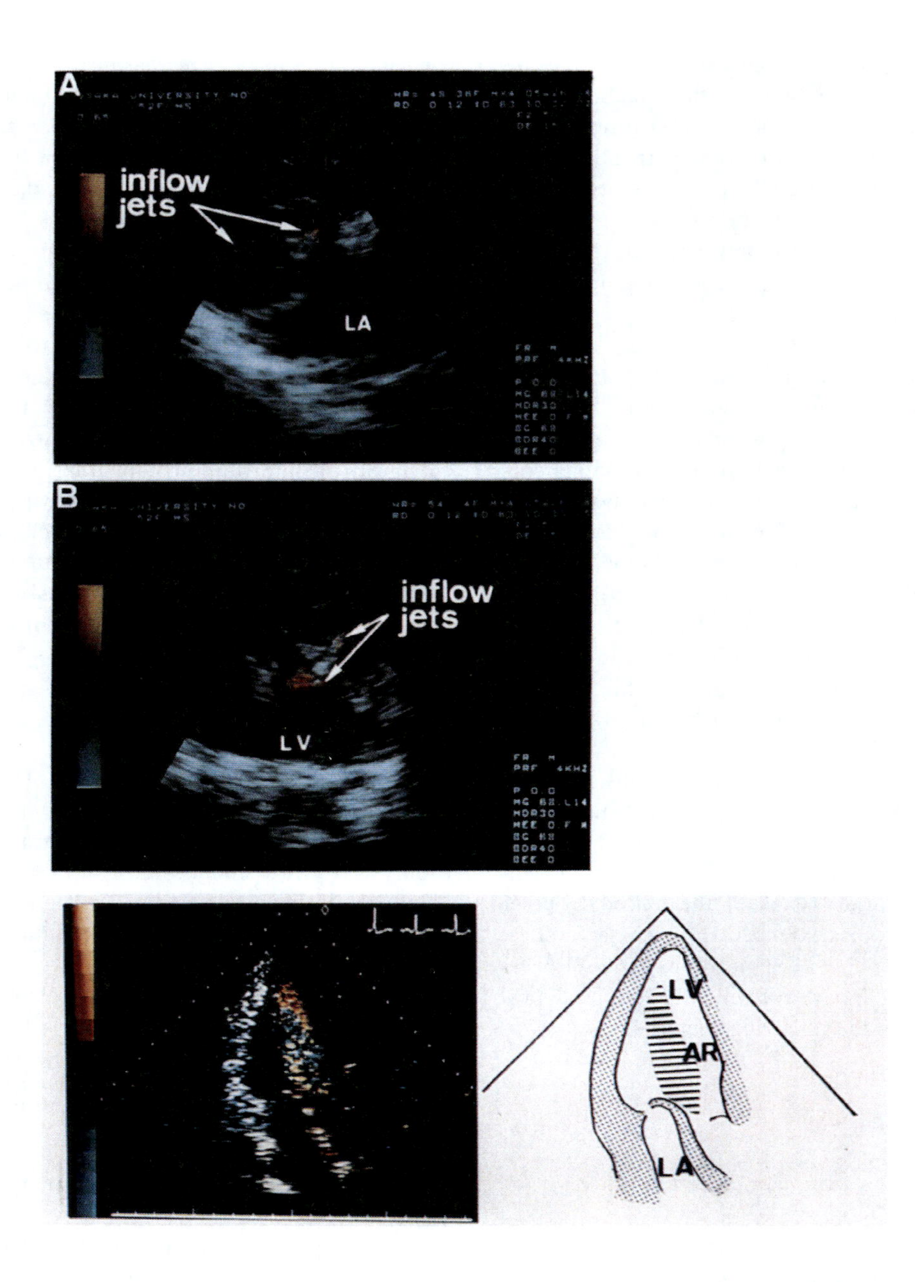

Figs 4 A & B. Mitral stenosis with the rupture of the anterior mitral leaflet (parasternal long axis view (A) and short axis view (B). The double mitral inflow jets may occasionally rarely be observed in patients with mitral stenosis. In this case, the one inflow jet spreads from the mitral orifice toward the central portion of the left ventricle. The other jet spurts from the echo interruption in the anterior mitral leaflet toward the outflow tract. The double inflow jets can be clearly identified by the Doppler flow imaging system. Abbreviations as in Fig. 1.

Fig. 5. Aortic regurgitation (apical iew). Aortic regurgitant jet (AR) represents the mosaic mixture of orange and green colors spreading from the aortic valve into the left ventricular cavity. Abbreviations as in Fig. 1.

Since the direction of the jet flow is regarded as that of the central zone representing the color reversal, we can perform the angle correction for Doppler flow velocity measurements within the plane of imaging. To know the direction of the jet flow also allows us to perform guided continuous wave Doppler examination to obtain maximal flow velocity. We can predict the pressure drop across the mitral stenosis from the maximal flow velocity, according to the simplified Bernoulli equation (2)($\triangle P = 4v^2$; where $\triangle P$ = pressure drop across the valve (in mmHg), v = stenotic jet flow velocity (in m/sec)).

We have occasionally experienced the double mitral inflow jets in patients with mitral stenosis since we begin the ultrasound examination with the color Doppler. Multiple inflow jets are likely caused by either the perforation of the mitral leaflet associated with mitral stenosis or the partial adhesion of the leaflets in the stenotic mitral orifice. Figs 4 A and B illustrate the color flow images of the left ventricle in the patient with mitral stenosis with the perforation of anterior leaflet stenosis. Double inflow jets are clearly depicted: one goes toward the central portion of the left ventricle and the other spurts toward the ventricular outflow tract. The inflow jet toward the ventricular outflow tract introduces flow disturbances which are sometimes hardly differentiated from the aortic regurgitant signals by the conventional pulsed Doppler technique. The dynamic distribution of double inflow jets have hardly been evaluated by the point by point flow mapping technique. However, the Doppler flow imaging system provides easy and useful approach to identify the spatial distribution of the double inflow jets and to help our better understanding of the flow abnormalities in the left ventricle.

3.3 Aortic regurgitation

The aortic regurgitant jet is expressed by the mosaic mixture of orange and green colors spreading from the aortic valve into the left ventricular cavity during diastole (Fig. 5). The sensitivity of the Doppler flow imaging system in the detection of aortic regurgitation was reported to be over 90% in reference to the cineaortographic findings [8].

At present, the mosaic mixture pattern shown in the color-coded flow display is interpreted to be the result of multiple frequency aliasing due to the high velocity regurgitant jet or to represent the spatial disorganization of the flow structure generated by the regurgitant jet. When the Doppler sample volume is placed in the area filled with the mosaic mixture pattern, the fast Fourier transform spectral analysis shows bidirectional spectral broadening during diastole which is the typical finding of the aortic regurgitation by the conventional pulsed Doppler technique. For this reason, the area filled with the mosaic mixture on the color flow image is considered to represent the spatial distribution of the aortic regurgitant flow.

In some cases, the regurgitant jet goes toward the central portion of the left ventricular cavity. In other cases, the regurgitant jet runs down along the interventricular septum generating the oscillation of the septum or along the anterior mitral valve leaflet generating the oscillation of the mitral valve. Thus, we can easily define the direction of the aortic regurgitant jet and investigate the mechanism of the oscillation of either the mitral valve or the interventricular septum by the color flow imaging.

The extent of the aortic regurgitant jet in the left ventricle is useful information for evaluating the severity of the aortic regurgitation. The maximal extent of the aortic regurgitant jet was reported to correlate with the aortic regurgitant fraction in dogs with experimentally produced aortic regurgitation [13]. In clinical study, either the maximal length or area of the regurgitant jet was demonstrated to correlate with semiquantitative cineaortographic grades [12]. However, some problems have been pointed out in the evaluation of the aortic regurgitation by the Doppler flow imaging technique. In patients with additional mitral stenosis, the mitral stenosis often introduces a parallel jet and may obscure the aortic regurgitant flow, so that spatial distribution of the regurgitant jet would be hardly identified (Fig. 6). It would be more problematic in case the aortic regurgitation is mild and mitral stenosis, severe. Such phenomenon may

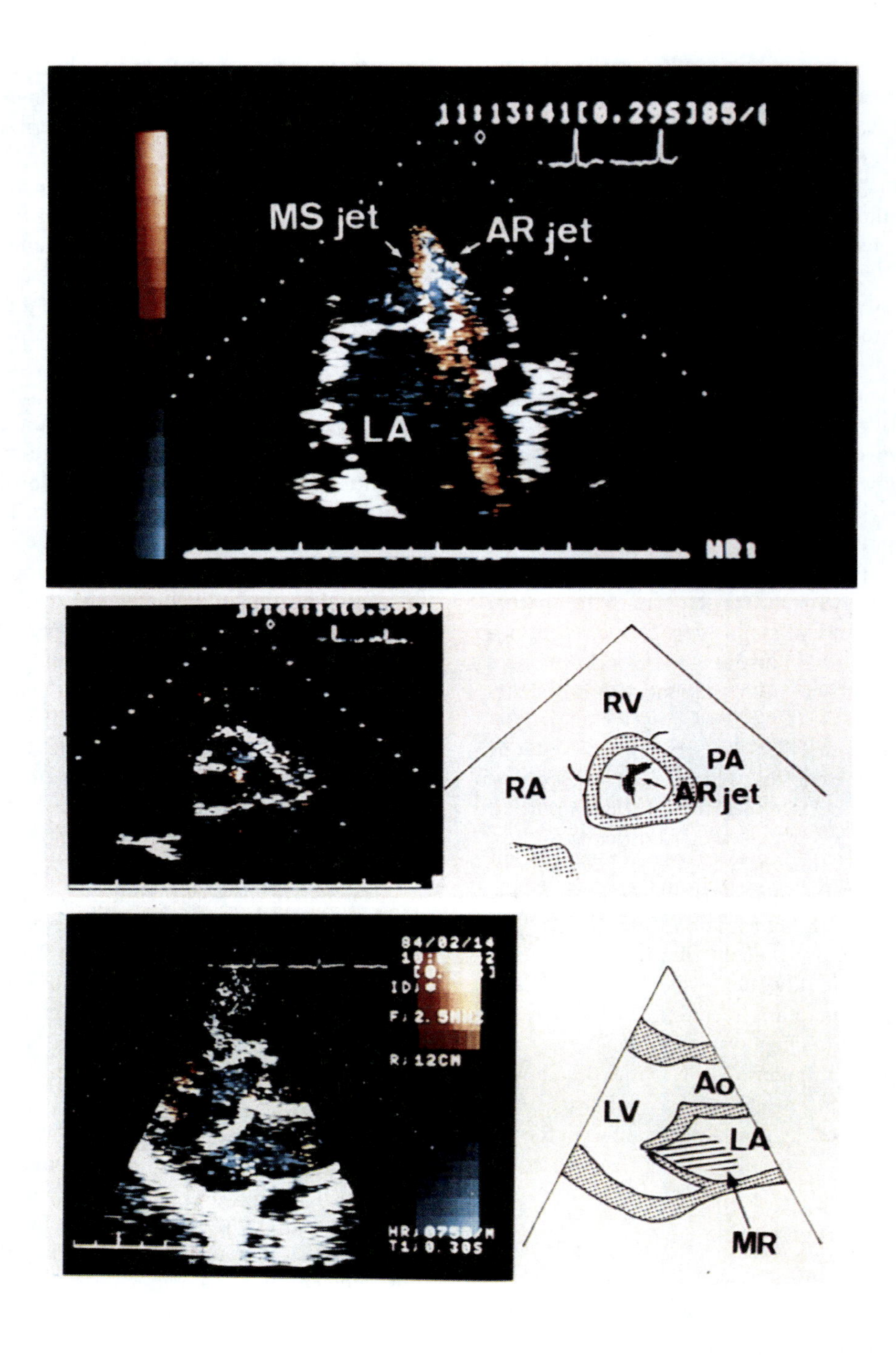
MS jet
AR jet
LA
RV
PA
RA
AR jet
Ao
LV
LA
MR

←

Fig. 6. Association of mitral stenosis with aortic regurgitation (apical view). The mitral stenotic jet (MS jet) introduces flow disturbances in the left ventricle during diastole, which obscure the identification of aortic regurgitant jet flow (AR jet). In such cases, we cannot evaluate the severity of aortic regurgitation merely from the spatial distribution of AR jet. Abbreviation as in Fig. 1.

Fig. 7. Identification of the cross sectional area of aortic regurgitant jet on the short axis view at the level of the aortic valve. The aortic regurgitation is shown by the mosaic mixture of orange and green colors appearing along the edge of the left coronary cusp during diastole in this case. The pathological changes in the left coronary cusp is considered to account for the cause of the aortic regurgitation. The cross section of the aortic regurgitant jet was refered to as the area filled with the mosaic mixture during diastole and was considered to be a useful discriptor for the evaluation of the aortic regurgitation. Abbreviations: AR jet = aortic regurgitant jet, PA = pulmonary artery, RA = right atrium, RV = right ventricle.

Fig. 8. Mitral regurgitation due to the prolapse of the anterior mitral leaflet (parasternal long axis view). In the patients with mitral regurgitation, the mitral regurgitant jet (MR) is expressed by the mosaic mixture of orange and blue spurting from the mitral orifice into the left atrial cavity during systole. In this case, the mitral regurgitant jet goes toward the posterior wall of the cavity. Abbreviations as in Fig. 1.

lead to the misjudgement of the severity of the aortic regurgitation.

The investigation of the aortic orifice on the short axis view provides other useful information for the evaluation of the aortic regurgitation, that is the cross sectional area of aortic regurgitant jet [5]. The cross section of aortic regurgitant jet is usually diplayed by the mosaic mixture of orange and green colors appearing along the edge of the semilunar cusps (Fig. 7) or in the echo defect during diastole. Employing this approach, we can assess anatomic localization of the pathological lesions. In the case of Fig. 7, the aortic regurgitant jet is localized along the edge of the left coronary cusp, and so the incompetence of the left coronary cusp is suspected. We can also evaluate the severity of the aortic regurgitation from the cross sectional area of aortic regurgitant jet. In our previous study, we found a significant correlation between the aortic regurgitant fraction and the cross sectional area of aortic regurgitant jet corrected for the aortic orifice area.

The Doppler flow imaging technique provides useful method in the examination of the prosthetic valve function after the aortic valve replacement. To differentiate the paravalvular leakage from the transvalvular one is clinically important in the diagnosis of the partial detachment of the artificial valve from the surrounding tissue and in determining the timing of re-operation. If the regurgitant jet is originated from the valvular ring outside of the artificial valve, the paravalvular leakage due to the detachment of the valve is suspected. On the other hand, the regurgitant jet is originated from the inside of the artificial valve ring in the case of the transvalvular leakage. Even in the cases of the transvalvular leakage, we have to know the severity of the regurgitation for the evaluation of the function of the artificial valve. In physiological regurgitation as found in the cases of the Björk-Shiley valve, the aortic regurgitation is trivial and well localized near the prosthetic valve in the ventricular outflow tract. However, in cases of the valve dysfunction, the more severe aortic regurgitation is usually found.

3.4 Mitral regurgitation

In patients with mitral regurgitation, the mitral regurgitant jet is expressed by in the mosaic mixture of orange and green colors spreading from the mitral orifice into the left atrium during systole (Fig. 8). The sensitivity of the Doppler flow imaging system for the detection of the mitral regurgitation was reported to be more than 90% in comparison with the cine left ventriculographic findings [8].

The spatial orientation of the mitral regurgitant jet can be visualized by the Doppler flow imaging technique. The regurgitant jet spurts toward the central portion of the left ventricle in a majority of cases of rheumatic mitral insufficiency. On the

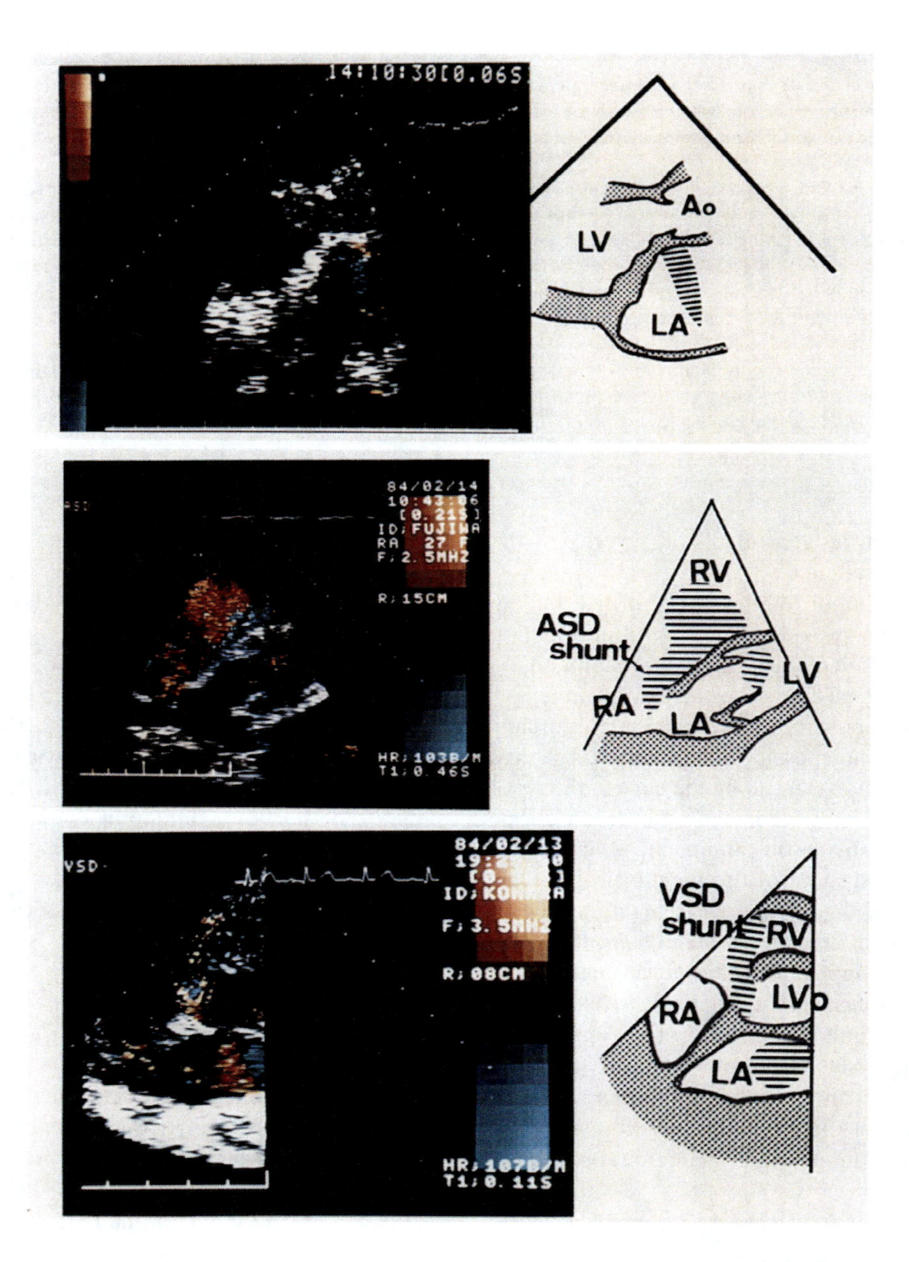

Fig. 9. Paravalvular leakage in the case of the mitral valve replacement (parasternal long axis view). The mitral regurgitant jet originates from the outside of the artificial valve ring and spreads toward the posterior wall of the left atrial cavity. Abbreviations as in Fig. 1.

Fig. 10. Atrial septal defect (parasternal four chamber view). The left-to-right shunting flow (ASD shunt) is expressed by the reddish color running from he left atrium to the right atrial outflow tract through the echo interruption observed in the interatrial septum. Abbreviations: LA = left atrium, LV = left ventricle, RA = right atrium, RV = right ventricle.

Fig. 11. Ventricular septal defect (membranous type; short axis view). The left-to-right shunting flow (VSD shunt) is expressed by the mosaic mixture of the orange and blue colors spurting from the echo defect observed in the high portion of the interventricular septum toward the right ventricular inflow tract. Abbreviations: LVo = left ventricular outflow tract, other abbreviations as in Fig. 8.

other hand, it tends to go toward the anterior wall of the cavity in the prolapse of the posterior mitral leaflet, and toward the posterior wall in the prolapse of the anterior mitral leaflet. Our previous study [3] suggested that the direction of the mitral regurgitant jet is closely related to the location where the systolic blowing murmur is audible. If the mitral regurgitant jet blows toward the anterior wall, the murmur can be heard on the precordium. On the other hand, the audible point may deviate toward the axilla region if the regurgitant jet goes toward the posterior wall of the atrial cavity. The direction of the regurgitant jet may vary with time even in one cardiac cycle. These time-related changes in the direction of the regurgitant jet have hardly been observed by the conventional pulsed Doppler technique.

The spatial mapping of the mitral regurgitant jet provides the semiquantitative approach to evaluate the severity of mitral regurgitation. The Doppler flow imaging technique is a quite promising technique to observe the changes in the instantaneous maximal extent of the regurgitant jet during one cardiac cycle. Either the maximal length or area of the mitral regurgitant jet was demonstrated to correlate well with semiquantitative grades based on cine left ventriculographic findings [9, 12].

The function of the artificial mitral valve can be assessed by the Doppler flow imaging system in a similar way as shown in the aortic valve replacement. The trans- or para-valvular leakage may be evaluated from the location of the origin of the regurgitant jet. Fig. 9 illustrates the color flow mapping in the case of the paravalvular leakage. The mitral regurgitant jet originates from the outside of the artificial valve ring, and the localized detachment of the artificial valve might be suspected. However, the detection of the mitral regurgitation is sometimes troublesome in these cases because the emitted ultrasound passing the artificial valve is mostly reflected by the hard artificial valve and the weak Doppler signals may be obscured. We should search for a better view for the visualization of the flow signals in the left atrial cavity avoiding the effect of the artificial valve.

3.5 Tricuspid and pulmonary regurgitation

The Doppler flow imaging technique also has advantages for the detection of flow abnormalities produced by tricuspid or pulmonary regurgitation. In patient with tricuspid regurgitation, the regurgitant flow is expressed by the mosaic mixture of orange and blue colors spreading from the coaptation of the tricuspid valve into the right atrial cavity during systole. In some cases, it spurts toward the central portion of the right atrial cavity. In other cases, it blows against the interatrial septum and changes its direction toward the center of the right atrium. In the patients with the pulmonary regurgitation, the regurgitant flow spurts from the pulmonary orifice into the outflow tract of the right ventricle during diastole. The maximal extent of the regurgitant jet was considered to be a useful indicator of the severity of the tricuspid and pulmonary regurgitation.

3.6 Congenital heart disease

The Doppler flow imaging system allows us the rapid orientation to the presence and position of atrial and/or ventricular septal defects. Potential significance is that it would provide a promising method to rapidly identify small or even multiple septal defects. The color Doppler findings in the septal defects are as follows.

Atrial septal defect. In patients with atrial septal defect, the left-to-right shunting flow is usually displayed by reddish color running from the left atrium to the right atrial outflow through the echo interruption in the interatrial septum [8, 14] (Fig. 10). The anatomical size of the septal defect might be semiquantitatively assessed as the width of the shunt flow imaging. The direction of the shunt flow is another useful piece of information to evaluate the presence or absence of the right-to-left shunt flow. Even changes in the instantaneous direction of the shunt flow can be judged by the Doppler flow imaging system. In the cases of the balanced shunt, the co-existence of the left-to-right and right-to-left shunt flows or the instantaneous changes in the direction of the shunt flow can be observed. The right-to-left shunting flow represented in a bluish color is mainly observed in the cases of Eisenmenger complex.

Ventricular septal defect. In patients with ventricular septal defect, the shunt flow through the septal defect produces well localized but highly disturbed flow in the right ventricle during systole [8, 14] (Fig. 11). Even though the echo interruption cannot be visualized in the interventricular septum by the two-dimensional echocardiography because of its limited resolution, the origin of the shunt flow visualized by the color flow imaging is considered to be the location of the defect. The localization of the defect is valuable information in determining the operative procedure.

The direction of the shunt flow may alter under the presence of the severe pulmonary hypertension. In cases of the balanced shunt, the direction of the shunt flow may momentarily vary even in one cardiac cycle. The instantaneous changes in the direction of the shunt flow can be determined by the Doppler flow imaging system.

4. Conclusion

As mentioned above, the real-time two-dimensional Doppler flow imaging technique provides a promising approach to the diagnosis and the evaluation of valvular lesions and congenital heart disease. Moreover, it has also added much other values to the Doppler capabilities and utilities in clinical cardiology.

1. Since it provides the color-coded flow mapping together with monochromatic echo image, we can relate the unusual flow pattern to the anatomic abnormalities of the cardiac structure.
2. Time-sequential changes in the two-dimensional flow structure, which cannot be obtained by the conventional pulsed Doppler technique, can be observed. This dynamic flow image has enhanced our better understanding of flow dynamics in the cardiovascular system in health and disease.
3. Since the total distribution map of the flow velocities on the sector image is continuously displayed, unexpected abnormal flow signals may be found out of the area of one's interest. This is quite helpful in the precise and complete Doppler diagnosis.
4. Examination time would be shortened because troublesome point by point flow mapping procedure can be eliminated.

The Doppler echocardiography including the Doppler flow imaging system is still being technically developed, and this development will further expand the capabilities and clinical applications of the Doppler technique.

References

1. Hatle L: Noninvasive assessment and differentiation of left ventricular outflow obstruction with Doppler ultrasound. Circulation 64: 381–387, 1981.
2. Holen J, Aaslid R, Landmark K, Simonsen S: Determination of pressure gradient in mitral stenosis with a noninvasive ultrasound Doppler technique. Acad Med Scan 199: 455–460, 1976.
3. Kitabatake A, Matsuo H, Asao M, Tanouchi J, Mishima M, Hayashi T, Abe H: Intra-atrial distribution of mitral regurgitation in mitral valve prolapse visualized by pulsed Doppler technique combined with electronic beam sector scanning echocardiography. J Cardiogr 10: 111–121, 1980 (in Japanese).
4. Kitabatake A, Masuyama T, Asao M, Tanouchi J, Morita T, Ito H, Hori M, Inoue M, Abe H, Chihara K, Sakurai Y: Colour visualization of two dimensional distribution of intracardiac flow abnormalities by multigate Doppler technique. In: MP Spencer (ed) Cardiac Doppler Diagnosis. Martinus Nijhoff Publishers, Boston, 1983, pp 309–318.
5. Kitabatake A, Ito H, Nakatani S, Tanouchi J, Ishihara K, Fujii K, Yoshida Y, Tominaga N, Hori M, Inoue M, Kamada T: Cross sectional visualization of aortic regurgitant jet is an effective approach to evaluate aortic regurgitation. J. Cardiogr (in press) (in Japanese).
6. Loeber CP, Goldberg SJ, Allen HD: Doppler echocardiographic comparison of flows distal to the four cardiac valves. J Am Coll Cardiol 4: 268–272, 1984.
7. Magnin PA, Stewart JA, Myers S, von Ramm O, Kisslo JA: Combined Doppler and phased-array echocardiographic estimation of cardiac output. Circulation 63: 388–392, 1981.
8. Miyatake K, Okamoto M, Kinoshita N, Izumi S, Owa M, Takao S, Sakakibara H, Nimura Y: Clinical application of a new type real-time two-dimensional Doppler flow imaging system. Am J Cardiol 54: 857–868, 1984.

9. Miyatake K, Izumi S, Okamoto M, Kinoshita N, Asonuma H, Nakagawa H, Yamamoto K, Takamiya M, Sakakibara H, Nimura Y: Semiquantitative grading of severity of mitral regurgitation by real-time two-dimensional Doppler flow imaging technique. J Am Coll Cardiol 7: 82–88, 1986.
10. Namekawa K, Kasai C, Koyano A: Real-time blood flow imaging system utilizing autocorrelation techniques. In: RA Lerski and P Morley (eds) Ultrasound '82. Peramon Press, Oxford, 1983, pp 203–208.
11. Namekawa K, Kasai C, Omoto R, Kondo Y, Katabaki T, Hidai T, Yoshioka Y, Tsukamoto Y, Yokote Y, Takamoto S, Koyano A: Real time two-dimensional blood flow imaging using ultrasonic Doppler. J Ultrasound Med 2: (Supp 65): 203–208, 1983.
12. Omoto R, Yokote Y, Takamoto S, Kyo S, Ueda K, Asano H, Namekawa K, Kasai C, Kondo Y, Koyano A: The development of real-time two-dimensional Doppler echocardiography and its clinical significance in acquired valvular diseases: with specific reference to the evaluation of valvular regurgitation. Jpn Heart J 25: 325–340, 1984.
13. Sahn DJ, Valdes-Cruz L, Scagnelli S, Tomizuka F, Elias W, Covell J: Two-dimensional Doppler color mapping for spatial localization and quantification of aortic insufficiency: validation of a new diagnostic modality using an open chest animal model. Circulation 70 (Supp II): II–38, 1984.
14. Sahn DJ: Real-time two-dimensional Doppler echocardiographic flow mapping. Circulation 71: 849–853, 1985.
15. Satomura S, Kanek Z: Ultrasonic blood rheograph. In: Proc 3rd Int Conf Med Electronics, 1960, p 254.

Address for offprints:
Akira Kitabatake, M.D.
The First Development of Medicine
Osaka University School of Medicine
1-1-50 Fukushima, Fukushima-ku
Osaka 553, Japan

Medical Progress through Technology 12 (1987) 101–115

Left ventricular image processing

Shigeru Eiho, Michiyoshi Kuwahara & Naoki Asada
Automation Research Laboratory, Kyoto University, Japan

Key words: left ventricular image processing, bound...y detection, 3-D reconstruction of the left ventricle, regional wall motion, 3-D functional image of the left ventricle

Summary

Left ventricular image processing methods of x-ray cineangiocardiograms and ultrasound echocardiograms are discussed. 3-D reconstruction methods of the left ventricle from ultrasound echocardiograms and magnetic resonance images are also discussed.

Boundary detction of the left ventricle and the quantitative analysis of the left ventricular function and wall motion are discussed.

To reconstruct 3-D shapes, we need several cross sectional shapes or silhouettes of the left ventricle. Several cross sectional echo images of apical long axis view are taken by changing the angles of rotation of the probe of echo transducer around its axis. Gated multi-phase MRI method is used to obtain each 2 cross sectional images in transverse, coronal and sagittal directions.

Some results of 3-D shapes of the left ventricle and myocardium reconstructed are shown and 3-D functional images which give us regional functions of the left ventricular wall on three dimensional shape are shown.

1. Introduction

Medical images, obtained by x-ray, ultrasound, radionuclides and others, have been used to diagnose various kinds of diseases for a long time. New kinds of imaging machines, such as digital subtraction angio machines, magnetic resonance imaging and so on, have appeared after x-ray CT machines and they are now clinically used in wide fields of medicine. Medical image processing has been of great interest but there were not so many methods developed and used clinically to produce quantitative data from medical images.

In this paper, some results of the research and development of digital image processing methods for left ventricular images obtained by x-ray, ultrasound and magnetic resonance imaging are discussed.

2. Image processing of cineangiocardiograms

Cineangiocardiography has been used as one of the highly helpful techniques to examine the cardiac functions. Manual techniques such as the tracing of the left ventricular boundary and planimetry have been often used by cardiologists to measure the volume change of the left ventricle. However, manual methods are very troublesome and time-consuming, especially when a large number of images are to be processed.

Some research groups have been working on automatic detection of left ventricular endocardial boundaries. Quantitative information such as volume change and wall motions of the left ventricle during a cardiac cycle can be obtained by detecting the boundary of the left ventricle on every frame of cineangiocardiograms [1, 2, 3, 8, 11].

One of the methods to detect the left ventricular

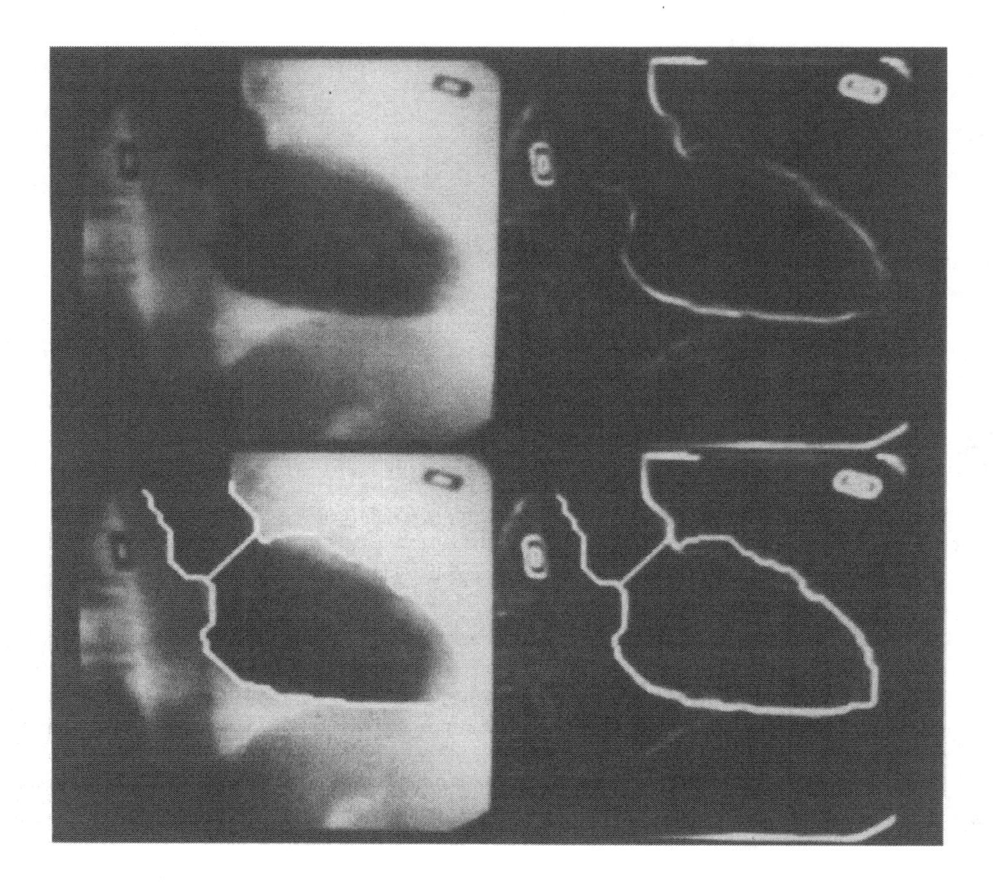

Fig. 1. Cine-leftventriculogram, gradient image and detected left ventricular boundary.

boundary is an automated heuristic tracing of the boundary [3] which uses each gradient image of the left ventriculogram. Fig. 1 shows an example of the original left ventriculogram, its gradient image and each with the detected edge. Fig. 2 shows some of the detected boundaries in a cardiac cycle.

Using consecutive boundary curves during a cardiac cycle thus obtained, we can easily calculate left ventricular volume, cardiac output and ejection fraction by applying the area-length method to those boundary curves. Fig. 3 shows the volume curve thus calculated, where × marks show the volume values obtained by the manual method. As shown in this figure, the curve is fitted to these × marks in a sense of the mean. Moreover the volume values obtained from the manual tracing have much noise. The main reason for this is that the cardiologist drew each curve by watching every still image independently. On the other hand, the volume curve obtained from boundaries drawn by the computer was smooth, because each boundary was detected by referencing the boundary obtained on the previous frame.

Several kinds of the regional wall motion analysis by using the boundary curves obtained will be discussed in Chapter 4.

3. Image processing of echocardiograms

Two dimensional echocardiographic examinations have been widely used as real time noninvasive diagnostic techniques in clinical medicine observing the motion of the left ventricle on various cross

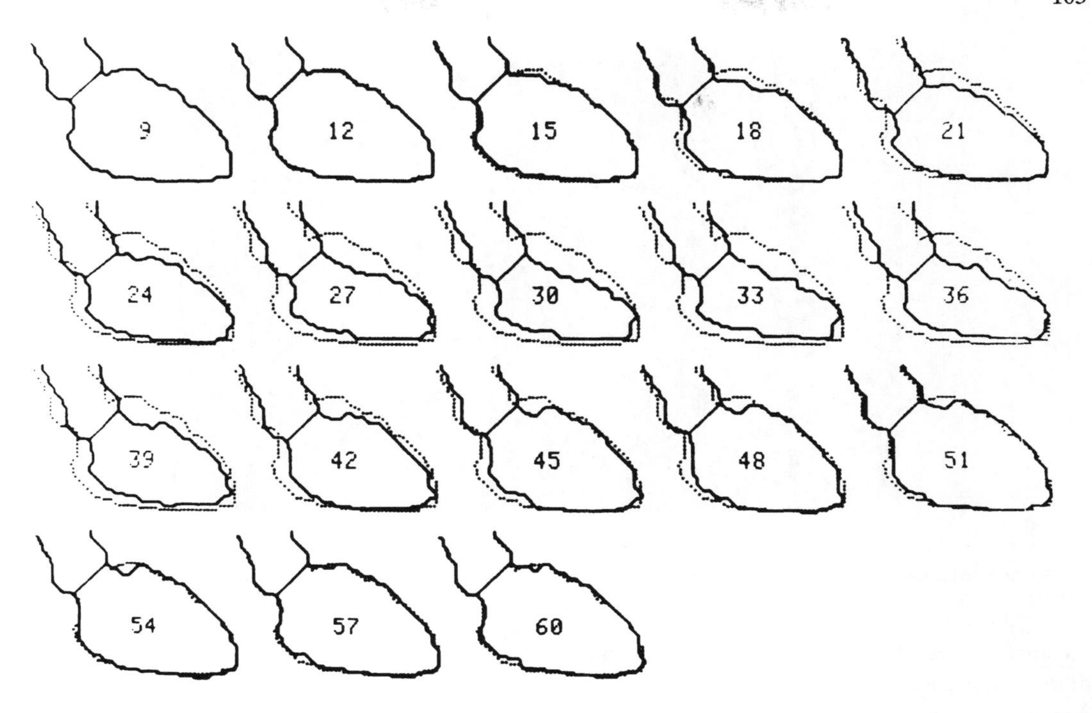

Fig. 2. Left ventricular boundaries in a cardiac cycle.

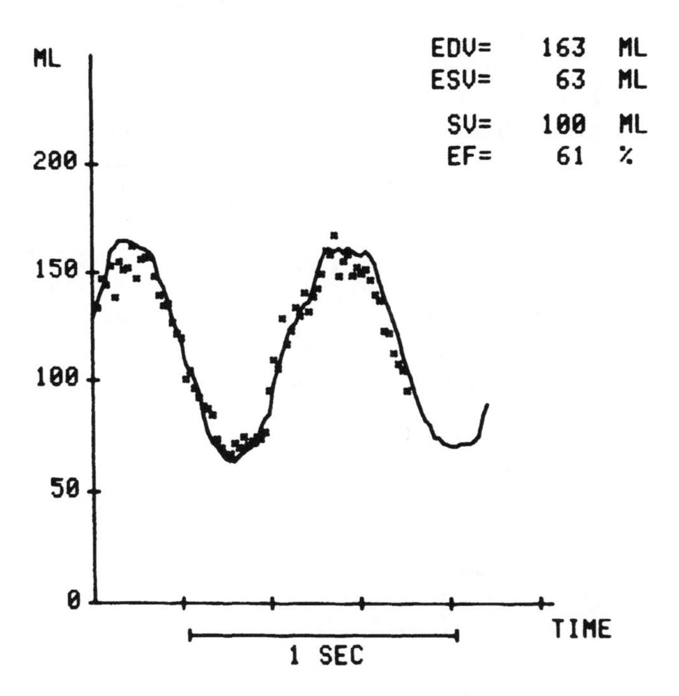

Fig. 3. Volume change of the left ventricle.

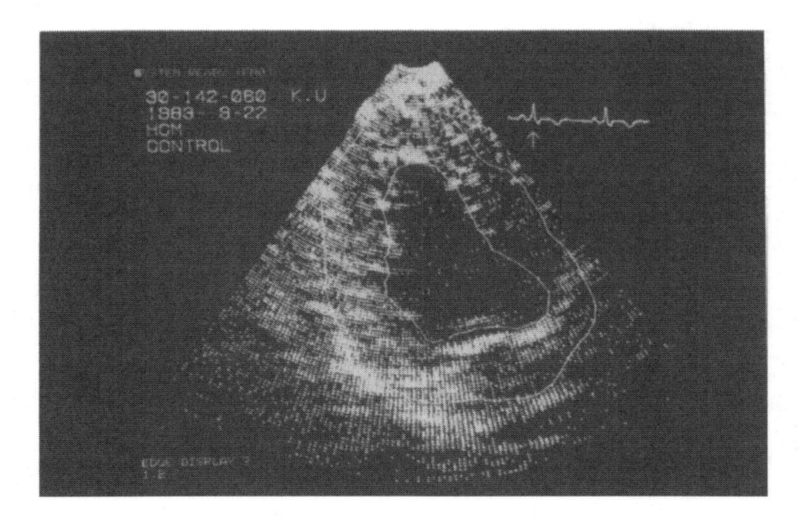

Fig. 4. Detected boundaries and original echocardiogram.

sectional planes. Moreover, various kinds of quantitative information useful for the diagnosis of cardiac diseases are obtainable through image processing of echo data by using a mini- or micro-computer system [5, 7, 9, 10].

Every frame of consecutive 2-D echocardiograms is digitized 128×110 byte data (sector format) with the ECG signal which indicates the cardiac phase of each frame. End diastolic frames are detected by processing the ECG signal and thus the frames in a cardiac cycle to be processed are fixed. The following steps are used for detecting the left ventricular boundaries during the cardiac cycle:

Step 1: Pick up about 10 points of the left ventricular boundary on a digitized image at ED phase. These points are connected by spline curves and used as the principal reference boundary.

Step 2: The echocardiogram in the sector format of the next frame is radially re-sampled at 64 points on 64 directions from the center of gravity of the reference boundary.

Step 3: The boundary point on each radial line is automatically obtained mainly by a thresholding method for endocardial boundary and a maximum-value detecting method for the epicardium. The range for each search is restricted within 5 points both sides of the left ventricular boundaries on the previous frame.

Step 4: The boundary points are smoothed both spatially and temporally by using the present, the previous and the principal reference boundary points.

Step 5: Repeat processing from step 2 to step 4 for frames within two-thirds of the cardiac phase.

Step 6: Again execute step 5 from next ED frame to the frame at one-third of the cardiac cycle backward.

Step 7: Average two boundaries in the middle one-third of the cardiac phase.

Fig. 4 shows an example of the detected endo- and epicardial boundaries superimposed on the original echocardiogram. Fig. 5 shows volume change of the left ventricular inner cavity calculated by the area length method over 64 frames with ECG signal.

4. Regional wall motion analysis

We can obtain various kinds of information related to the cardiac function from detected left ventricular boundaries. Fig. 6 shows an example of the wall movements between end diastole (ED) and end systole (ES) which are given by the change of the length from the center of gravity of ED boundary

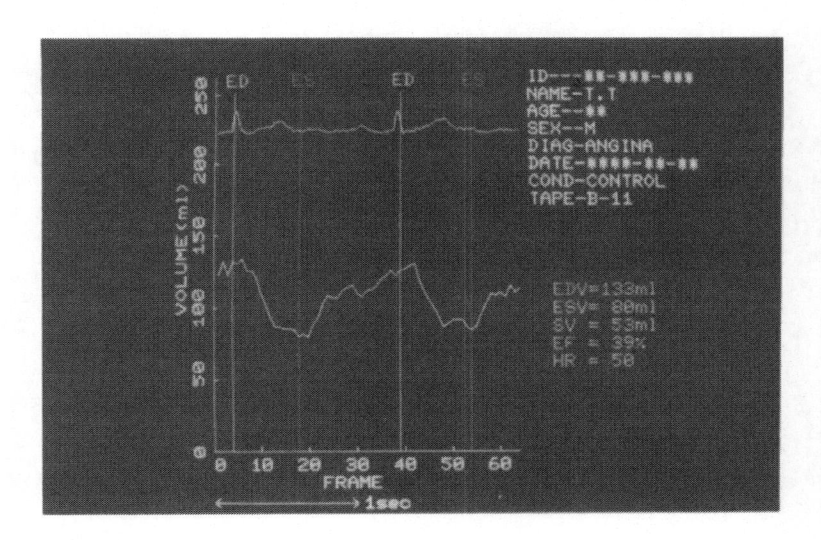

Fig. 5. Volume change obtained from echocardiograms.

to each point on the wall. The left-hand side is for rested condition (control) and the right-hand side is after an anginal attack induced by rapid pacing of the right atrium (pacing). Fig. 7 gives the percentage shortening of the same patient, which is calculated by dividing the length of each line segment in Fig. 6 by the length from the center of gravity of the left ventricle to the point on the wall at ED phase.

Fig. 8 gives motions of 3 points picked up on the left ventricular wall where three curves on the left-hand side show the movements of the left ventricular wall segments in control and those on the right-hand side show the movements after dosing nitroglycerine (NTG) to extend capillaries. Fig. 9 shows the wall motion around the left ventricle from the anterior wall to the inferior wall through the apex.

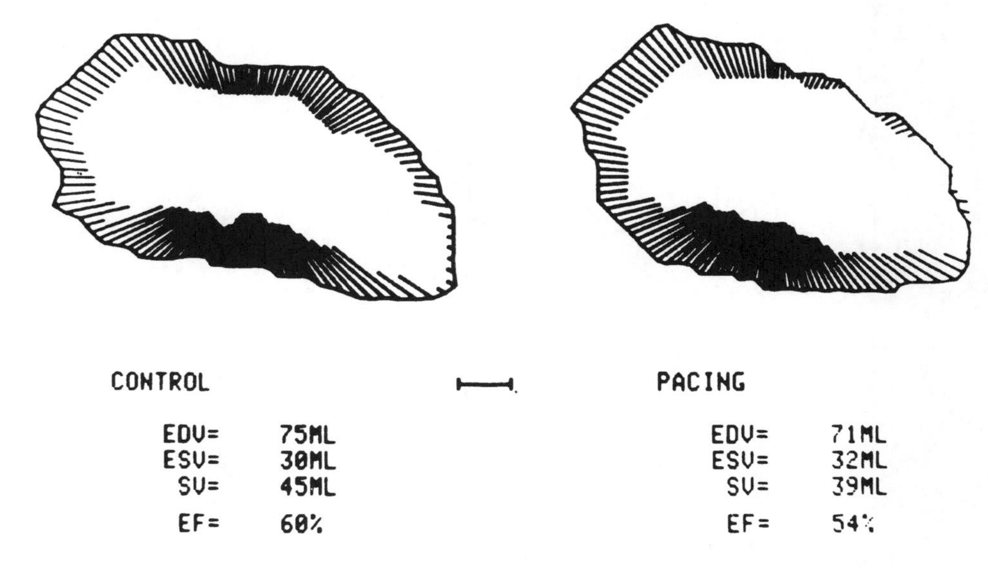

Fig. 6. Left ventricular wall movements between ED and ES phases.

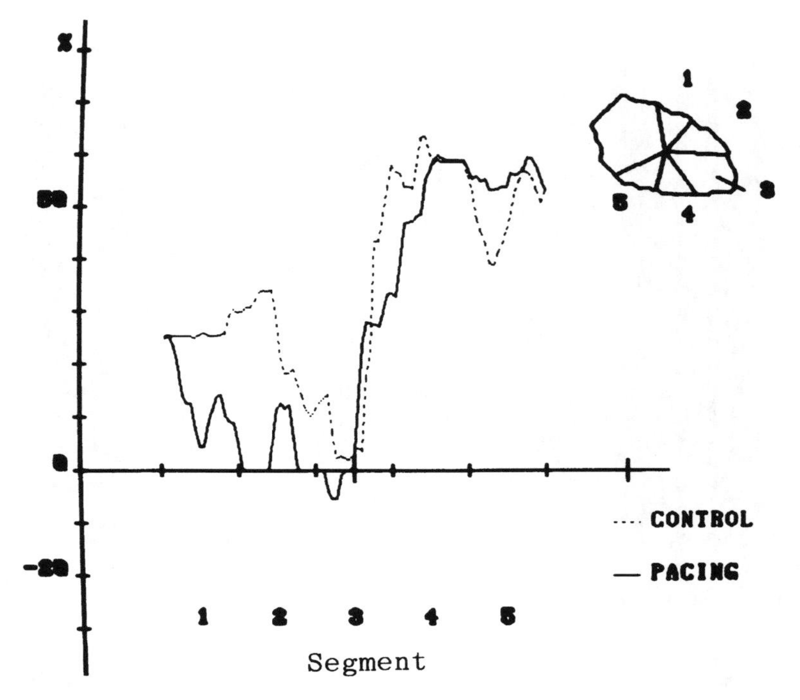

Fig. 7. Percentage shortening of the left ventricle.

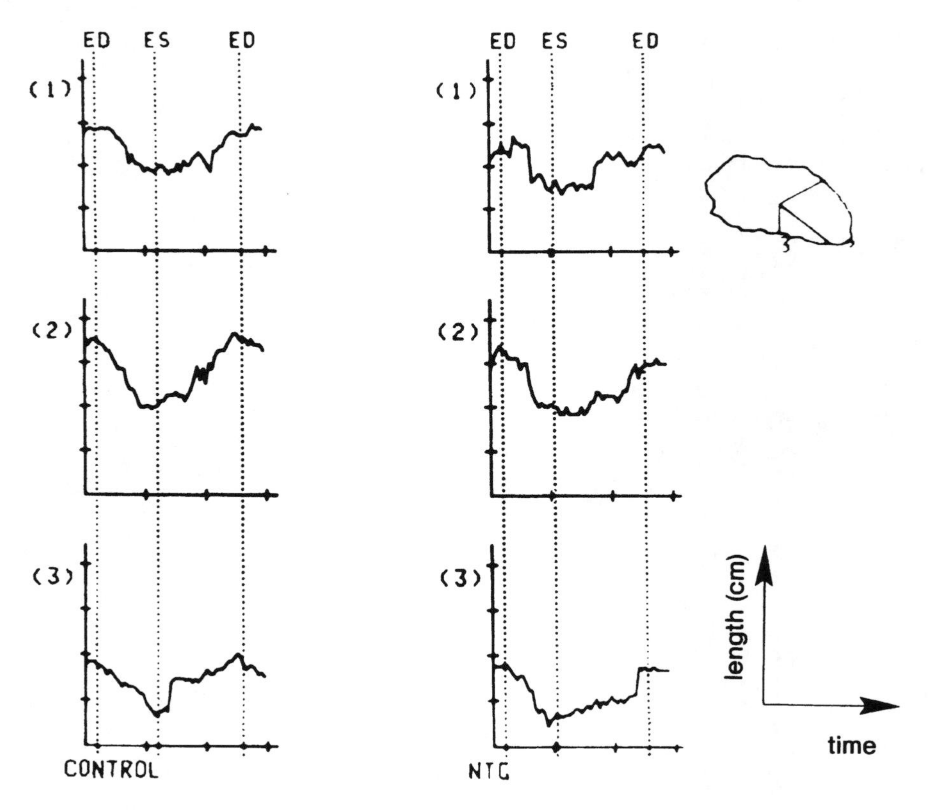

Fig. 8 Motions of 3 points on the left ventricular wall.

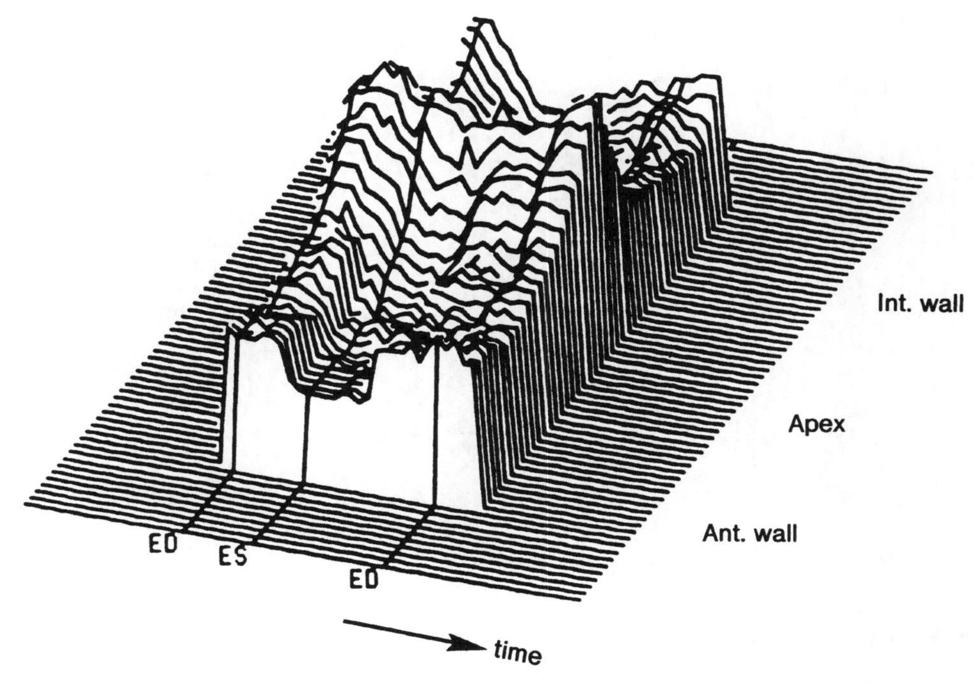

Fig. 9. 3-dimensional display of the wall motion.

From these figures, we can observe the wall motion in various conditions and we can easily grasp the abnormal area and its degree of abnormality.

The above examples were obtained from cineangiocardiograms. We can get the similar results from echocardiograms. The following results were obtained by using the microcomputerized system just mentioned in Chapter 3: Fig. 10 shows an example of regional wall motion of the endocardium and Fig. 11 is an example of the change of regional wall thickness. Fig. 12 shows the %-shortening.

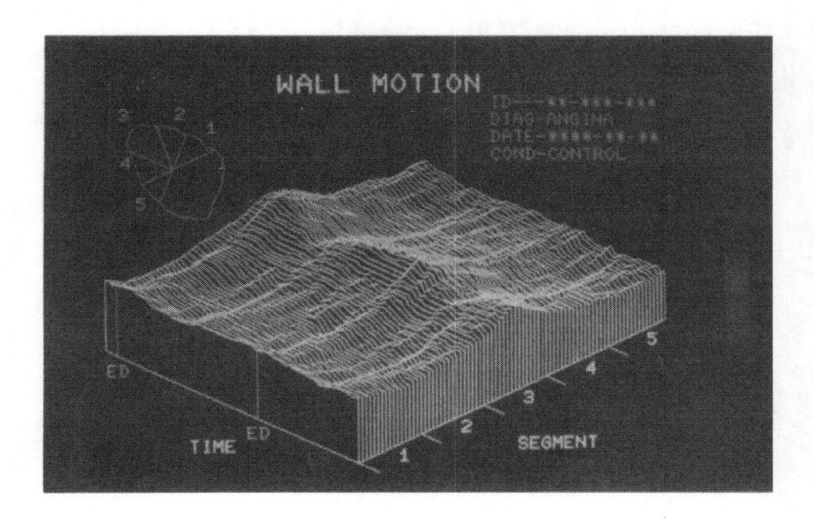

Fig. 10. Regional wall motion obtained from echocardiograms.

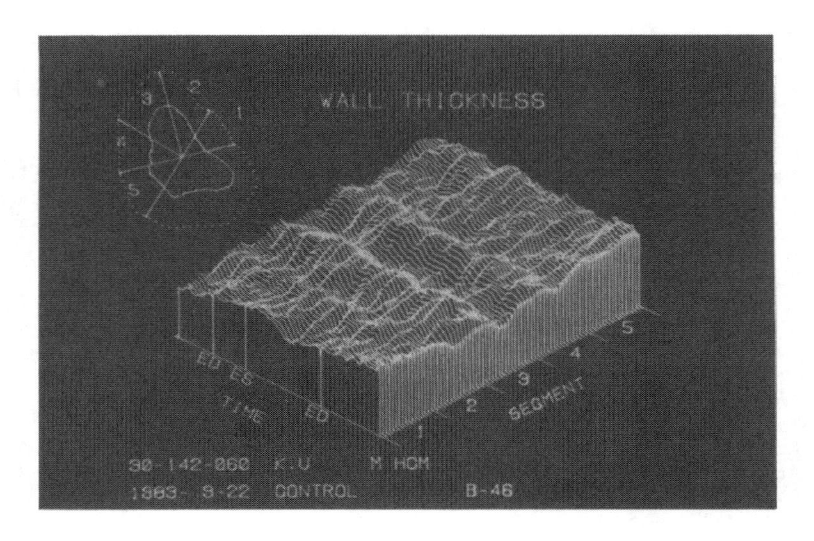

Fig. 11. Change of wall thickness obtained from echocardiograms.

5. 3-D reconstruction of the left ventricle

We can observe some performances of the left ventricle by using 2-D images such as x-ray cineangiocardiograms or echocardiograms. But it is impossible to know the regional function of the wall motion on the whole area of the left ventricle from these images. If 3-D shapes of the left ventricle are observable, then the left ventricular wall motion will be analyzable more easily and more precisely. We cannot obtain 3-D shapes of the left ventricle directly by using any method at present. But we can reconstruct 3-D shapes of the left ventricle by using several cross sectional shapes or silhouettes of the left ventricle.

A conventional method to reconstruct 3-D images of the left ventricle is to use bi-plane cineangiocardiograms and to reconstruct 3-D images

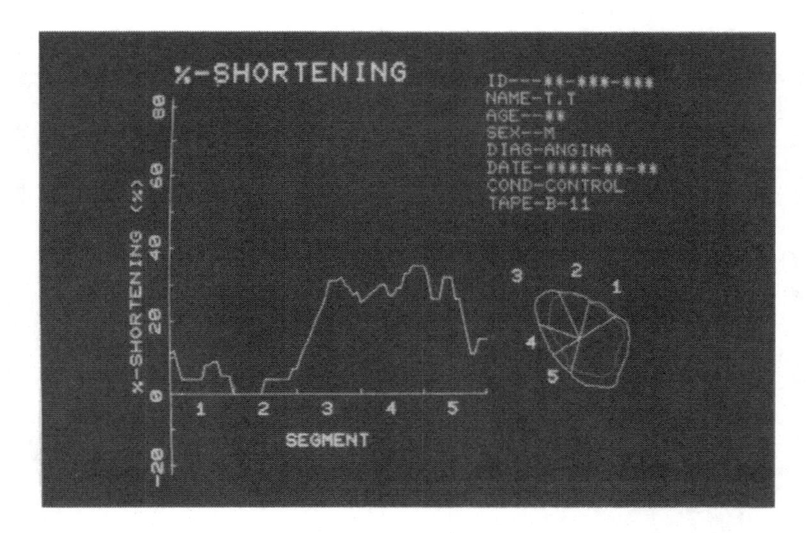

Fig. 12. Percentage shortening obtained from echocardiograms.

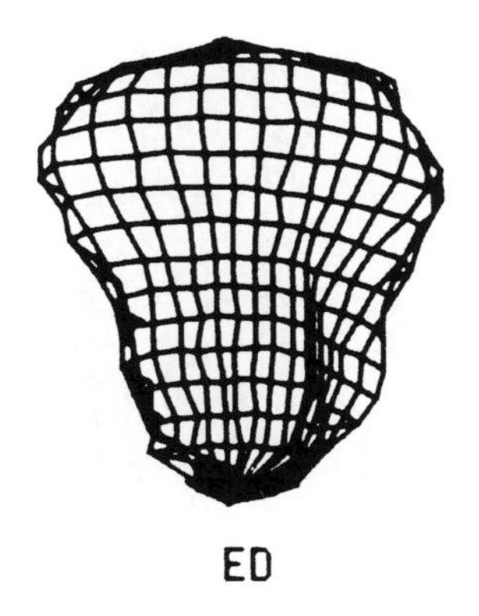

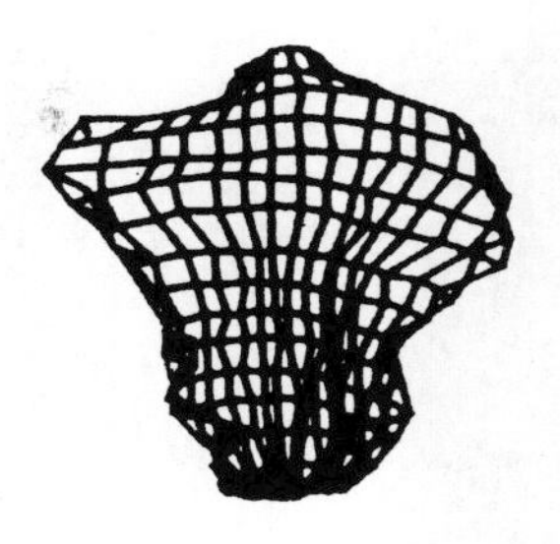

Fig. 13. Reconstructed left ventricle at ED and ES phases.

from the set of left ventricular boundaries on two orthogonal silhouettes [4]. The more angles of silhouettes are used to reconstruct the left ventricle, the more accurate the image we can obtain. A new method has been proposed by authors' group to obtain silhouettes of the left ventricle by continuously rotating the pair of x-ray source and its detector of monoplane cineangiographic device from 0° to 180° for several seconds during one usual dose injection, by which 3 or 4 silhouettes of the different angles at the same cardiac phase were obtainable [6].

5.1 3-D reconstruction from echocardiograms

One can observe various cross sectional images of the left ventricle by the echocardiography and 3-D shapes of the left ventricle can be reconstructed by using some series of 2-D echocardiograms. We can take two ways for this reconstruction: One is to get the short axis images by changing the position of ultrasound probe on the chest wall and the other is to take long axis images at several angles by rotating the probe whose tip is fixed at the same direction and position on the chest wall. We have been using this latter method because of easiness of 3-D reconstruction without precise measuring of the positions and angles of the probe [5, 7].

2-D echocardiograms on several (usually 6) cross sectional planes are taken by rotating the ultrasound probe at the same position on a chest wall. A 3-D left ventricular shape is reconstructed by the following steps:

Step 1: Pick up the left ventricular boundary curves at the same cardiac phase.

Step 2: Rearrange them at their angles.

Step 3: Cut these curves by 16 planes which are perpendicular to the axis of rotation of the probe.

Step 4: Connect the 12 cross points on each plane with a spline curve and sample the curve at 32 points.

Step 5: Store these 16 × 32 (512) points as the 3-D shape of the left ventricle.

Fig. 13 shows an example of the reconstructed left ventricle at ED and ES phases.

By using two sets of 3-D boundary data of endocardium and epicardium, we can observe cross sections of the left ventricular myocardium. Fig. 14 shows longitudinal cross sections of the myocardium at ED and ES.

5.2 3-D reconstruction from magnetic resonance image (MRI)

Magnetic resonance imaging method gives us several cross sectional images like x-ray CT. MRI is a noninvasive method and we can set the cross sectional planes more freely than with x-ray CT. The quality of the images has been improved in recent years. Several sets of images in a cardiac cycle are

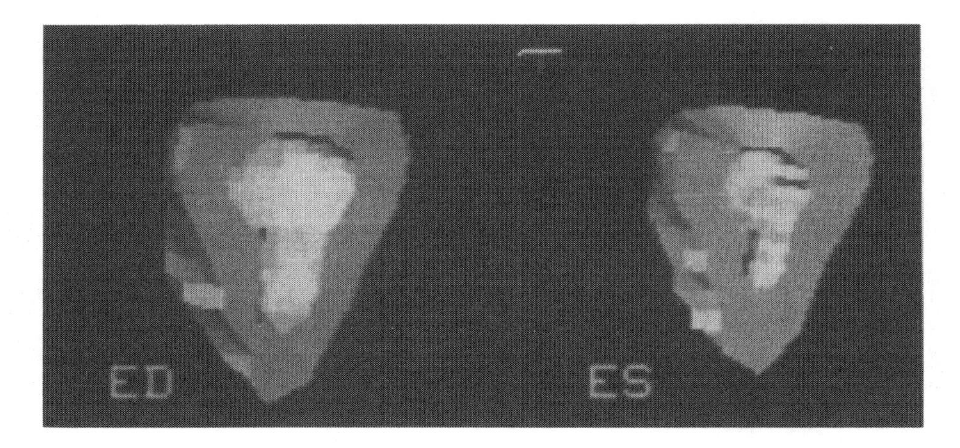

Fig. 14. Longitudinal cross sections of the myocardium.

taken by the multi-phase MRI method gated by ECG.

Fig. 15 shows an example of 6 cross sectional images of MRI and ED phase: 2 transverse (Z-plane), 2 coronal (Y-plane) and 2 sagittal (X-plane) images. Each image has 128×128 pixels. We can get these sets of images at 4 cardiac phases by 6 times of scanning of 0.2 Teslar resistive MRI. The lines on each image show the places of the planes of other cross sections, i.e., the lines on sagittal images show 2 coronal and 2 transversal planes. The left ventricular boundaries (inner and outer) on each image are traced manually by using a track ball. A boundary curve traced on a plane intersects at 2 points on another plane perpendicular to this plane. Thus a boundary traced on a plane

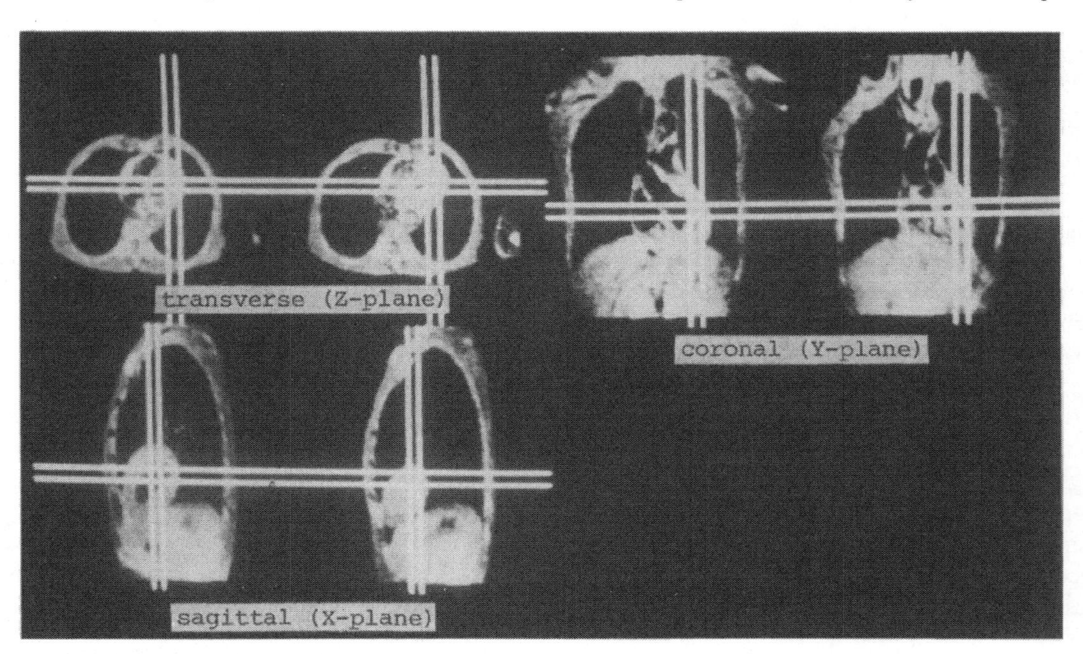

Fig. 15. An example of 6 cross sectional images of MRI.

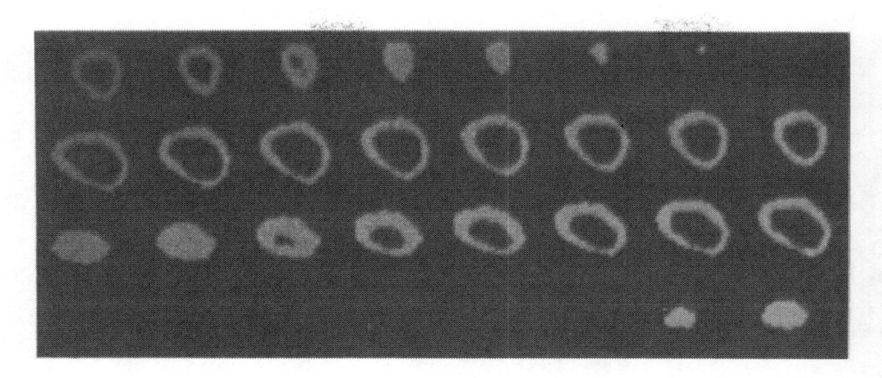

Fig. 16. Voxel data reconstructed.

intersects with 4 cross sections at most 8 points. By displaying these points as bright dots on the images on 4 cross sections, we can easily check the correctness of the traced boundary. These dots are useful also for drawing the boundary on rather unclear image. By using these 6 inner and outer boundaries, the 3-D shape of the left ventricle is reconstructed as the voxel data.

$32 \times 32 \times 32$ voxels are used for the reconstruction of 3-D shape of the left ventricle. The steps for 3-D voxel reconstruction are as follows:

Step 1: Draw boundary curves in the voxel space. If we cut the voxel space in Z direction, we get 32 planes and almost every plane has 8 boundary points.

Step 2: Connect these points with spline curves and digitize these curves at each voxel element.

Step 3: Fill the inner part of the boundary. Thus we get several cross sectional shapes of the left ventricle on every Z-plane.

Step 4: Execute the same procedure to X and Y planes.

Step 5: Smooth these X-, Y- and Z-plane 3-D shapes in their 3-D space (size for smoothing is $3 \times 3 \times 3$), sum up in one 3-D voxel space and cut

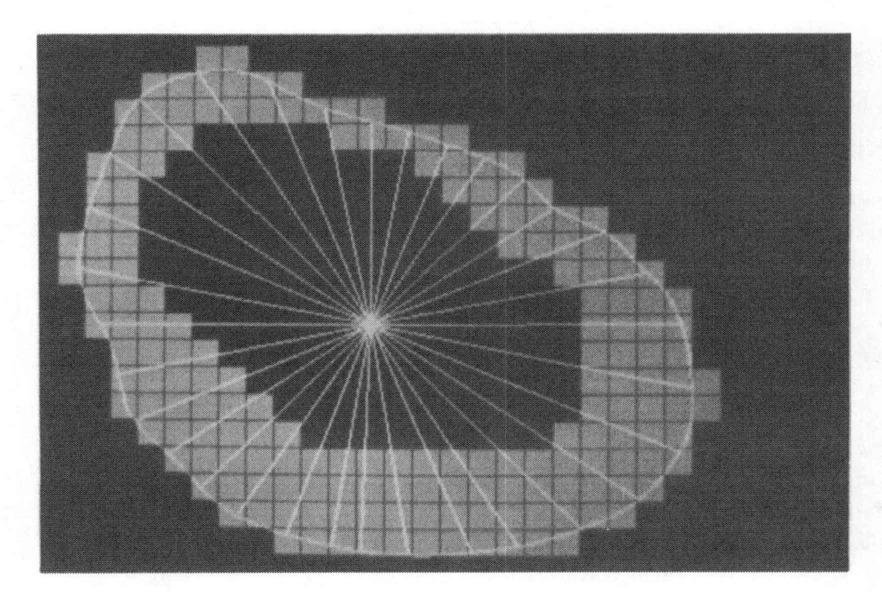

Fig. 17. Re-sampling of Voxel data.

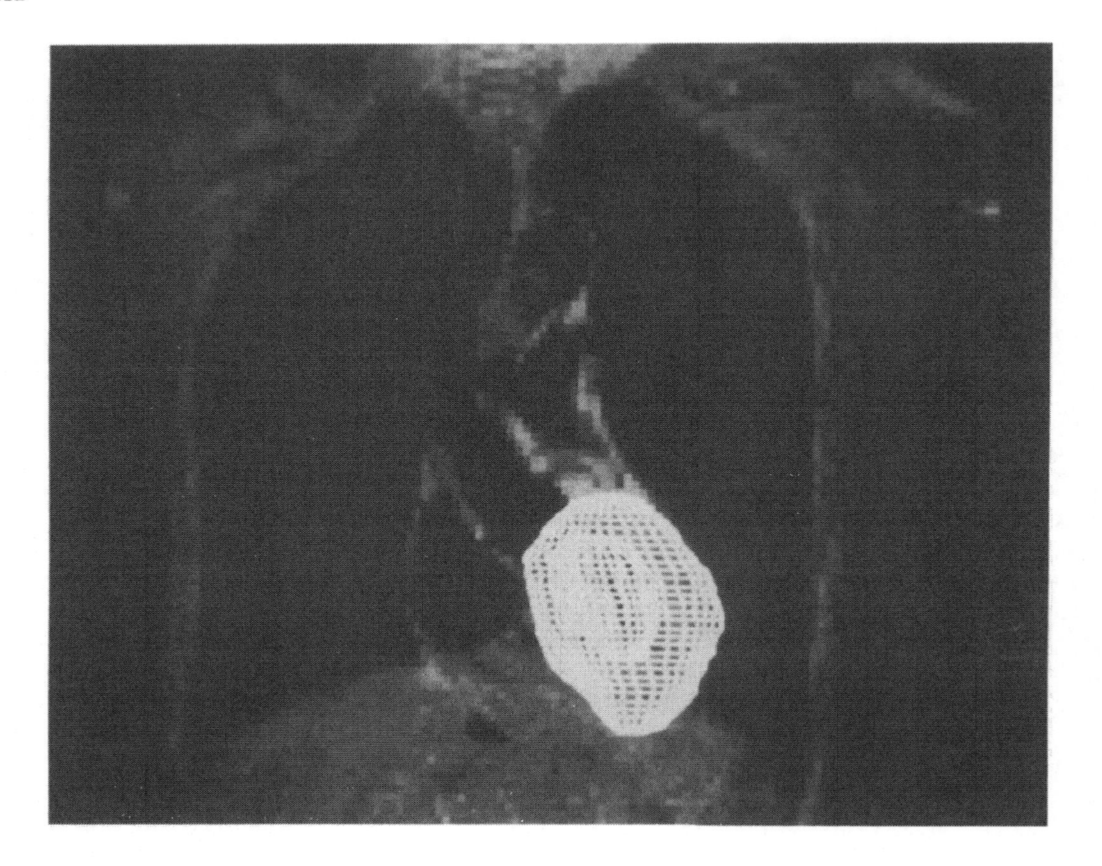

Fig. 18. 3-D left ventricle superposed on the original MRI.

by a threshold value. Then we can get 3-D voxel shape of the left ventricle.

Fig. 16 shows an example of the voxel data of myocardium on every Z-plane thus obtained. The voxel data on each Z-plane are changed to a smooth curve and sampled at 32 points as shown in Fig. 17.

Fig. 18 shows 3-D inner and outer shapes of the left ventricle drawn on the original magnetic resonance image, and we found that reconstructed shapes were closely fit to the original image.

Various kinds of 3-D shapes are obtainable from these 3-D data. Fig. 19 is a myocardium cut by a horizontal plane with inner and outer parts of the left ventricle where a wire framed epicardium is superposed.

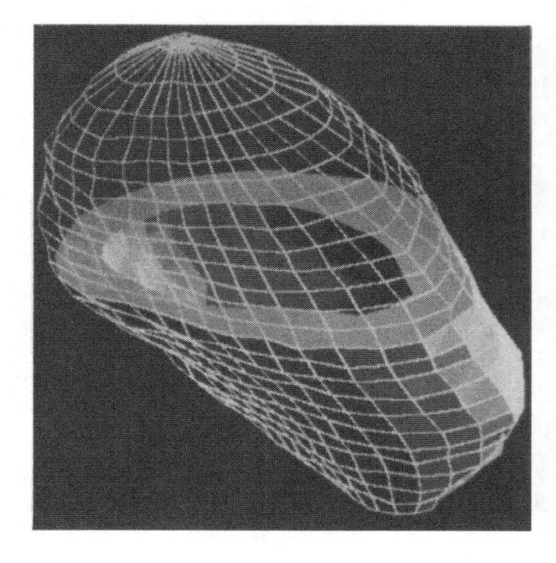

Fig. 19. An example of myocardium, endo- and epicardium.

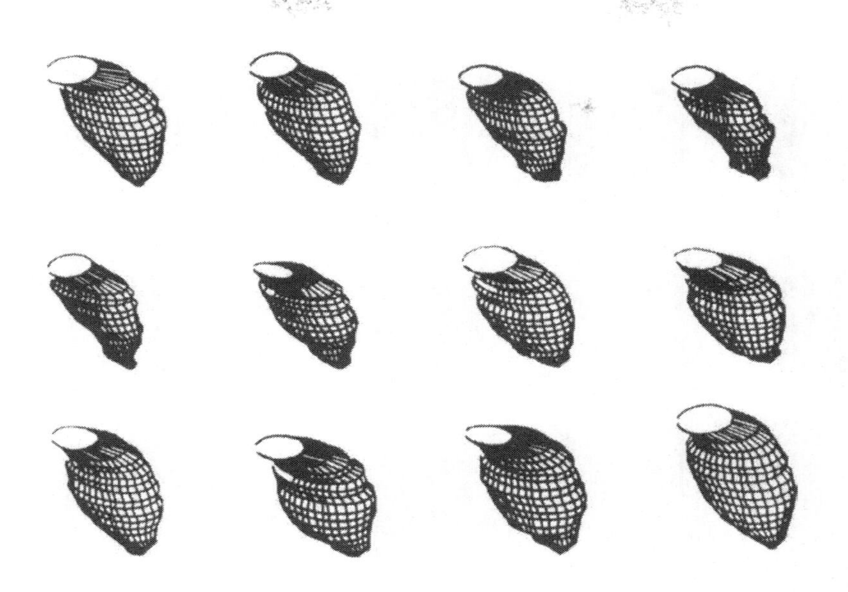

Fig. 20. 3-D left ventricular shapes in a cardiac cycle.

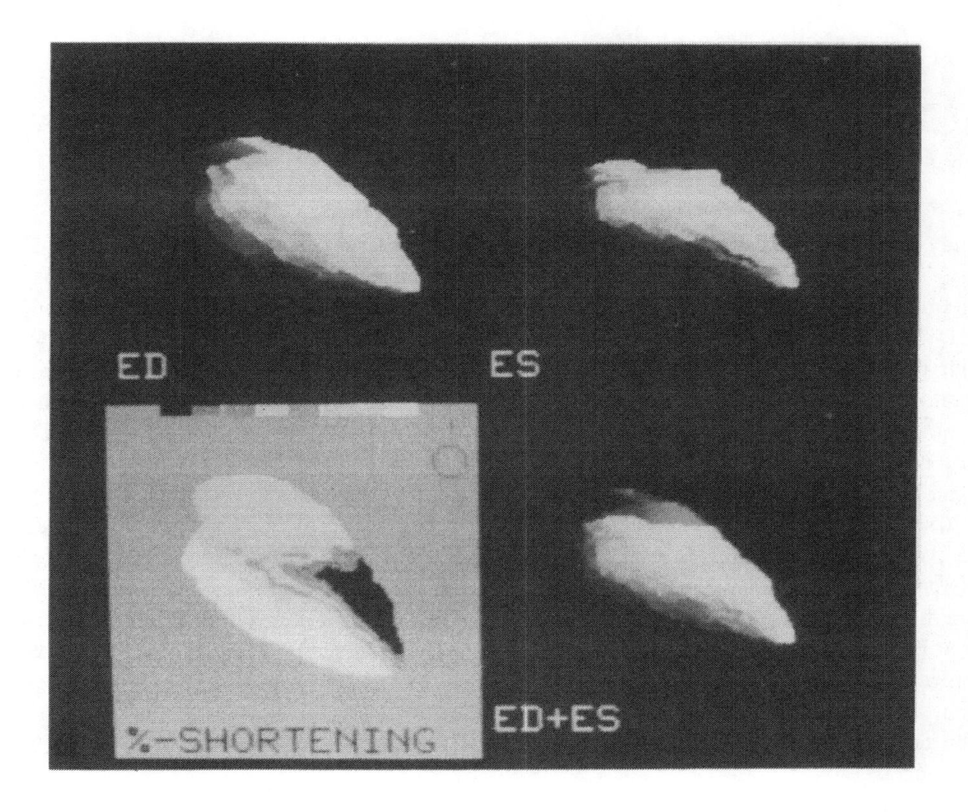

Fig. 21. 3-D percentage shortening and 3-D left ventricular shapes at ED and ES phases.

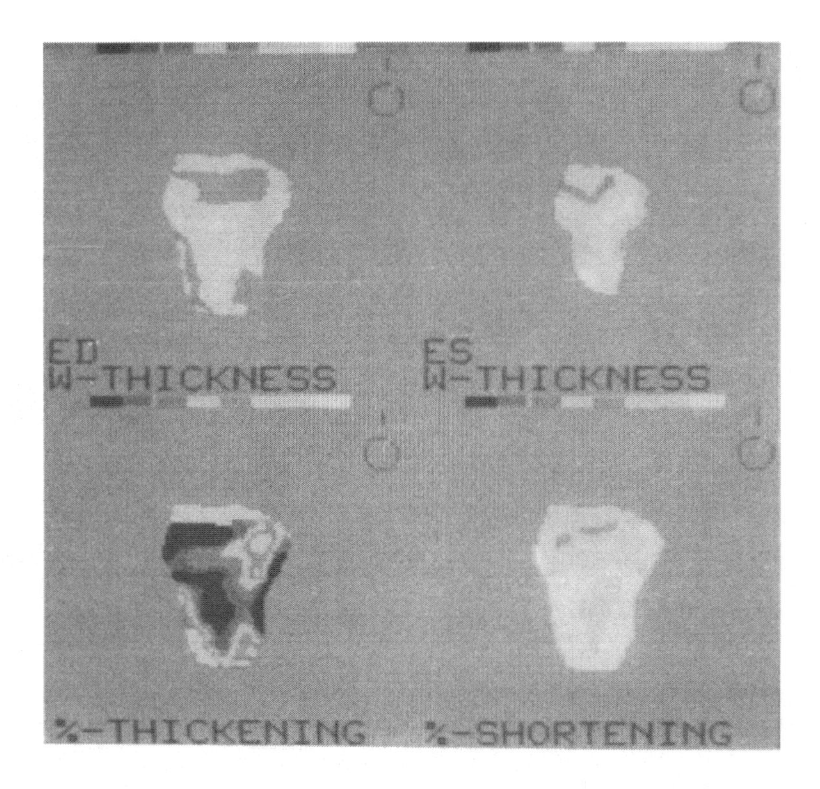

Fig. 22. Wall thickness, %-shortening and %-wall thickening obtained from echocardiograms.

6. Display of 3-D functional images

We can observe motion of 3-D left ventricle in the cardiac cycle by displaying 3-D sequential shapes in a cardiac cycle repeatedly and we can check the abnormality of the motion of the regional wall from such a motion display. We can also obtain various kinds of cardiac functions from these 3-D data which can be shown as 3-D functional images.

Fig. 20 shows 3-D shapes of the left ventricle in a cardiac cycle. These shapes were obtained from bi-plane cineangiocardiograms of a patient suffering from the variant angina. By comparing two 3-D images at ED and ES phases, we can calculate 3-D percentage shortening by the following equation:

$$\%\text{-shortening} = (Ld\text{-}Ls)/Ld \times 100\ [\%]$$

where Ld and Ls are the distance measured from the center of gravity of the ED image along the same direction to two points on the 3-D left ventricular walls at ED and ES phases. Fig. 21 shows an example of 3-D percentage shortening with ED and ES shapes. The color code is assigned to every 5%. Black and red regions show negative values during a contractile period. These color values are put on in place of shading values on 3-D shape left ventricle at ED phase.

Fig. 22 shows an example of functional images obtained from echocardiograms. Upper 2 images of Fig. 22 show wall thickness at ED (left) and ES (right). The values of wall thickness are put on the 3-D endocardium where each 2 mm increase in the wall thickness is coded by a different color starting from an offset thickness of 8 mm. Lower left-hand side of Fig. 22 shows 3-D %-shortening and right-hand side %-wall thickening in pseudo color.

7. Conclusions

We discussed left ventricular image processing and 3-D reconstruction of the left ventricle by using various kinds of imaging techniques; x-ray cineangiocardiography, echocardiography and MRI.

Original image quality of x-ray cineangiocardiograms is the highest among above three methods but sometimes it is difficult to get boundaries on a certain angles of silhouettes.

Echocardiography is very easy method of obtaining 2-D data and 3-D reconstruction is not so difficult if appropriate 2-D data are taken with good quality of images. By using the microcomputerized on-line image processing system, we can get the boundary sequence of the left ventricle in quite a short time and get various kinds of left ventricular functions. 3-D left ventricular inner cavity and myocardium are also obtainable from several cross sectional 2-D echocardiograms. But to utilize the 3-D shapes from echocardiograms in a more quantitative measurement of the cardiac functions, the echo data should be measured with position and angle of the probe.

MRI is the most simple method of reconstructing the left ventricle. The problem is that we can get only a small number of left ventricle images in a cardiac cycle; 4 images in a cardiac cycle in our case. For ease of 3-D reconstruction, MRI method should be the easiest way for 3-D reconstruction of the heart, not only left ventricle but also the left atrium, the right ventricle, the right atrium and so on.

Regional wall motion analyses in 2- and 3-dimensional cases discussed in this paper give us a useful quantitative evaluation of the ischemic area and the motion of the left ventricle.

References

1. Barrett WA, Clayton PD, Warner HR: Determination of left ventricular contours: A probabilistic algorithm derived from angiographic images. Computers and Biomedical Research 13: 522–548, 1980.
2. Chow CK, Kaneko T: Automatic boundary detection of the left ventricle from cineangiograms. Computers and Biomedical Research 5: 388–410, 1972.
3. Eiho S, Kuwahara M, Fujita M, Sasayama S, Kawai C: Automatic processing of cineangiographic images of left ventricle. Proc of 4th International Joint Conference on Pattern Recognition: 740–742, 1978.
4. Eiho S, Yamada S, Kuwahara M: 3-dimensional display of left ventricle by biplane X-ray angiocardiograms and assessment of regional myocardial function. Medinfo 80: 1093–1097, 1980.
5. Eiho S, Kuwahara M, Asada N, Sasayama S, Takahashi M, Kawai C: Reconstruction of 3-D images of pulsating left ventricle from two-dimensional sector scan echocardiograms of apical long axis view. Computers in Cardiology 1981: 19–24, 1982.
6. Eiho S, Kuwahara M, Shimura K, Wada M, Ohta M, Kozuka T: Reconstruction of the left ventricle from X-ray cineangiocardiograms with a rotating arm. Computers in Cardiology 1983: 63–67, 1984.
7. Eiho S, Kuwahara M, Asada N, Yamashita K: A microcomputerized image processor for 2-D echocardiography and 3-D reconstruction of left ventricle. Computers in Cardiology 1985: (to appear).
8. Heintzen PH (ed): Roentgen-, cine- and videodensitometry. Stuttgart, Georg Thieme Verlag, 1971.
9. Kuwahara M, Eiho S, Kitagawa H, Asada N, Ohtsuyama K. Ogawa H: A micro-computerized on-line image processing system for sector scan echocardiography. Computers in Cardiology 1983: 105–108, 1984.
10. Kuwahara M, Eiho S, Asada N, Osakada G, Kawai C: 3-D images of left ventricular myocardium reconstruction from 2-D echocardiograms. Computers in Cardiology 1984: 505–508, 1985.
11. Slager CJ, Reiber JHC, Schuurbiers JCH, Meester GT: Contourmat: A hard-wired left ventricular angio processing system. I. Design and application. Computers and Biomedical Research 11: 491–502, 1978.

Address for offprints:
Shigeru Eiho
Automation Research Laboratory
Kyoto University, Uji
Kyoto 611, Japan

Medical Progress through Technology 12 (1987) 117–122

Body surface potential mapping – its application to animal experiments and clinical examinations

Kenichi Doniwa, Takuya Kawaguchi & Mitsuhara Okajima
Lab. of Med. Eng. & Computer Sci., Fujita-Gakuen Health University School of Medicine, Toyoake, Aichi 470-11, Japan

Key words: body surface mapping, ventricular activation, multi A-C amplifiers, inverse problem, forward problem

Introduction

Potential distributions of electrocardiogram (ECG) on the body surface had already been drawn schematically with the isopotential lines supposing an electromotive force of the heart as the single dipole in as early as 1888 by Waller [19]. However, for its practical application in a clinical environment a computer was indispensable to collect electrocardiographic signals from numerous spots on the body surface and to process them to derive isopotential contour lines. This has developed in accordance with progress of the computer technology [11, 12]. Particularly in the 1970's a clinically applicable system was devised as a result of the advanced development of microcomputers. Here we take as an example the most frequently used mapping system in Japan, developed by us, and discribe its outlines as well as its application to experimental studies and clinical examinations.

Microcomputer-based mapping system

The device is composed of: (1) the input unit; (2) the main unit; and (3) the output unit. The electrocardiographic signals obtained from 96 lead-points placed on the body surface are amplified at the input unit simultaneously and fed into the microcomputer in the main unit wherein they are processed to derive a map of potential distributions on the body surface. Whenever necessary, the map is displayed on the cathode ray tube (CRT) or drawn on the hard copy through a thermal dot printer. Of course, the maps can also be stored in a floppy disk attached to the main unit, etc. (Fig. 1).

The unipolar precordial lead-points, 87 in number, including 59 in the anterior chest and 28 in the posterior chest, are relatively equally spaced on the body surface. Including nine more to prepare the standard twelve lead electrocardiogram and Frank lead vectorcardiogram simultaneously, a total of 96 leads were recorded at the same time.

Firstly electrocardiograms are amplified 500 times in magnitude through 96 AC amplifiers set in parallel in the input unit, then acquired into the main unit via the multiplexing module and A-D converters with a sampling rate at 1, 2 or 4 ms interval for each channel. In sampling 96 channels in multiplexing mode, a time lag of about 400 μs exists between the first and the last (96th) channel. However, in ordinary electrocardiograms such a difference has no significance. A-D conversion is conducted at each sampling interval, and in the cases of 1 and 2 ms the samples are moving-averaged to obtain a value for the 4 ms interval. Waves of the electrocardiograms eventually sampled at intervals of 4 ms are held for 8 seconds' duration for each channel. Consequently, five to ten consecutive heart beats are preserved for processing, which makes it possible to eliminate noises by selecting a non-noisy beat by observer's eye in the

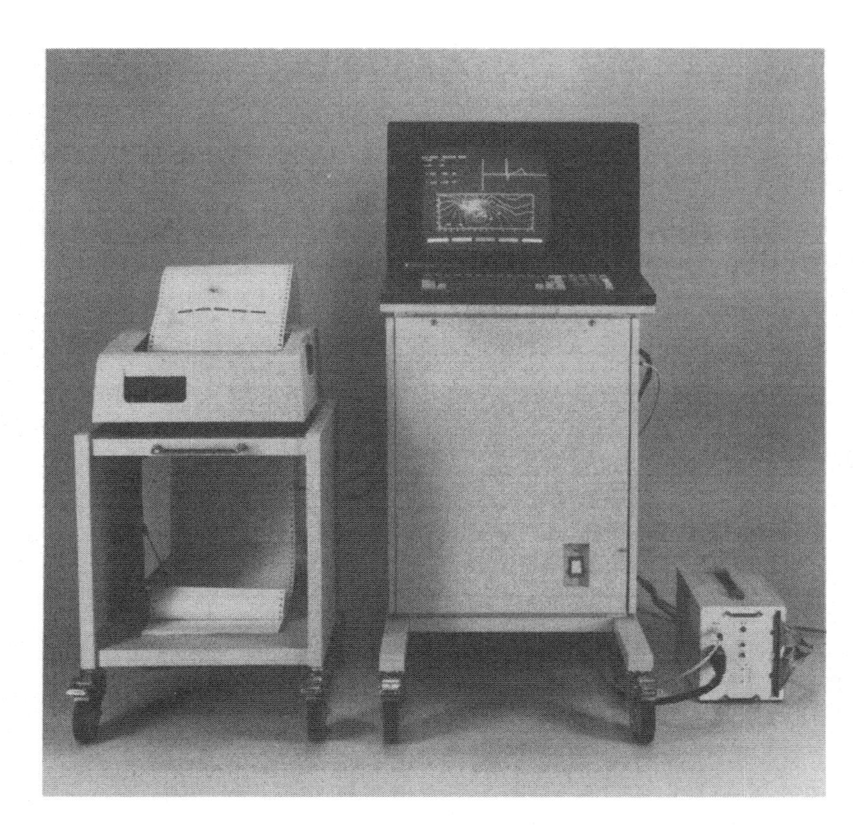

Fig. 1. The body surface mapping system developed by the participation of the authors. It consists of thermal dot printer, main unit and input box (left to right). These three components are required for data aquisition and processing.

respective lead, and whenever necessary, to pick up sporadically occuring ventricular extrasystole beats.

The electrocardiograms induced from the body surface may reveal the baseline fluctuations (drift of potential) caused by respiratory motions and polarization of electrodes and so on. These can be corrected by indicating the zero point of electrocardiogram at two spots on CRT by the operator. The baseline drift is then adjusted by linear interpolation of these two spots. The unusable noisy records on some lead points are replaced by a synthesized one obtained by linear interpolation of potentials of the adjacent lead-points [16, 18, 20] (Fig. 2).

From thus processed electrocardiograms an isopotential map is drawn by computer. The potentials on the spots located midway among the lead points are obtained mathematically by linear interpolation.

Experimental studies and clinical applications

This microcomputer-based mapping system has been utilized to investigate the cardiac potential distributions to the best of accuracy. Unlike the electrocardiograms of conventional twelve leads, the positive and negative potential areas, maximum and minimum potentials as well as the zero potential in reference to the Wilson's central terminal can be obtained and displayed visually with this mapping system, thus enabling collection of the electrical information from the whole of the body surface most efficiently.

It is therefore useful to know the intramuscular or epicardial potential distributions. Making use of such an advantage numerous experimental studies on the microcomputer-based mapping system have been conducted referring to the epicardial poten-

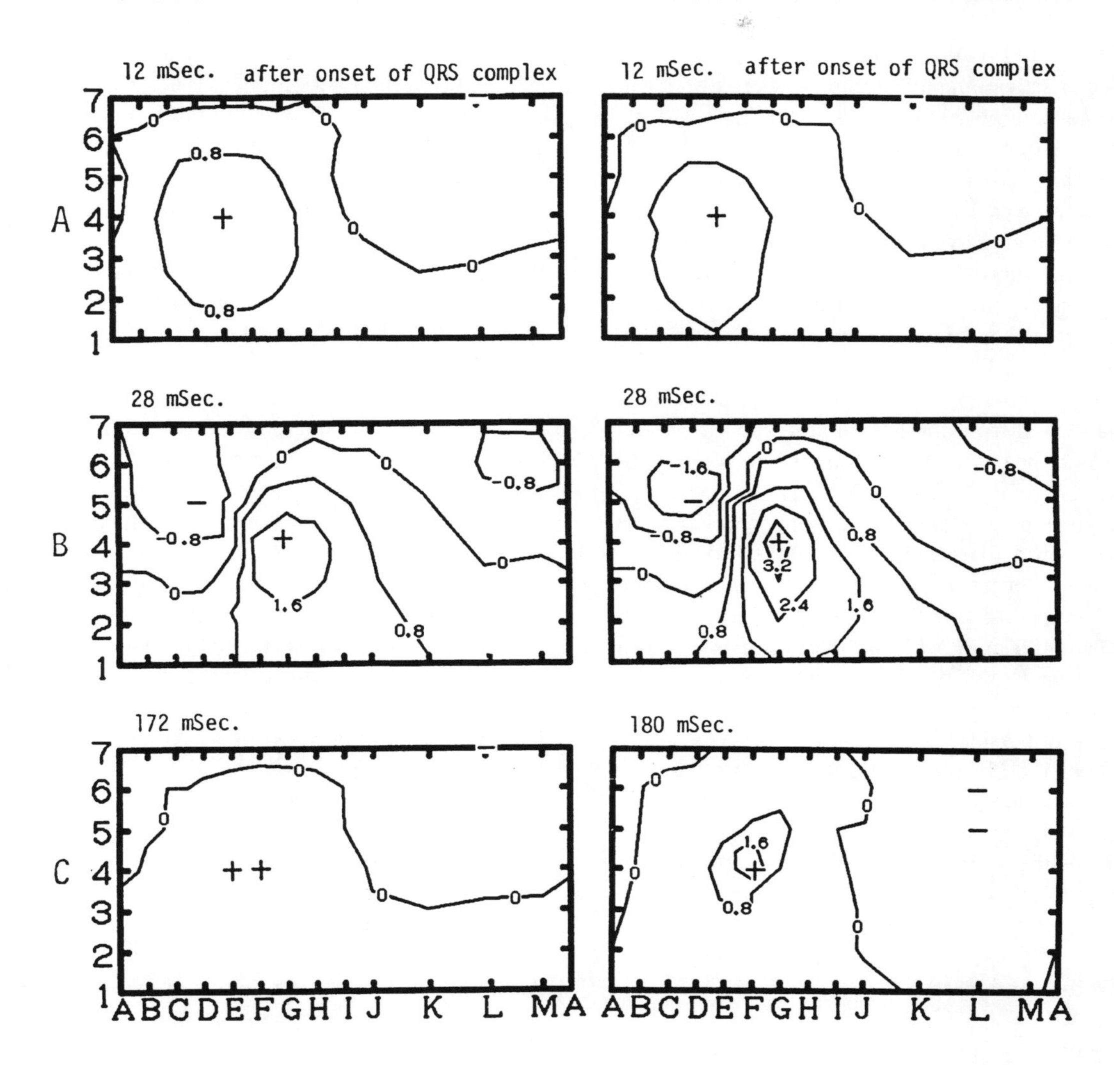

Fig. 2. Changes of body surface isopotential map by occlusion of a coronary artery branch in a dog experiment. The left panels depict control (before occlusion) and the right ones are for five minutes after occlusion.

A: initial stage of ventricular depolarization (QRS); B: middle stage of ventricular depolarization (QRS); C: middle stage of repolarization (ST-T).

Occlusion brought about relatively small changes in maps of depolarization phases (A and B) but prominent alteration in repolarization phase (C).

tials in addition to that of the body surface [13, 15].

Specially, there are a good number of studies available on myocardial ischemia [2], yocardial infarction [1, 5, 10, 14], WPW syndrome [6], intraventricular conduction disturbances [3], ventricular hypertrophy and arrythmias [4]. Explanations are made here on the maps of the normal subject as well as myocardial infarction and arrhythmias.

Normal subject

In the initial stage of 15 ms after the onset of ventricular activation the anterior chest is covered with the positive potential area and the back with the negative one. Potential of the anterior chest is then elevated gradually. These phenomena depict progress of the excitation from the left side to the right one through the ventricular septum.

Furthermore, in the midst of excitation it arrives at the right ventricular epicardium while the excitation in another direction proceeds from the right to the left in the left ventricle. On the body surface the latter is reflected by the positive potential area transferred from the left anterior area to the left area on the chest. At this time the maximum positive potential also moves in the same way.

When the excitation wave-front is broken at the right ventricular epicardium (breakthrough), the minimum occurs at the center of the anterior chest frequently bringing about a niche on the isopotential contour lines, while another niche may appear referring to the breakthrough of excitation proceeding through the left ventricular free wall from inside to outside.

Up to the final stage the excitation remains on the posterior wall of the left ventricle and on the conus of pulmonary artery. These are noted on the map as the positive potential areas at the superior part of the anterior chest and the back.

Myocardial infarction

The object of making diagnosis of myocardial infarction by means of the microcomputer-based mapping system is to predict the size and site of infarct quantitatively. It is ideal if a map of the patient had been obtained earlier before onset of myocardial infarction as control, which is unfortunately not the case in most of the patients. Hence, a diagnosis is usually made by refering to the mean value and its standard deviation of the potentials on the map derived from a number of normal subjects.

Disappearance or diminution of electromotive force due to myocardial necrosis can be shown by subtraction on maps of the normal and infarction in the initial, middle and final stages of the QRS duration (subtraction map). For example, in anterior myocardial infarction, there is no or very little electromotive force observed in the anterior chest at the initial and middle stages of the QRS duration [8, 17]. In the same manner disappearance or diminution of electromotive force is observed in the inferior chest at the initial and middle stages of the QRS duration in case of inferior myocardial infarction, and on the back at the middle and final stages of the QRS duration in case of posterior myocardial infarction.

The ventricular gradient expressed by the area surrounded by baseline and electrocardiographic curve for the period beginning at the QRS onset and ending at T wave terminal is believed to show no or very little change even when activation sequence alters significantly.

However, it is known for this ventricular gradient to undergo significant changes in case of myocardial infarction. Making use of this phenomenon, special studies on ventricular gradient map for myocardial infarction complicated with bundle branch block and intraventricular conduction disturbance are being carried out [9].

The above refers mainly to myocardial infarction of the chronic stage, and as to the acute stage, specially on ST-T changes a series of studies are being made [7].

Arrhythmias: Search for origin of extrasystole and localization of A-V accessory pathway

It is important to know the origin of extrasystole especially in case of the ventricular tachycardia among others. Clinical inference of the origins as well as experimental detection of reentrant circuits of ventricular premature beat, ventricular tachycardia and supraventricular premature beat are studied by many. Furthermore, as an application of the mapping system a non-invasive localization of the accessory pathway in the Wolff-Parkinson-White syndrome is being discussed [21].

In many cases for diagnosis of arrhythmias by mapping in the directions mentioned above, an isochronal map is more useful than an ordinary isopotential map. The former is composed of contour lines for the ventricular activation time of QRS complex obtained from numerous lead points on the body surface. In this system the origin of ectopic the beat and course of reentrant circuit can be shown with ease.

Similarly a good number of the basic studies are being carried out in measuring activation sequences of electrocardiogram simultaneously to clarify onset mechanisms of arrhythmias and establishment of the therapy.

For example, it is a well known fact that when the ventricular arrhythmia is observed with time after producing an experimental myocardial infarction, it reveals onset of various ventricular arrhythmias immediately after infarction and several days later. Referring to such arrhythmias, origin of onset and reentrant circuit are estimated from the activation sequence, and then characteristics of ventricular arrhythmias with different mechanisms are estimated.

Experimental studies in our laboratory

It is important to know degrees and ranges of myocardial ischemia in the acute phase of myocardial infarction as well as in various stress tests in consideration of the treatment to be determined and its prognosis. Thus much is studied upon the experimental occlusion of coronary artery. In open chest experiments the exposure of the heart to the open air frequently resulted in significant alteration in ST-T portion of electrocardiogram. In order to avoid such a trouble, a close chest coronary occlusion has to be produced with a balloon catheter to proceed with the test under the physiological conditions as far as possible. Simultaneously, the body surface isopotential map is to be evaluated.

In our laboratory seven mongrel dogs weighing 10 to 20 kg were anesthesized intravenously and fixed in the supine position. Electrodes were spaced with nearly equal distance between each other at 87 spots on the body surface. For occlusion of the coronary artery a special metal catheter was inserted from the neck through the carotid artery up to the inlet of coronary artery, through which a balloon catheter was passed through into the left main coronary artery. The placement was confirmed by the coronary angiography. After occlusion of coronary artery for 20 minutes with the inflated balloon the catheter was withdrawn.

Here a case wherein of the stages of experiment were accomplished with success will be described in some detail. Before coronary occlusion the width of QRS complex of body surface electrogram was 44 ms, and the map was noted normal. Five minutes after occlusion the width of QRS complex became 48 ms, showing however nearly the same positive and negative potential areas as that of the normal on the body surface map. The width of the QRS complex 15 minutes after coronary occlusion was a little prolongated to 52 ms, while the body surface potential map indicated nearly the same process. Thus, there was no special difference noted in potential distribution of the QRS complex. However, the R waves in the left anterior chest were a little higher, and the maximum potential was transferred a little to the right upon occlusion.

Meanwhile, changes of the ST-T interval are explained. Five minutes after coronary occlusion at the end of the QRS complex the positive potential area in the left chest remained unchanged as that of the ST segment, which gradually prolonged to the anterior chest and the supra-anterior chest. Fifteen minutes after coronary occlusion such trend was noted further remarkable, and the maximum potential occurred at the superior part of the anterior chest and the minimum potential at the inferior part of the left anterior chest a little to the left.

After a consecutive occlusion of the coronary artery for 20 minutes the balloon was removed and a reperfusion was conducted. The map of about 20 minutes after reperfusion showed nearly the same pattern as that before occlusion.

Partly, ventricular tachycardia was noted after releasing of the coronary occlusion.

Due to the above mentioned transfer of the maximum potential as well as due to the delayed activation sequence of the ventricle, an increased electromotive force of the QRS complex is seen following coronary occlusion. On the other hand it is known that there was little change in activation sequence at the right ventricle, since no influence was noted on breakthrough therein.

References

1. Flowers NC, Horan LG, Sohi GS, Hand RC, Johnson JG: New evidence for infero-posterior myocardial infarction on surface potential maps. Am J Cardiol 38: 576–581, 1976.
2. Fox KM, Selwyn A, Oakley D, Shillingford JP: Relation between the precordial projection of S-T segment changes after exercise and coronary angiographic findings. Am J Cardiol 44: 1068–1075, 1979.
3. Fujino T: On genesis of RBBB pattern in electro- and vectorcardiogram as studied by simulation of ventricular propagation process and reconstruction of QRS patterns. Jap Circ J 32: 1533–1541, 1968.
4. Hayashi H, Ishikawa T, Uematsu H, Takami K, Kojima H, Yabe S, Ohsugi S: Identification of the site of origin of ventricular premature beats by body surface map in patients with or without cardiac disease. In: Yamada K, Harumi K, Musha T (eds) Advances in body surface potential mapping. Nagoya, The University of Nagoya Press, 1983, pp 257–264.
5. Horan LG, Flowers NC, Johnson JC: Significance of the diagnostic Q wave in myocardial infarction. Circulation 43: 428–436, 1971.
6. Koike Y: Correlation between areas of ventricular pre-excitation and types of WPW QRS patterns by means of computer simulation of ventricular activation sequence. Jap Heart J 18: 462–472, 1977.
7. Kubota I, Watanabe Y, Tsuiki K, Yasui S: Body surface distribution of exercise-induced ST depression in patients with angina pectoris. Jap Heart J 24: 853–862, 1983.
8. Mirvis DM: Body surface distributions of repolarization potentials after acute myocardial infarction. II. Relationship between isopotential mapping and ST segment potential summation methods. Circulation 63: 623–631, 1981.
9. Niimi N, Sugiyama S, Wada M, Sugenoya J, Oguri H, Toyama S, Okajima M, Yamada K: Genesis of body surface potential distribution in right bundle branch block. J Electrocardiology 10: 257–266, 1977.
10. Ohta T, Kinoshita A, Ohsugi J, Isomura S, Takatsu F, Ishikawa H, Toyama J, Nagaya T, Yamada K: Correlation between body surface isopotential map and left ventriculograms in patients with old inferoposterior myocardial infarction. Am Heart J 104: 1262–1270, 1982.
11. Okajima M, Fujino T, Kobayashi T, Yamada K: Computer simulation of the propagation process in excitation of the ventricles. Circ Res 23: 203–211, 1968.
12. Okajima M, Doniwa K, Ishikawa T, Niimi N, Koike Y: On body surface VAT 'isochrone' maps generated by computer using simulated excitation sequences in ventricular model. Comp in Cardiol, IEEE Computer Society, 1980.
13. Spach MS, Barr RC: Ventricular intramural and epicardial potential distributions during ventricular activation and repolarization in the intact dog. Circ Res 37: 243–257, 1975.
14 Sugiyama S, Wada M, Sugenoya J, Toyoshima H, Toyama J, Yamada K: Experimental study of myocardial infarction through the use of body surface isopotential maps: Ligation of the anterior descending branch of the left coronary artery. Am Heart J 93: 51–59, 1977.
15. Taccardi B: Distribution of heart potentials on the thoracic surface of normal human subjects. Circ Res 12: 341–352, 1963.
16. Tatematsu H, Wada M, Okajima M, Yamada K On-line conversational mode processing system for body surface mapping. Adv in Cardiol 10: 20–25, Karger, Basel, 1974.
17. Tonooka J, Kubota I, Watanabe Y, Tsuiki K, Yasui S: Isointegral analysis of body surface maps for the assessment of location and size of myocardial infarction. Am J Cardiol 52: 1174–1180, 1983.
18. Toyama J, Ohta Y, Yamada K: Newly developed body surface mapping system for clinical use. In: Yamada K, Harumi K, Musha T (eds) Advances in body surface potential mapping. Nagoya, The University of Nagoya Press, 1983, pp 125–133.
19. Waller AD: The electromotive properties of the human heart. Brit Med J 2: 751–754, 1888.
20. Watanabe T, Toyama J, Toyoshima H, Oguri H, Ohno M, Ohta T, Okajima M, Naito Y, Yamada K: A practical microcomputer-based mapping system for body surface, precordium and epicardium. Computers and Biomed Res 14: 341–354, 1981.
21. Yamada K, Toyama J, Wada M, Sugiyama S, Sugenoya J, Toyoshima H, Mizuno Y, Sotohata I, Kobayashi T, Okajima M: Body surface isopotential mapping in Wolff-Parkinson-White syndrome. Non-invasive method to determine the localization of the accessory atrioventricular pathway. Am Heart J 90: 721–734, 1975.

Address for offprints:
K. Doniwa
Fujita-Gakuen Health University
Toyoake
Aichi 470-11, Japan

Medical Progress through Technology 12 (1987) 123–143

Noninvasive measurement of arterial blood pressure and elastic properties using photoelectric plethysmography technique

Ken-ichi Yamakoshi & Akira Kamiya
The Research Institute of Applied Electricity, Hokkaido University, N12, W6, Kita-ku, Sapporo 060, Japan

Key words: noninvasive measurement, photoelectric plethysmography volume-oscillometric method, arterial blood pressure, arterial elastic property, human fingers and rabbit forelegs

Abstract

The objective of this paper is to review our developed method for measuring noninvasively the arterial blood pressure as well as the mechanical properties of the vascular system in a thin portion of the biological segment such as human fingers or small animal extremities like rat tails and rabbit forelegs. This measurement is based on a principle called the 'volume-oscillometric method'. During the gradual change in cuff pressure, the amplitude of consecutive arterial volume pulsations associated with pulse pressure shows change characteristically due to the nonlinearity of arterial pressure-volume(P-V) relation. Arterial pressure can be accurately determined by detecting this characteristic change in the amplitude, while the arterial elastic properties such as P-V relationship and volume elastic modulus can be noninvasively obtained as a function of arterial transmural pressure, provided that the arterial volume changes are quantitatively determined during this pressure measurement. The validity and accuracy of this pressure and elasticity measurement with photoelectric plethysmography technique for detecting arterial volume changes are clearly demonstrated on the in vitro and in vivo experiments. Considering the simplicity and practicability of this measurement using the photoelectric plethysmography, we present a new portable instrument for the long-term ambulatory monitoring of indirect arterial pressure and a handy fully-automatic instrument for the noninvasive measurement of arterial elastic properties, and a few examples obtained by each instrument are also described.

1. Introduction

The arterial blood pressure as well as the mechanical properties of the vascular system will provide some of the most valuable and useful information for the evaluation of hemodynamic conditions in such cardiovascular diseases as hypertension, arteriosclerosis and so on. To date, in daily clinics and basic medicine as well, there is an eager requirement for a simple and practicable instrument which allows noninvasive and accurate measurement of arterial pressure and vascular elasticity.

We have previously proposed a new sphygmomanometry called 'volume-oscillometric method' for the noninvasive measurement of arterial pressure using photoelectric plethysmography technique, and demonstrated its accuracy and validity through in vitro and in vivo studies using excised arterial segments and human fingers [24, 25]. From the considerations of its practical use [25], we have also presented a new portable instrument equipped with a microprocessor for the long-term ambulatory monitoring of arterial pressure in the human finger using this method [27].

In this method, the arterial pressure can be accurately determined by detecting the characteristic change in the amplitude of arterial volume pulsations during the application of counterpressure

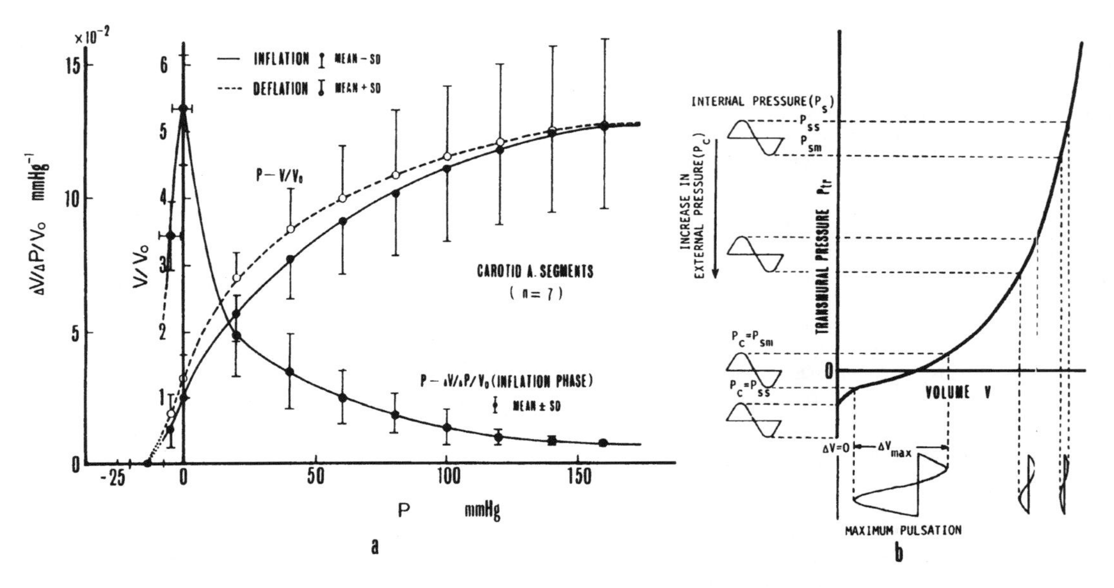

Fig. 1. (a) Volume ratio (V/Vo in percent) and volume compliance ($\Delta V/\Delta P/Vo$ in $mmHg^{-1}$) plotted against internal pressure (P in mmHg) obtained from seven carotid arteries. (b) Graphical representation elucidating the mechanism of the occurrence of maximum volume pulsation, showing the principle of the volume-oscillometric method for the determination of systolic and mean arterial pressure. For symbols and details see text.

(cuff pressure). This characteristic change has been revealed to be due to the nonlinearity of pressure-volume relationship of the artery [24]. From this evidence it is suggested that if the arterial volume changes can be quantitatively determined during the pressure measurement by this method, the arterial elastic properties such as pressure-volume relationship and volume elastic modulus can be noninvasively obtained as a function of arterial transmural pressure.

From this standpoint, we have successfully developed a new method for the noninvasive measurement of the elastic properties in human fingers or rabbit forelegs based on the volume-oscillometric method using electrical admittance [18] or photoelectric plethysmography technique [10, 11, 16].

This paper describes a brief review of the principle and evaluation of accuracy of our developed methods for measuring arterial pressure and elastic properties using photoelectric plethysmography technique. Outlines of newly designed instruments based on these measurements and some examples obtained through animal and human experiments are also presented.

2. Arterial pressure measurement

2.1 Principle

The principle of the volume-oscillometric method capable of measuring systolic and mean arterial pressure noninvasively is based on the nonlinear characteristics of pressure-volume relation in the artery [24]. Fig. 1(a) shows the static relationship between internal pressure (P in mmHg) and volume ratio (V/Vo; Vo, unloading volume or volume at $P = 0$) obtained in the in vitro experiments using common carotid arterial segments (about 4 cm long and 1.5–2.3 mm inner diameter) excised from seven anesthetised mongrel dogs (see Ref. 24 for the experimental setup and details on the experimental procedures). The P-V/Vo relationship showed curvilinear and hysteresis at inflation-deflation cycle. The volume compliance ($\Delta V/\Delta P/Vo$ in $mmHg^{-1}$) was calculated from the P-V/Vo curve at the inflation phase and also plotted against P in Fig. 1 (a). It was revealed by this curve that the volume compliance increased as P decreased within the range $P > 0$, while it decreased as P decreased within the

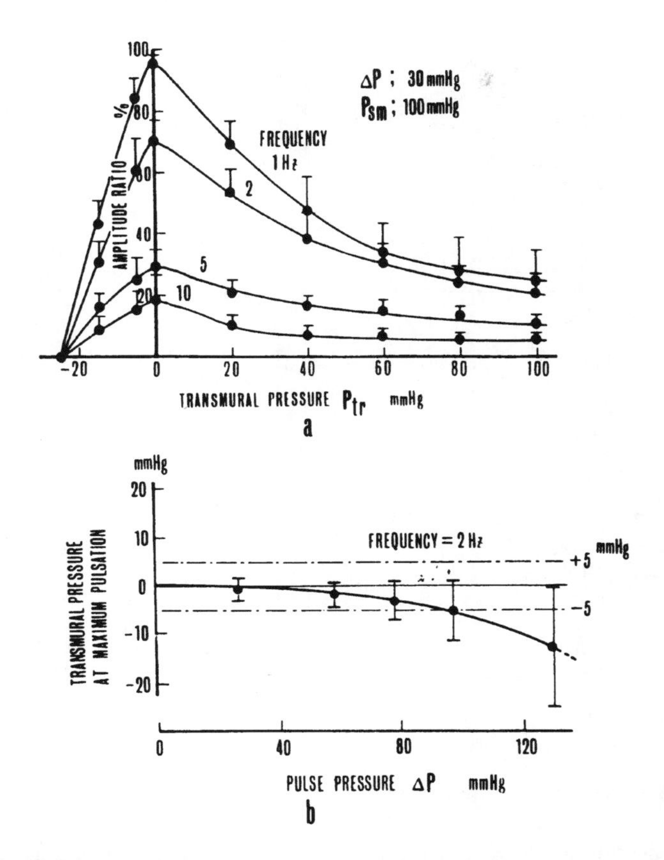

Fig. 2. (a) Ratio of amplitude of volume pulsation to that of the maximum volume pulsation determined from the static pressure-volume relationship in each artery at various frequencies plotted against transmural pressure (Ptr in mmHg). Note that each curve shows a peak at Ptr = 0, although the peak becomes less predominant as increasing the frequency. (b) Transmural pressure at maximum volume pulsation versus the amplitude of pulse pressure ($\triangle$P in mmHg). Note that the shift of the point of the maximum pulsation following the change in $\triangle$P is within 5 mmHg if the $\triangle$P is less than about 100 mmHg.

range $P < 0$; it reached the maximum at zero pressure (*unloaded state* of the arterial segment).

Fig. 1(b) is a graphical representation of the transmural pressure (Ptr; the difference between the mean internal (Psm) and external pressure (Pc), Ptr = Psm - Pc) versus arterial volume which was redrawn from Fig. 1(a). Ptr can be controlled by the external pressure (counterpressure; Pc). It is clearly demonstrated that the amplitude of the arterial volume pulsation ($\triangle$V) produced by the pulse pressure ($\triangle$P) gradually increases with decreasing Ptr (or increasing Pc) due to the increase in the volume compliance of the artery. Thus, the maximum volume pulsation ($\triangle$Vmax) would occur at the point where the Pc reached the mean internal pressure (Psm), i.e. Ptr = 0. The pulsations disappear when the Pc is further increased beyond the peak internal pressure (Pss) (systolic pressure).

In Fig. 2(a) the ratio of amplitude of the volume pulsation to that of the maximum volume pulsation ($\triangle$Vmax; see Fig. 1(b)) determined from the static pressure-volume relationship in each arterial segment was plotted against transmural pressure (Ptr in mmHg). The amplitude of sinusoidal pulse pressure ($\triangle$P) and mean internal pressure (Psm) were 30 and 100 mmHg, respectively, and frequency of the pulse pressure was controlled at 1, 2, 5 and 10 Hz. Therefore, this graph represents the dynamic characteristics of arterial volume compli-

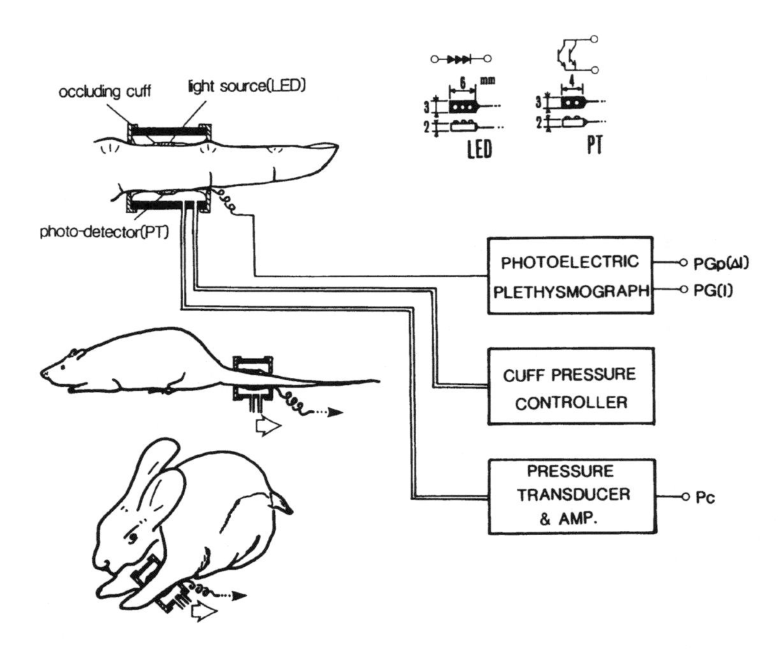

Fig. 3. Schematic diagram of the device for the noninvasive measurement of arterial pressure by the volume-oscillometric method with photoelectric plethysmography in the human finger, rat's tail or rabbit foreleg. The arrangement of a photoelectric transducer (LED and PT) is shown in the inset.

ance. All four curves showed the maximum peak at Ptr = 0. In other words, the occurrence of the maximum volume pulsation at Ptr = 0 was little affected by the change in frequency of the pulse pressure, although its existence became less predominant with increasing the frequency, which would be due to the viscoelastic property of the arterial wall [4].

The shift of the point of the maximum pulsation following the change in the amplitude of pulse pressure was also small; the error caused by this factor was within 5 mmHg if the pulse pressure was less than about 100 mmHg as shown in Fig. 2(b).

This evidence can strongly suggest that during the gradual change in the counterpressure (Pc) the Pc values corresponding to the point of the maximum amplitude and to the disappearance (or appearance) point of the volume pulsations are given as indirect mean and systolic pressure, respectively.

2.2 Evaluation: Methods and results

To evaluate the validity and accuracy of this method, comparison experiments with the direct measurement were made using rats, rabbits and human subjects. Fig. 3 shows a schematic diagram of the device for the noninvasive measurement of arterial pressure. The root of a human finger, a rat's tail or a rabbit foreleg was used as a measuring site. A transmittance type infrared photoelectric plethysmograph [25] was used to detect the arterial volume change in the biological segment. A light source (LED; TLN 104, Toshiba Co.) and a photodetector (PT; TPS 605, Toshiba Co.) were placed respectively on the skin opposite each other using pieces of adhesive tape. The arrangements of this photoelectric transducer (LED and PT) are shown in the inset of Fig. 3.

An annular occluding rubber cuff was installed in a light-shielded black acrylic chamber. The chamber had two side connections; one for counterpressure (cuff pressure; Pc), the other for a Statham P37 pressure transducer. The cuff was placed around the segment to cover the photoelectric transducer at its middle part. The cuff width was determined according to the theoretical and experimental considerations of Alexander et al. [1]: The applied cuff pressure is accurately transmitted throughout the segment when the cuff width is greater than 1.2 times the diameter of the segment concerned. Therefore, several kinds of the cuff whose width had 1.3–1.5 times the diameters of the segments employed were prepared in this experiment.

In the animal experiments, five normotensive (Wistar-Kyoto) and three spontaneously hypertensive (SHR; Aoki-Okamoto strain) rats, weighing 250–400 g, and seven rabbits (New Zealand albino), weighing 2.2–3.5 Kg, were anesthetized with sodium pentobarbital, 25–30 mg/Kg ip. Femoral arterial pressure in the rat and carotid arterial pressure in the rabbit were measued directly using a Statham P23ID pressure transducer and an indwelling arterial catheter made of polyethylene tubing (0.5–1 mm inner diameter and 12–18 cm long; Hibiki Co.). The rats were warmed for about 10 min in a temperature-controlled chamber at 39° C to allow the detection of the photoplethysmographic signal in the tail. The measurements were carried out after the animals lightly recovered from anesthesia. At least five measurements were made for each rat and rabbit, and fifty and eighty pairs of the simultaneous data measured by the direct and indirect method were obtained in the rats and in the rabbits, respectively, in response to resting, bleeding and transfusion.

On the other hand, the simultaneous comparison with the direct measurement was performed on six normotensive (20–36 years old) and six hypertensive (21–45 years old) subjects with an indwelling arterial catheter for routine care. The catheter (18 gauge thin-wall needle) was inserted into the left brachial artery at the medial side of the cubital fossa (the catheter tip in the artery was placed 4–5 cm proximal to the insertion point) and connected to a Statham P37 pressure transducer. The subjects were supine on a bed with their left arms held horizontally at heart level and the left index, middle or ring finger was used as a measuring site. At least five measurements were done for each subject, and seventy five pairs of the simultaneous data were obtained.

Cuff pressure (Pc), photo-plethysmogram (PG: or transmitted light intensity; I) and pulsatile component of PG (PGp: or pulsatile component of I; ΔI), along with direct arterial pressure (Pb), were simultaneously recorded on a multichannel penwriter (Polygraph; model 142, San-Ei Co.).

Fig. 4 is an example of the simultaneous recordings of direct brachial arterial pressure Pb, its mean pressure Pbm, cuff pressure Pc, photo-plethysmogram PG and its pulsatile component PGp obtained from the index finger of a normotensive subject. Following the gradual increase in the Pc, the amplitude of the PGp gradually increased and then decreased until the PGp pulsations at last disappeared. The Pc value revealing the maximum pulsation amplitude was found to show a close agreement with the corresponding direct mean arterial pressure (Pbm), while that at the disappearance point of the pulsation was nearly equal to the direct systolic pressure (Pbs). However, both the indirect systolic (Pcs) and mean pressure (Pcm) determined by this method at the root of the finger were slightly lower than those recorded simultaneously in the brachial artery directly. The difference may be caused by the difference in the recording sites [23, 25, 26].

It was also demonstrated from Fig. 4 that during the range of low Pc level the rapid downward shift of the PG was first observed and then the similar but slower downward shift was recognized during the range of higher Pc level. It is suggestive that the difference of this slope following the change in the Pc was caused by the difference of the elastic properties of venous and arterial vessels [23]. Therefore, the venous and arterial compartment could be separated from this characteristic change in the PG (see Fig. 4). This evidence could be utilized to measure arterial elastic properties noninvasively, which will be described later.

Fig. 5 presents graphs of the values of systolic (left part) and mean (right part) pressure, showing the relationships between the simultaneous data obtained from the indirect and direct measurements in human subjects (upper pannel), rats (middle pannel) and rabbits (lower pannel). A fairly

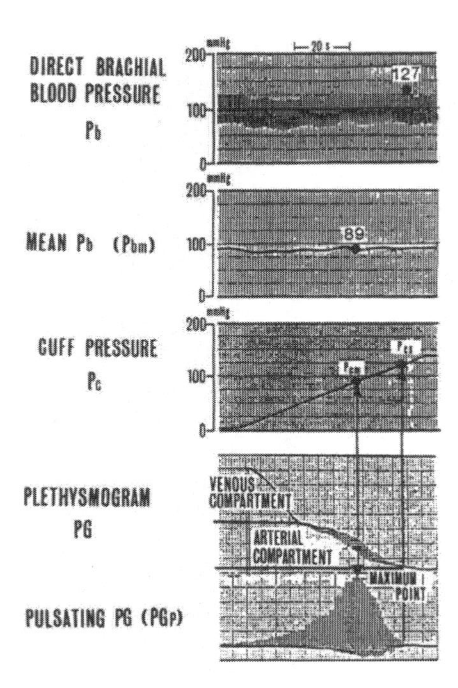

Fig. 4. An example of simultaneous recordings of direct brachial arterial pressure (Pb), its mean pressure (Pbm), cuff pressure (Pc), photoelectric plethysmogram (PG) and its pulsatile component (PGp) obtained from the index finger of a normotensive subject. The arrows directed upward with the solid lines indicate the pressure values (Pcs and Pcm) corresponding to the systolic end point and to the point of the maximum amplitude of PGp. Note that the venous and arterial compartment can be clearly separated from the difference of the slope in the PG signal.

good linear correlation between the pairs of the simultaneous data was obtained in each object over a wide range of mean arterial pressure as well as systolic pressure.

These results clearly indicate that the noninvasive measurement of arterial pressure by the volume-oscillometric method would be applicable not only to the human subjects but to any other animals, and that this is expected to be considerably more reliable and accurate than the conventional cuff-sphygmomanometric techniques [see Ref. 2, 7] which have some practical and/or seriously unsolved problems in the measurement principle [12, 14, 19, 23–26].

2.3 Application to ambulatory monitoring

Since the volume-oscillometric technique with photoelectric plethysmography is simple and reliable, an instrument based on this method can be constructed more simply and compactly compared with conventional commercially available arm-encircling cuff sphygmomanometers.

From this standpoint, we have recently designed a new portable instrument equipped with a microprocessor for the long-term ambulatory monitoring of indirect arterial pressure in the human finger at desired intervals. (More recently, a commercially available system similar to this has been produced (BP-100, M.E. Commercial Co.).)

The details of operation and evaluation of this instrument have been reported elsewhere [27]. Briefly, it consists of (i) a volume-sensing and cuff pressure control (VSCP) unit; (ii) a microprocessor-based central processing & recording (MCPR) unit with interactive software for sequential control and data storage; and (iii) a data reproducing & analysing unit using a conventional personal computer. The former two units are carried by a subject during the measurement as shown in Fig. 6. Usually the left fourth finger is adopted as a measuring site. The cuff pressure is controlled hydraulically, and a water-filled tube (0.5 mm inner diameter) from the cuff is led to the VSCP unit. This VSCP unit containing a pressure transducer is carried in a breast pocket of the subject which is fixed at heart level. Thus, the change in hydrostatic pressure due to the difference in the height between the measuring site and the heart can be corrected to obtain the arterial pressure at heart level.

A schematic block diagram of the instrument is shown in Fig. 7. In this instrument, all the necessary procedures are performed automatically as follows (see also Fig. 8): (1) programmed control of cuff pressure (Pc); (2) detection of systolic end point (SEP) and the point of maximum amplitude (MAP) of volume pulsations (PGp); (3) reading of the Pc values corresponding to these to points; (4) its processing and (5) recording of the systolic (Pcs) and mean pressure (Pcm) together with heart rate (HR) on a digital-memory IC (CMOS RAM).

The VSCP unit is for controlling the Pc and for

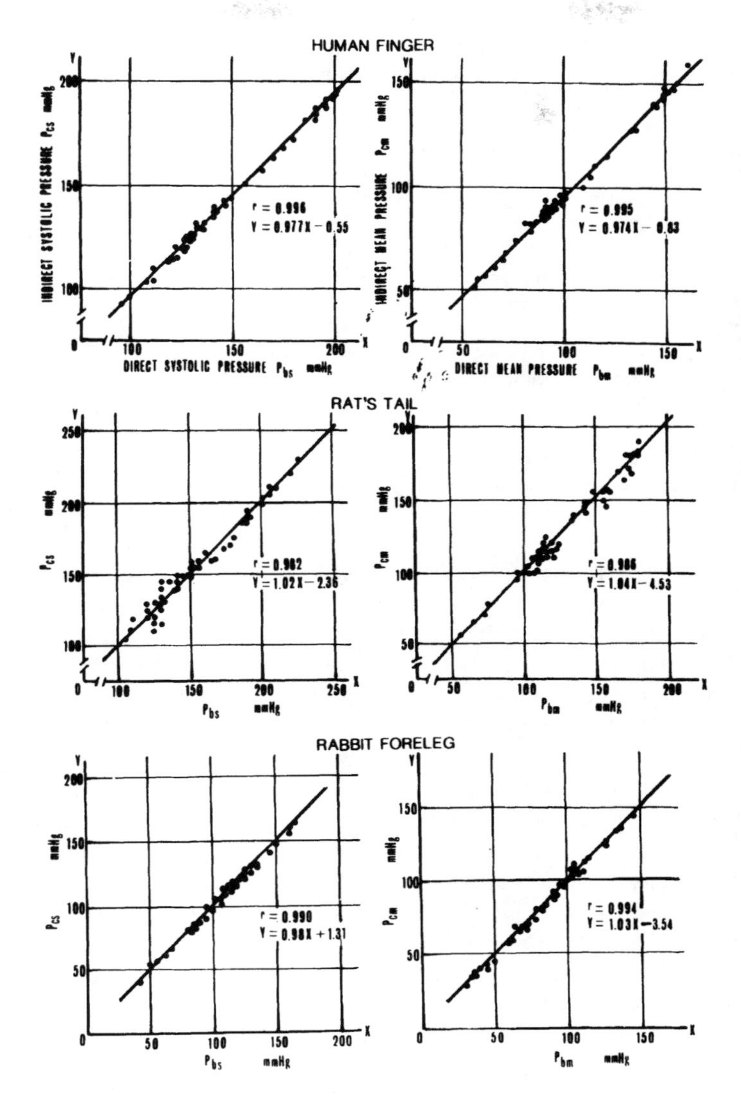

Fig. 5. Comparison of direct and indirect simultaneous measurements of systolic pressures (left part) and mean pressures (right part) obtained in the human subjects (upper pannel), rats (middle pannel) and rabbits (lower pannel). Indirect systolic (Pcs) and mean (Pcm) pressures determined by the volume-oscillometric method are plotted against the corresponding direct systolic (Pbs) and mean (Pbm) pressures recorded by intra-arterial catheters. A solid line in each diagram indicates the regression line.

detecting the PGp, comprising (a) the cuff filled with water; (b) a hydraulic micro-roller pump; (c) a pressure transducer with an appropriate amplifier and (d) a photo-plethysmograph. The MCPR unit performs the following functional roles: (a) A/D conversion of the Pc and PGp signals by an A/D converter (ADC; sampling time, 10 ms); (b) detection of the amplitude of beat-to-beat PGp; (c) data processing by the sequential procedures; (d) detection and discrimination of the SEP and MAP; and (e) storing the results (Pcs, Pcm and HR) on the memory IC. Interactive software for these procedures using a CPU (Z80 CMOS) and a PROM is provided in this unit. To curtail the current consumption in the VSCP unit (about 60 mA), this unit also contains a power supply controller (PSC).

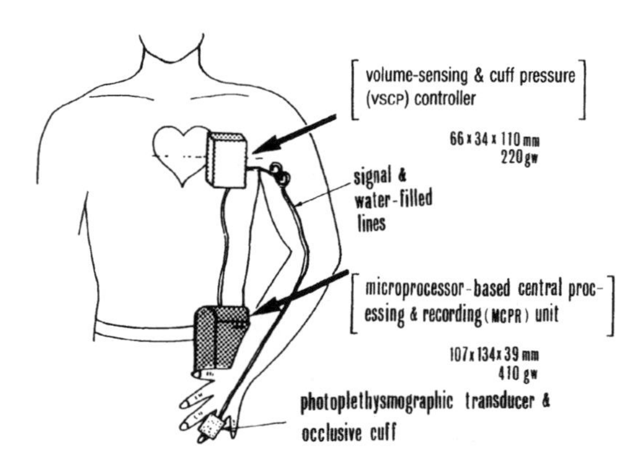

Fig. 6. Outline of the portable instrument for the long-term ambulatory monitoring of indirect arterial pressure carried by a subject.

The operative sequence of the instrument is illustrated by the timing chart shown in Fig. 8. This figure represents a decreasing-mode operation (increasing-mode operation is also available). During the stage of gradual decrease in the Pc at a rate of 2–4 mmHg per heart beat, the SEP and the MAP are detected and the Pc values corresponding to these two points (Pcs and Pcm) are stored as the systolic and mean pressure, respectively. When the SEP and/or the MAP cannot apparently be discriminated due to the artefacts caused by activities such as the strong and sharp movement of the hand, the measurement is stopped to hold the initial mode until the start of the next measurement. The HR is calculated by the processing time from the determination of the SEP to that of the MAP as well as the number of heart beats during this time. Less than thirty seconds are required for each measurement. The measurement interval can be preset at 1, 2, 5 or 10 minutes.

Up to the present time, more than 24-hour continuous monitoring with this instrument has been successfully carried out in over 500 subjects including hypertensive and diabetic patients and patients with cardiac diseases. Through a number of measurements, immeasurable data due mainly to motion artefacts occasionally appeared in the results. However, it was not so disadvantageous in practical long-term monitoring [27]. The details of these clinical applications will be reported elsewhere.

Fig. 9 shows an example of the 24-hour's trend chart of the simultaneous comparison between direct systolic (Pbs) and mean pressure (Pbm) in the left radial artery (upper tracing) and indirect systolic (Pcs) and mean pressure (Pcm) (middle tracing) together with heart rate (HR) (lower tracing) obtained from the left fourth finger in a catheterization subject with hypertension. The measurement interval was 5 minutes. In this experiment, the subject carried the portable instrument along with a cassette data-recorder (RCD-712S, Minebea Co.) for recording the direct arterial pressure signal. After the measurement, the recorded pressure signal was reproduced and analysed by a playback system to obtain the trend chart. It was clearly shown that the transient changes and momentary

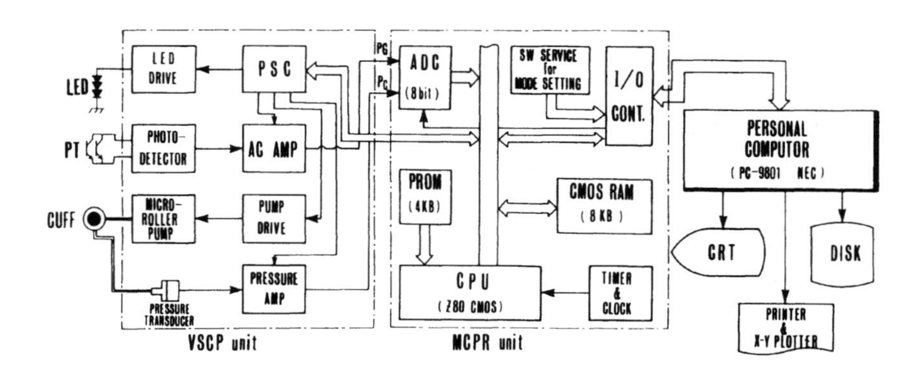

Fig. 7. Schematic block diagram of the instrument. The volume sensing and cuff pressure control (VSCP) unit and microprocessor-based central processing and recording (MCPR) unit are surrounded by broken lines. Data reproducing and analysing was performed by a conventional personal computer. For symbols and functional roles in each block see text.

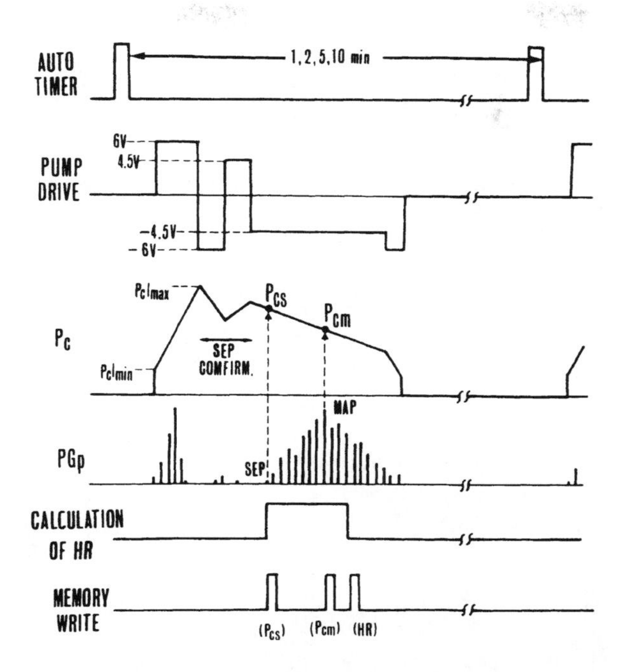

Fig. 8. Timing chart of the sequential procedure of the instrument. See text for further details.

variations of indirect finger pressure measured by the instrument corresponded well with those of the direct arterial pressure at respective times.

Fig. 10 is a typical example of clinical application showing a 24-hour monitoring (5-min interval) of Pcs and Pcm as well as HR obtained in a patient with pheochromocytoma. The patient was sometimes attacked with paroxysm, and at that time paroxysmal hypertension indicated by the arrows at the top could be well recorded by the instrument.

Since the finger was adopted as the measuring site for the long-term monitoring, the measurements were done in the subjects being scarcely affected by a discomfort. In addition, as the digital-memory IC was used to store the data, a conventional personal computer could be available to reproduce the data and to perform necessary data analyses promptly. In this sense this instrument seems to be more practicable and advantageous than another method for the long-term monitoring using an arm-encircling cuff [8, 15].

From these investigations, the instrument using the volume-oscillometric technique appears to provide a helpful and useful means for the long-term ambulatory monitoring of momentary variations of arterial pressure not only in clinics but in research laboratories.

3. Measurement of arterial elastic properties

3.1 Principle

Fig. 11 is a schematic diagram illustrating the principle of the elasticity measurement in the human finger based on the volume-oscillometric technique with photoelectric plethysmography.

When the finger inserted into an occluding cuff is gradually compressed by raising cuff pressure (Pc), the changes in the transmitted light intensity (I and ΔI) will occur as depicted in Fig. 11(b). Since the tissues other than the vascular systems are considered to be incompressible, the venous system is first collapsed at low Pc level, and then the blood volume in the arterial system gradually decreases according to the vascular compliances (see the upper part of Fig. 11(b) and also Fig. 4). When the Pc reaches above systolic pressure, the arterial system would be completely collapsed and no volume

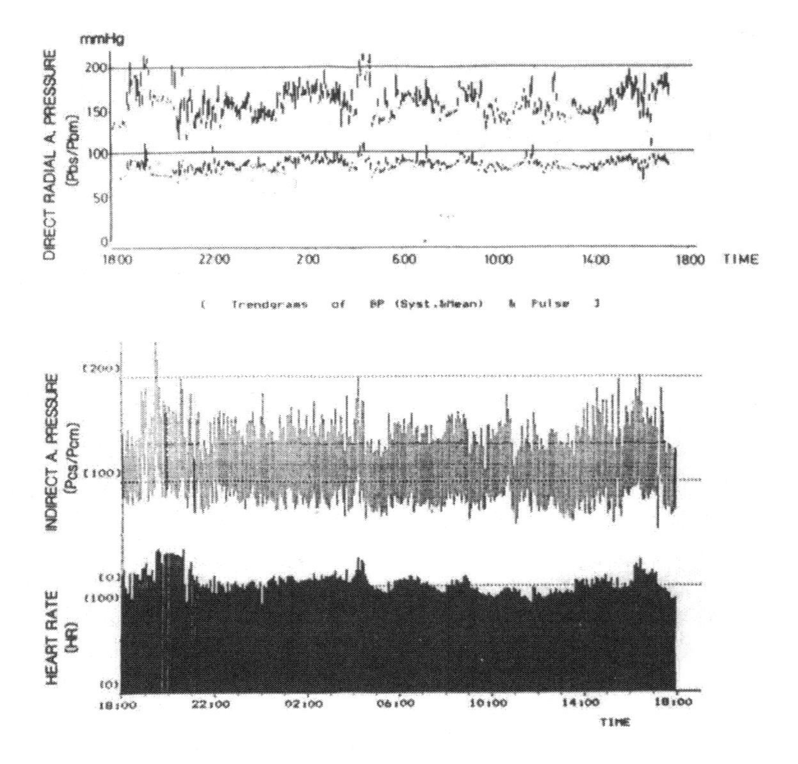

Fig. 9. An example of the 24-hour's trend chart of the simultaneous comparison between direct systolic (Pbs) and mean pressure (Pbm) in the left radial artery (upper tracing) and indirect systolic (Pcs) and mean pressure (Pcm) (middle tracing) together with heart rate (HR) (lower tracing) obtained from the left fourth finger in a catheterization subject with hypertension, showing the volume-oscillometric method used in this instrument to permit accurate tracking of arterial pressure.

changes will occur. The vascular volume change (V) caused by the compression of the segment can be calculated from the mean output signal of the photo-detector (I) under the assumption that the optical model expressed by the Lambert-Beer's law may hold in the finger segment [28],

$$V = -\alpha \cdot \log(I/I_t) \quad (1)$$

where I_t is the transmitted light intensity across the incompressible tissues and α is an absorption rate of the arterial blood or the extinction coefficient peculiar to the substance.

As have been described before, the indirect systolic (Pcs) and mean pressure (Pcm) can be determined from the characteristic changes in the amplitude of the pulsatile components superimposed on I ($\triangle$I). Therefore, the arterial transmural pressure (Ptr) at a certain Pc level is given by,

$$Ptr = Pcm - Pc \quad (2)$$

Taking Io as the mean transmitted light intensity corresponding to the maximum amplitude of $\triangle$I, the relative volume change (V/Vo) is given from Eq. (1) as,

$$V/Vo = \log(I/I_t)/\log(Io/I_t) \quad (3)$$

where Vo is the mean arterial volume corresponding to Io, which indicates the unloading volume at zero transmural pressure.

The volume elastic modulus (Ev), which is usually described as 'bulk modulus' and one of the most widely and practically used indices for expressing arterial elasticity, is defined as [see Ref. 3],

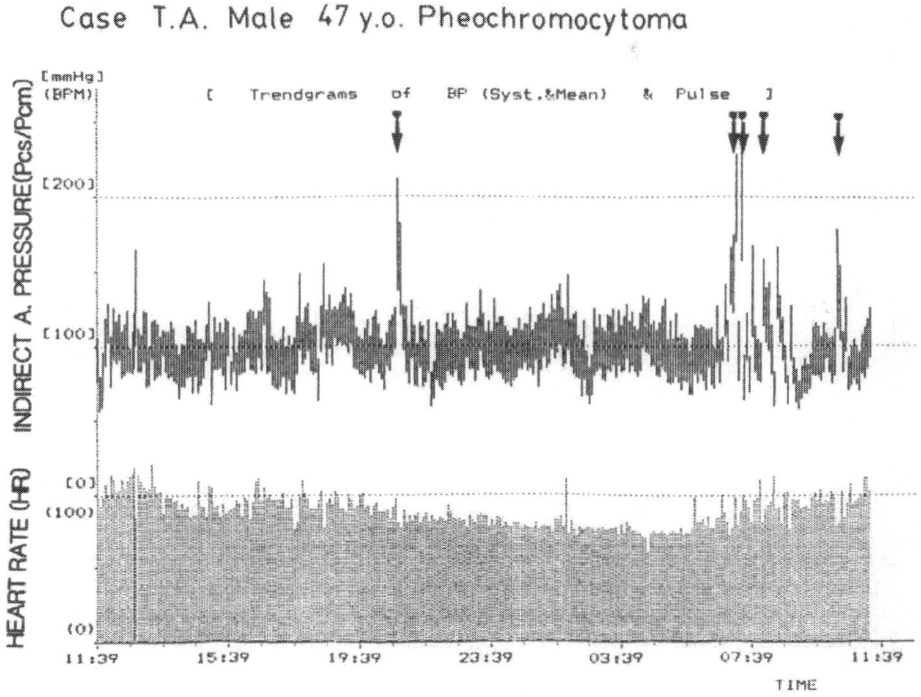

Fig. 10. A typical example of clinical application showing a 24-hour monitoring of indirect systolic (Pcs) and mean pressure (Pcm) together with heart rate (HR) obtained in a patient with pheochromocytoma. This monitoring was carried out at 5-min intervals. The arrows at the top indicate the paroxysmal attack of the patient.

$$Ev \equiv \triangle P/(\triangle V/V) \quad (4)$$

where $\triangle P$ is the arterial pulse pressure, which is also indirectly obtained from the values of Pcs and Pcm; it is approximately calculated as 3/2 (Pcs–Pcm) [see Ref. 5] provided that the significant changes in peripheral resistance does not occur during the measurement. The pulsatile volume change ($\triangle V$), which can be assumed to be extremely smaller than the vascular volume change (V), is given by differentiating Eq. (1) with respect to I as,

$$\triangle V = -\alpha \cdot \triangle I/I \quad (5)$$

By using Eqs. (1) and (5), the relative value of volume ratio ($\triangle V/V$) is given as,

$$\triangle V/V = (\triangle I/I)/\log(I/I_t) \quad (6)$$

This indicates that the $\triangle V/V$ can be calculated from the output signals of the light intensity ($\triangle I$, I and I_t; see Fig. 11(b)) from the photo-detector. Thus, Eq. (4) is rewritten as,

$$Ev = 3/2(Pcs - Pcm)/(\triangle I/I)/\log(I/I_t) \quad (7)$$

From these expressions, the transmural pressure v.s. relative volume (Ptr - V/Vo) relationship can be noninvasively obtained by Eqs. (2) and (3), and Ev in dyn/cm^2 (or mmHg) by Eq. (7) as a function of Ptr. Thus, by this method, the arterial elastic properties obtained from individual subjects whose arterial pressure levels are much different can be compared with each other.

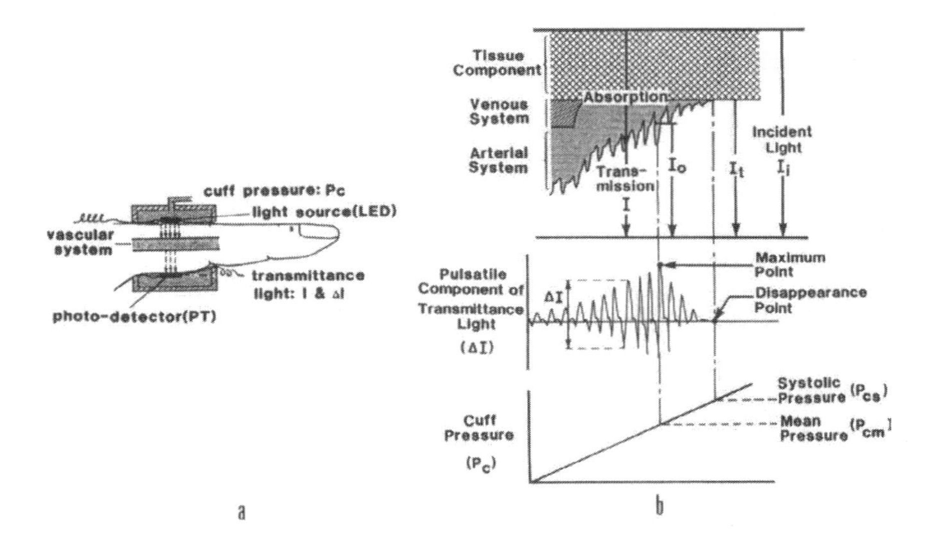

Fig. 11. Schematic diagram illustrating the principle of the non-invasive measurement of arterial elasticity based on the volume-oscillometric method with photoelectric plethysmography. (a) Arrangement of a photoelectric transducer (LED and PT) and an occluding cuff in the human finger. (b) Changes in the transmitted light intensity (I and △I) following the gradual increase in cuff pressure (Pc). I_i, I_t and Io; the intensity of the incident light, the mean transmitted light intensity across the tissue and that corresponding to the maximum amplitude of △I, respectively.

3.2 Evaluation: Methods and results

In vitro model experiment using six canine carotid arterial segments was made to evaluate the validity and accuracy of this elasticity measurement. The experimental setup was almost the same as that used for the evaluation of the volume-oscillometric method [24]. Briefly, the arterial segment was stretched to its in situ length and mounted on a plastic base. Both the segment and the base were surrounded with chicken meat. This model was then covered with a Penrose tube (19 mm inner diameter). The light source (LED) and the photo-detector (PT) were fixed on the tube opposite each other at the middle part of the model. Two stiff polyethylene catheters were cannulated into the arterial segment; one was connected to a Statham P23ID pressure transducer, and the other to a 1 ml glass syringe, the piston of which was controlled by an electro-magnetic shaker (G-002S, Shinken Co.) and a power amplfier to produce stepwise or sinusoidal changes in the internal pressure of the segment. The position of the piston was sensed by a displacement transducer (DCH-101TH, Shinko Denshi Co.). Thus, the actual volume changes in the segment (V and △V) could be obtained from the output of this transducer. Fresh heparinized dog blood was used as a perfusate.

Fig. 12 is a result showing the Ptr–V/Vo (a) and Ev–Ptr relationship (b) obtained in the model experiment. Data points denoted by the closed circles in this figure represent the actual values obtained by the actual volume changes and the direct internal pressure, while those by the closed triangles represent the measured values determined by the photo-plethysmographic measurement. It was clearly shown that the actual and measured data agreed well with each other within about 5–10% error both in the Ptr–V/Vo and the Ev–Ptr relationships.

Because it is too difficult to evaluate directly the accuracy of this method in vivo, we tentatively compared this method with the elasticity measurement using electrical admittance plethysmography technique [6, 9, 17, 20, 22]. Through our previous investigations, the electrical admittance method permits the noninvasive and accurate measurement of limb volume changes and blood flow in

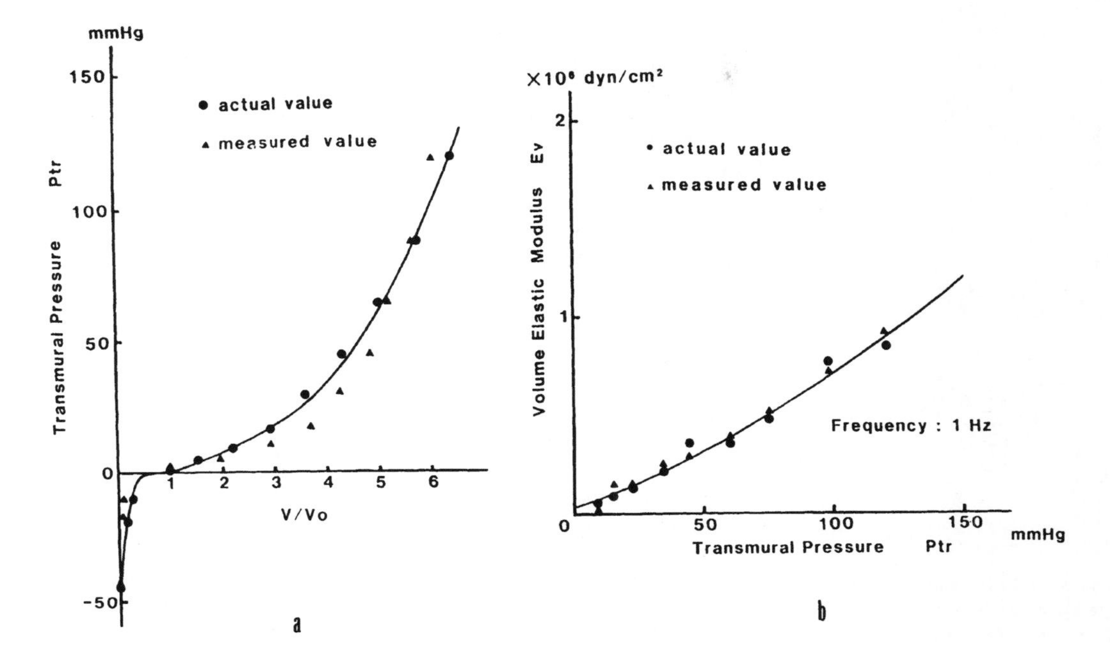

Fig. 12. Relationships between transmural pressure (Ptr in mmHg) and volume ratio (V/Vo)(a) and between volume elastic modulus (Ev in dyn/cm^2) and Ptr at 1 Hz of pulse pressure obtained in the in vitro model experiment. Data points denoted by the closed circles indicate the actual values obtained by the actual volume changes and the direct internal pressure, while those by the closed triangles represent the measured values determined by the photo-plethysmographic measurement.

human forearms and legs [6, 17, 20] as well as arterial volume changes in human fingers [22]. Thus, we consider this to be one of the most advantageous methods of measuring the volume changes noninvasively and quantitatively.

The comparative study aiming especially at the noninvasive measurement of Ev in the finger was performed on six healthy subjects (21–41 years old; four males and two females). The Ev values in the finger arteries measured by the photo-plethysmographic method (PT method) were compared with those determined by the electrical admittance method (ADM method) simultaneously carried out in the same fingers. The tetrapolar method [13] was used for measuring the electrical admittance signal; fine aluminium wires were used for the electrodes with ECG paste. A 1 mA constant current at 50 KHz, which was supplied from a current source, was passed through the finger via a pair of electrodes (current electrodes) around the wrist and fingertip. The voltage drop across the other pair of electrodes (voltage electrodes) around the distal and proximal end of the basal phalanx of this finger was detected, amplified and demodulated to obtain the impedance signal. The spacing between the voltage electrodes was about 1 cm. The occluding cuff was placed to completely cover the finger segment between the voltage electrodes. The admittance signal was obtained by inverting the impedance signal with an IC divider. The total admittance (Y) and its pulsatile change ($\triangle$Y) were obtained through a DC and AC amplifier, respectively. Further details of the electrical admittance method have been reported previously [9, 20–22].

The arterial volume pulsation ($\triangle$Vy) at each cuff pressure level was calculated from the $\triangle$Y signal as [22],

$$\triangle Vy = \varrho_b \cdot L^2 \cdot \triangle Y \qquad (8)$$

where ϱ_b(Ωcm) is the blood resistivity, which can be calculated from hematocrit value of the blood

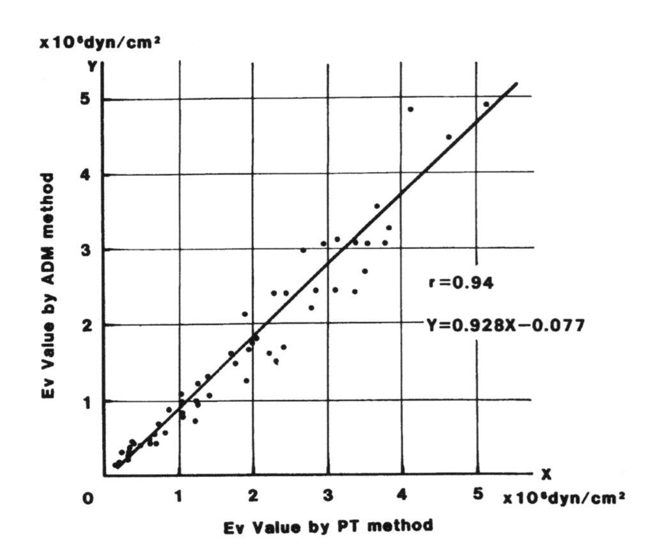

Fig. 13. Scatter diagram comparing the values of volume elastic modulus (Ev in dyn/cm²) in the finger arteries determined by the photoplethysmographic method (PT method; *abscissa*) with those by the electrical admittance method (ADM method; *ordinate*) collected at different levels of transmural pressure obtained in six healthy subjects. A solid line indicates the regression line.

using the empirical equation [20, 22], and L(cm) is the distance between the voltage electrodes. The mean arterial volume in the segment concerned ($\overline{V}y$) was calculated by the following procedures [18]. First, the volume of the blood pooled in the venous compartment was expelled from the segment at a very low cuff pressure (about 15–20 mmHg). Then, the mean Y signal ($\overline{Y}$) decreased with the further increase in the cuff pressure. At this time, the volume of the blood in the arterial compartment was linearly related to the $\overline{Y}$ signal. The $\overline{Y}$ signal at the moment when the $\triangle Y$ signal completely disappeared on increasing the cuff pressure just above systolic arterial pressure denotes the total admittance of the bloodless compartment of the segment ($\overline{Y}s$). Therefore, $\overline{V}y$ was calculated from the equation:

$$\overline{V}y = \varrho_b \cdot L^2 \cdot (\overline{Y} - \overline{Y}s) \tag{9}$$

From Eqs. (8) and (9), the Ev was calculated as,

$$Ev = \triangle P/(\triangle Vy/\overline{V}y) = \triangle P/(\triangle Y/(\overline{Y} - \overline{Y}s)) \tag{10}$$

The characteristic change in the amplitude of the $\triangle Y$ following the gradual change in the cuff pressure was almost similar to that obtained by the PT method (see Fig. 4). Fig. 13 shows a scatter diagram comparing the Ev values determined by the PT method (in dyn/cm²; *abscissa*) with those by the ADM method (in dyn/cm²; *ordinate*) at the same transmural pressure levels. These data were simultaneously collected at different levels of the transmural pressure ranging from 0 to 90 mmHg. A fairly good correlation between the pairs of the data from these two methods was obtained.

From these results, using the photoelectric plethysmography technique the arterial elastic properties can be noninvasively determined as a function of transmural pressure together with arterial pressure. Taking simplicity, safety and ease measurement into consideration, this should be practicable and useful for evaluating changes in arterial elasticity.

4. Automatic instrument and measuring results

A new handy fully-automatic instrument has re-

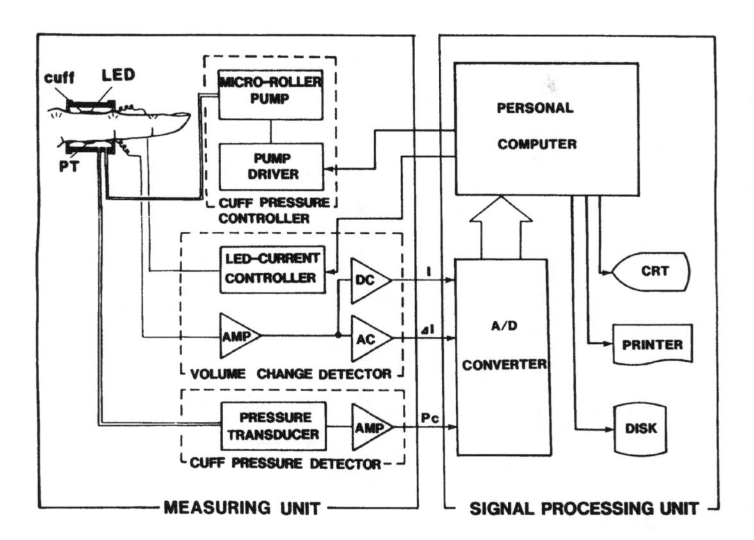

Fig. 14. Schematic block diagram of the instrument for the non-invasive automatic measurement of arterial elasticity. For symbols and functions of a measuring and signal processing unit see text.

cently been designed for the noninvasive measurement of arterial elastic properties using the photoelectric plethysmography technique and a conventional personal computer [11]. Fig. 14 is a schematic diagram of the instrument, comprising (i) a measuring unit and (ii) a signal processing unit. The former is almost the same as the VSCP unit in the portable instrument described above (see Fig. 7) except that it can measure the total transmitted light intensity (I) via a DC amplifier. The latter is for operating the following three functions: (a) sequential control of each parts of the measuring unit; (b) A/D conversion of the signals (I, ΔI and Pc) by an A/D converter (12 bits; sampling time, 10 ms); and (c) processing the data to obtain the indirect systolic (Pcs) and mean pressure (Pcm) together with heart rate (HR), and the Ptr–V/Vo and Ev–Ptr relationship calculated from Eqs. (2), (3) and (7) using a personal computer (PC-9801M2, NEC).

The sequence of operation of the instrument is illustrated by the timing chart shown in Fig. 15. This represents an increasing-mode operation (decreasing-mode operation is also available). Following a start signal, an adequate current for the LED is supplied from a LED-current controller until the intensity of the photo-current detected by the PT reaches a desired preset level (0.3–0.5 mA). Immediately after the adequate LED current was set, the Pc is gradually raised. During this stage, the A/D conversion of the Pc, I and ΔI signals is carried out, and then these digital values are fed into the computer to perform the necessary data processing using a computer program. At the end of the data analysis, the computed results are listed on a CRT display together with a hard copy using a printer before being stored on a floppy disk. About 2 minutes are required for the processing time from the start of the measurement to the display of the analysed data. The further details of this instrument have been reported previously [11].

With this instrument, we have successfully measured the arterial elastic properties in human fingers and in rabbit forelegs suspected to be developed the experimental atherosclerosis by feeding cholesterol-rich diet.

Twenty four rabbits (New Zealand albino; 3.0 ± 0.2 Kg body wt.) were used, the ages of which were about 10 weeks. These had been treated by feeding with 1% cholesterol diet to cause the experimental hyperlipemia. This process was followed by repeating the measurement using this instrument in the forelegs at every two or four weeks under light anesthesia by pentobarbital,

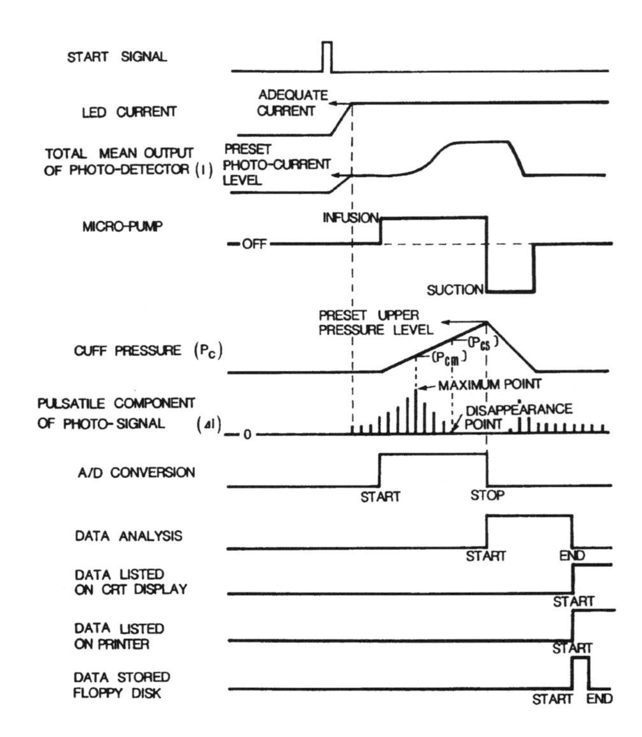

Fig. 15. Timing chart of the sequential procedure of the instrument. See text for further details.

20 mg/Kg iv. Two of these 24 rabbits which survived during this progressive period of the diet load over 10 weeks were fed with an ordinary cholesterol-free diet in order to observe the regression process.

Fig. 16 is an example showing a representative time course of the changes in the Ptr–V/Vo (a) and Ev–Ptr relationship (b) during the progressive (solid lines) and regressive process (dashed lines) obtained in the foreleg of a rabbit. It was revealed that during the progressive process up to 10 weeks these curves showed counter-clockwise shifts towards the sclerosis, followed thereafter by clockwise shifts towards the control curve during the regression process. These changes were not caused by the alterations in the arterial pressures as indicated in Fig. 16 (b).

Fig. 17 summarizes the results showing the progressive changes in the Ev–Ptr relationship obtained in the forelegs of 22 rabbits being treated with 1% cholesterol diet during 18 weeks. Data points and vertical bars in this figure represent mean ± SD calculated at every 10 mmHg of the transmural pressure (Ptr). These data are classified into 5 groups for the rabbits; before feeding cholesterol diet (control), after feeding it for less than 1 month, from 1 to 2 months, from 2 to 3 months, and over 3 months. The levels of significance of difference (p-value; *t*-test) between the Ev values in control and those in each period of the diet load are also indicated in this figure. It was demonstrated that a significant increase in the Ev values ($p < 0.01$–0.001) in the groups over 1 month was observed at any Ptr level compared with those in the control group.

On the other hand, the elasticity measurement in human fingers were carried out in over 100 subjects. Mostly the basal phalanx of the right index finger was used as a measuring site. During the measurement the subjects were sitting at rest on a chair with their right arms put on a table and held at heart level.

Fig. 18 shows an example of the accute changes in the Ev–Ptr relationship obtained from a patient

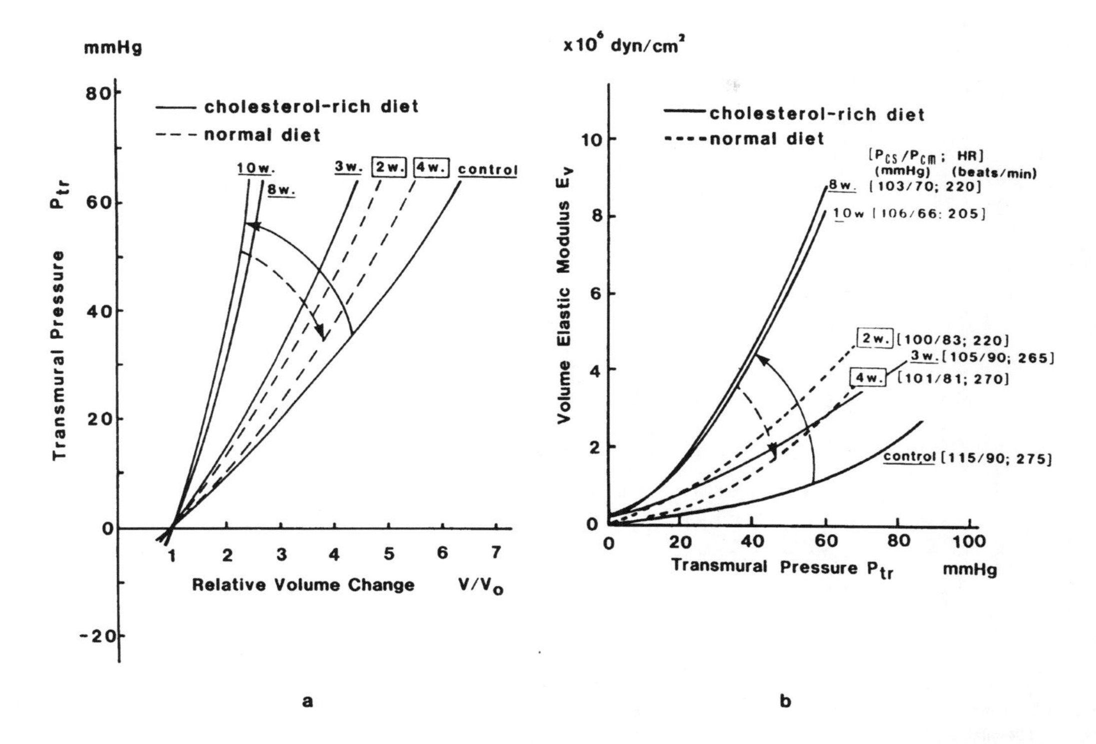

Fig. 16. An example of representative time course of the changes in the relationships between transmural pressure (Ptr in mmHg) and relative volume change (volume ratio; V/Vo(a) and between volume elastic modulus (Ev in dyn/cm^2) and Ptr(b) during the progressive (solid lines) and regressive process (dashed lines) obtained in the foreleg of a rabbit. Numbers indicated in the curves and in the solid line frames represent the period, in weeks, after the onset of cholesterol diet load and regression period after returning to the normal diet respectively. Systolic (Pcs in mmHg)/mean arterial pressure (Pcm in mmHg) and heart rate (HR in beats/min) at respective periods are also shown in (b).

(56 years old, female) with valvular heart disease after the sublingual administration of vasodilator (Isosorbide dinitrate; ISDN, 5 mg/tablet). After the administration of ISDN, the Ev values were distinctly lowered at each Ptr level, and then reached the minimum values at 10 minutes later. Thereafter the Ev values were gradually recovered to the level before the administration. This suggests that the extensibility of the arterial wall would increase due to the administration of ISDN, and that this efficacy on the arterial elasticity would continue during more than 60 minutes.

Fig. 19(a) summarizes the statistical result of the Ev–Ptr relationship obtained in 68 normal male-subjects aged from 18 to 90 years old, indicating the age effect on the arterial elasticity. The solid lines represent the Ev values of mean ± SE calculated at every 10 mmHg of the Ptr. Data are clustered in four groups for the subjects aged from 18 to 29, from 30 to 39, from 40 to 59, and over 65 years old, respectively. It is shown that the mean Ev values tend to increase as the age advances. While in Fig. 19(b), is shown the summarized statistical result of the Ev–Ptr relationship obtained in normal male and female subjects, indicating the difference between the sexes in the arterial elasticity. Data are calculated in two groups for the younger (18–24 years old; 10 males and 9 females) and old aged generation (over 65 years old; 26 males and 16 females). Both in the younger and older generations the Ev values of male subjects appeared to be higher than those of female.

Through these investigations, the instrument using the photo-electric plethysmography tech-

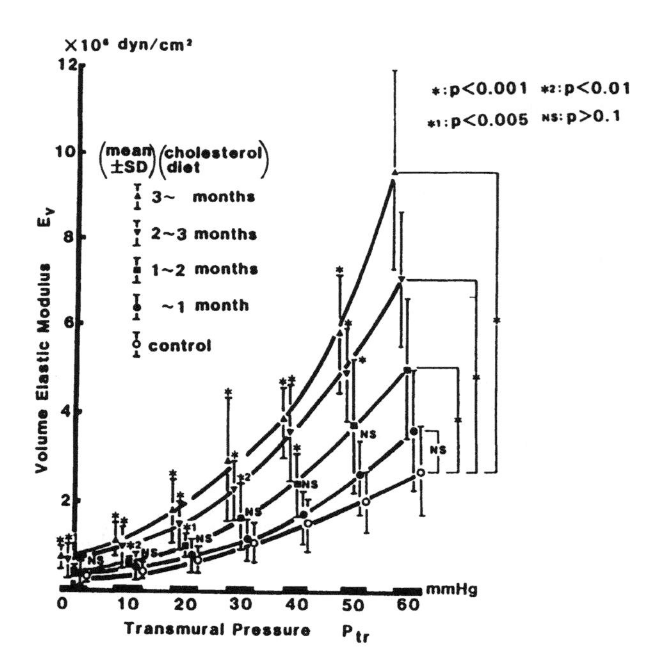

Fig. 17. Summarized results showing the progressive changes in volume elastic modulus (Ev in dyn/cm²) v.s. transmural pressure (Ptr in mmHg) relationship obtained in the forelegs of 22 rabbits being treated with cholesterol-rich diet during 18 weeks. Data points and vertical bars represent mean ± SD calculated at every 10 mmHg of Ptr. Note that a significant increase in the Ev values in the groups over 1 month is observed at any Ptr level compared with those in the control group.

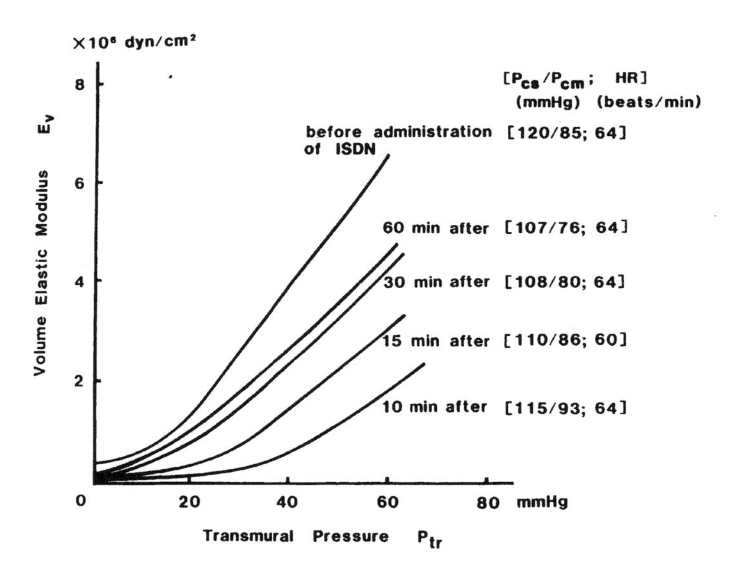

Fig. 18. An example of the accute changes in volume elastic modulus (Ev in dyn/cm²) v.s. transmural pressure (Ptr in mmHg) relationship obtained from the index finger of a patient with valvular heart disease after sublingual administration of Isosorbide dinitrate (ISDN). Note that the effect of ISDN on the Ev-Ptr relationship is clearly observed.

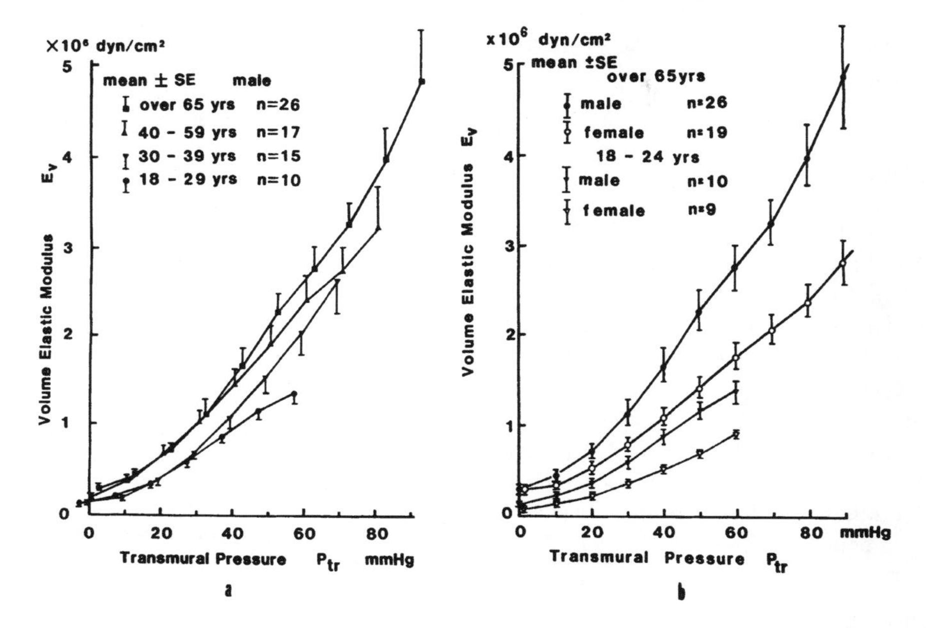

Fig. 19. Summarized statistical results of volume elastic modulus (Ev in dyn/cm²) v.s. transmural pressure (Ptr in mmHg) relationships obtained in 68 normal male subjects aged from 18 to 90 years old (a) and in 36 normal male and 28 normal female subjects (b). The graph (a) indicates the age effect on the arterial elasticity, while the graph (b) indicates the difference between the sexes in the arterial elasticity. For further details see text.

nique permits the adequate measurement for the noninvasive tracking of an accute or chronic change in arterial elastic properties in terms of 'static pressurevolume relationship' and 'dynamic characteristic curve (Ev–Ptr curve)'. This will be easily applicable both in clinics and in basic vascular research using experimental animal models.

5. Conclusion

The main points reviewed in this paper are conclusively listed as follows:

1. A new 'volume-oscillometric method' based on the nonlinear characteristics of arterial pressure-volume relationship has been developed for the noninvasive measurement of arterial pressure as well as arterial elastic properties.
2. The volume-oscillometric technique with photoelectric plethysmography permits the reliable and accurate identification over a wide range of systolic and mean arterial pressure. This appears to be quite available for the noninvasive arterial pressure measurement not only in human subjects but in any animals.
3. A new automated portable instrument based on this method, which was designed for the long-term ambulatory monitoring of indirect arterial pressure in the human finger, promises to be applicable not only in health screening and testing but also in other wide clinical practice.
4. A new noninvasive method for measuring arterial elastic properties based on the volume-oscillometric technique with photoelectric plethysmography has been developed.
5. The validity and accuracy of this elasticity measurement are successfully examined through in vitro model experiments and in vivo comparative study using electrical admittance plethysmography technique.
6. A handy fully-automatic instrument based on the elasticity measurement described herein is expected to be a helpful and useful means for the noninvasive tracking of accute or chronic changes in arterial elasticity not only in clinics

but also in basic vascular research using experimental animal models.

Acknowledgement

We are grateful to Prof. K. Tsuchiya, Department of Mechanical Engineering, Waseda University, Prof. T. Togawa, Institute for Medical and Dental Engineering, Tokyo Medical and Dental University, Prof. H. Ito, Department of Physiology, Kyorin University School of Medicine, for their valuable criticisms and comments, Assistant Prof. H. Shimazu, Department of Physiology, Kyorin University School of Medicine, Dr. A. Kawarada, Dr. J. Ando, for their useful discussions, data analysis and experimentation, and Dr. Y. Imai, Department of Internal Medicine, Tohoku University, for his generous contributions of clinical data and interest.

References

1. Alexander H, Cohen ML, Steinfield LS: Criteria in the choice of an occluding cuff for the indirect measurement of blood pressure. Med & Biol Eng & Comput 15: 2–10, 1977.
2. Cobbold RSC: Transducer for biomedical measurement; principle and applications. John Wiley & Sons, New York, 1974, pp 486.
3. Dinnar U: Cardiovascular fluid dynamics. CRC Press Inc. Boca Raton, Florida, 1981, pp 252.
4. Dobrin PB: Mechanical properties of arteries. Physiol Rev 58: 397–460, 1978.
5. Folkow B, Neil E: Circulation. Oxford University Press Inc, New York, 1971, pp 593.
6. Fukuoka M, Kawakami K, Shimada T, Shimazu H, Yamakoshi K, Ito H: Venous occlusive RN plethysmography; Comparison with electrical admittance plethysmography. J Biomed Eng 6: 141–145, 1984.
7. Geddes LA: The direct and indirect measurement of blood pressure. Year Book Publishers, Chicago, 1970, pp 196.
8. Hinman AT, Engel BT, Bickford AF: Portable blood pressure recorder; accuracy and preliminary use in evaluating intradaily variations in pressure. Am Heart J 63: 663–668, 1962.
9. Ito H, Yamakoshi K, Togawa T: Transthoracic admittance plethysmography for measuring cardiac output. J Appl Physiol 40: 451–454, 1976.
10. Kawarada A, Shimazu H, Yamakoshi K, Kamiya A: Noninvasive measurement of the arterial elasticity in terminal vascular beds with photoelectric plethysmography. Proc 14th Int Conf Med Biol Eng Espoo, 999–1000. 1985.
11. Kawarada A, Yamakoshi K, Kamiya A, Shimazu H: Noninvasive automatic measurement of arterial elasticity in human fingers and rabbit forelegs using photoelectric plethysmography. Med & Biol Eng & Comput (in press), 1986.
12. Kirkendall WM, Burton AC, Epstein FH, Freis ED: Recommendations for human blood pressure determination by sphyggmomanometers. Report of the Central Committee for Medical and Community Program of the American Heart Association. 3–24, 1967.
13. Nyboer J: Electrical impedance plethysmography; a physical and physiologic approac to peripheral vascular study. Circulation 2: 811–821, 1950.
14. Ramsey M. III: Noninvasive automatic determination of mean arterial pressure. Med & Biol Eng & Comput 17: 11–18, 1979.
15. Schneider RA, Kimmell GO, Van Meter RP Jr: An improved fully automatic portable blood pressure recorder. J Appl Physiol 37: 776–779, 1974.
16. Shimazu H, Kawarada A, Yamakoshi K, Kamiya A: Noninvasive measurement of sclerotic changes in rabbit forearm artery. Proc 13th Int Conf Med Biol Eng. Hamburg, 2–05, 1982.
17. Shimazu H, Yamakoshi K, Togawa T, Fukuoka M, Ito H: Evaluation of the parallel conductor theory for measuring human limb blood flow by electrical admittance plethysmography. IEEE Trans Biomed Eng BME-29: 1–7, 1982.
18. Shimazu H, Fukuoka M, Ito H, Yamakoshi K: Noninvasive measurement of beat-to-beat vascular viscoelastic properties in human fingers and forearms. Med & Biol Eng & Comput 23: 43–47, 1985.
19. Smith CR, Bickely WH: The measurement of blood pressure in the human body. SP-5006, NASA 1–34, 1964.
20. Yamakoshi K, Shimazu H, Togawa T, Ito H: Admittance plethysmography for accurate measurement of human limb blood flow. Am J Physiol 235: H821–H829, 1978.
21. Yamakoshi K, Shimazu H, Bukhari ARS, Togawa T, Ito H: Clinical evaluation of an electrical admittance blood flow monitor. J Clin Eng 4: 341–346, 1979.
22. Yamakoshi K, Shimazu H, Togawa T, Fukuoka M, Ito H: Noninvasive measurement of hematocrit by electrical admittance plethysmography technique. IEEE Trans Biomed Eng BME-27: 156–161, 1980.
23. Yamakoshi K, Shimazu H, Togawa T: Indirect measurement of instantaneous arterial blood pressure in the human finger by the vascular unloading technique. IEEE Trans Biomed Eng BME-27: 150–155, 1980.
24. Yamakoshi K, Shimazu H, Shibata M, Kamiya A: New oscillometric method for indirect measurement of systolic and mean arterial pressure in the human finger. Part I; model experiment. Med & Biol Eng & Comput 20: 307–313, 1982.
25. Yamakoshi K, Shimazu H, Shibata M, Kamiya A: New

oscillometric method for indirect measurement of systolic and mean arterial pressure in the human finger. Part II; correlation study. Med & Biol Eng & Comput 20: 314–318, 1982.

26. Yamakoshi K, Kamiya A, Shimazu H, Ito H, Togawa T: Noninvasive automatic monitoring of instantaneous arterial blood pressure using the vascular unloading technique. Med & Biol Eng & Comput 21: 557–565, 1983.
27. Yamakoshi K, Kawarada A, Kamiya A, Shimazu H, Ito H: Long-term ambulatory monitoring of indirect arterial blood pressure using a volume-oscillometric method. Med & Biol Eng & Comput 23: 459–465, 1985.
28. Yoshiya I, Shimada Y: Non-invasive spectrophotometric estimation of arterial oxygen saturation. In: Rolfe P (ed) Non-invasive physiological measurements Vol. 2. Academic Press Inc, London, 1983, pp 383.

Address for offprints:
Ken-ichi Yamakoshi, Ph.D.
The Research Institute of Applied Electricity,
Hokkaido University
N12, W6, Kita-ku
Sapporo 060, Japan

Medical Progress through Technology 12: 145–157 (1987)

Solid-state micro sensors

Masayoshi Esashi & Tadayuki Matsuo
Department of Electronic Engineering, Faculty of Engineering, Tohoku University. Sendai, Japan

Key words: micro sensor, chemical sensor, ISFET, biosensor, pressure sensor, sensing system

Summary

Recent research activities on solid state micro sensors in Japan are reviewed. Many kinds of micro sensors for chemical and physical quantitative analysis have been developed for biomedical instrumentation.

Many of these sensors are fabricated with the advanced art of semiconductor technology, which is called micromachining. This technology enables fabrication of sensors so small that they can be used in catheter tubes etc. Moreover, it has brought out integrated sensing systems or multi sensors.

In the field of chemical sensors, the development of ISFETs, i.e. ion sensitive field effect transistors, has been much advanced. These have been applied not only as ion sensors but also as biosensors or dissolved gas sensors.

On the other hand, the major research activities on micro sensors for physical quantities have been on pressure sensors for measurements in blood vessels etc.

1. Introduction

Micro sensors are indispensable to get accurate biomedical information for diagnosis or for basic physiological or medical research. They should be small enough to minimize invasion and to enable local measurements of chemical or physical quantities. In many cases, micro sensors are used mounted on the tip of a catheter tube or implanted in an object with a telemetry system.

The present advanced technology for integrated circuit fabrication can be the most powerful means for the fabrication of micro sensors. Silicon is the most prevalent material in solid state micro sensors. This application of semiconductor technology is called micromachining. This technology gives rise to the following excellent features of micro sensors.

1. Small size and good dimensional accuracy.
2. Low fabrication cost by batch processing leading to disposable sensors.
3. Integration of plural sensors or of electronic circuits on the sensor chip. Array sensors or intelligent sensors can be fabricated and additionally the assembly cost can be reduced.
4. Active effects of semiconductor materials are applicable for sensors. For example, the field effect is essential for ion sensitive field effect transistors and the piezoresistive effect for pressure sensors.

There are two important requirements for biomedical micro sensors. One is stability and the other is suitable packaging.

Degradation of the sensor and unwanted influences on the sensor can be sources of its instability. Semiconductor devices can sense different physical and chemical phenomena. However, one sensor must have sensitivity to only one parameter, or in other words, it must have a high selectivity. There are some biomedical sensors which are used exposed to an electrolyte. To eliminate unwanted influences from such a severe environment as an electrolyte, the passivation methods for the sensor chip are very important.

The second requirement, i.e. the packaging should be suitable for biomedical purposes from the following points of view. The reliability, that is, the stability depends on the encapsulation. If a sensor should be assembled at the tip of a flexible catheter tube for example, the packaging method should guarantee not only the performance of the sensor but also the lead wire attachment, the mechanical protection, the electrical stability and the biocompatibility. Furthermore, the catheter must be able to stand a sterilization.

Recent research activities on solid state micro sensors in Japan will be described in this paper.

Micro sensors for chemical quantities have been studied to an appreciable extent. Many of these sensors are based on the ion sensitive FET (ISFET). Ion sensors, biosensors and gas sensors have been developed.

Major research activities on micro sensors for physical quantities have been on pressure sensors mainly because of the great demand for such a sensor.

Some sensing systems, including telemetry systems, have also been developed.

2. Chemical sensors

Micro chemical sensors are desired to obtain information about local chemical compositions. One important clinical demand is to measure the concentration of some chemical species in blood. Indwelling or catheter tip micro sensors are suitable to monitor these continuously in vivo, i.e. in a blood vessel. Micro sensors also contribute to reduction of the necessary blood sample volume when the blood is analyzed in vitro. Traditional chemical sensors such as ion selective electrodes are not suitable for such purposes because of their high electrode impedances.

The Ion Sensitive Field Effect Transistor (ISFET) is an attractive integrated device composed of a conventional ion selective electrode and an Insulated Gate FET (IGFET) [8]. The structure and the principle of the ISFET are shown in Fig. 1.

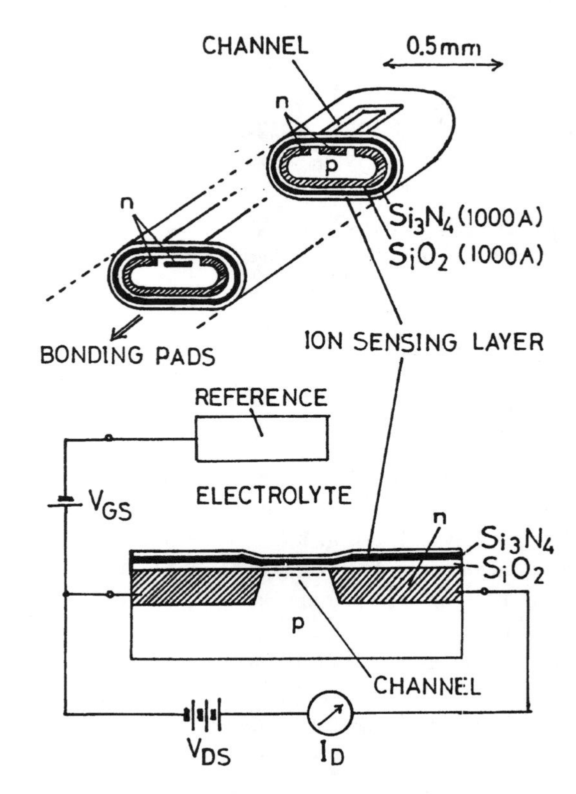

Fig. 1. Structure and principle of the ISFET.

The gate insulator surface is the ion sensing layer and the interface potential between the electrolyte and this layer is converted to a low impednce electrical signal by the FET. Practical reliability for long term use was given by the micromachined probe type structure shown in Fig. 1. The whole surface of the probe was covered with multiple layers of insulators including a chemically inert silicon nitride layer. The active gate region of the FET was located at the tip of the probe, and the n type drain diffusion layer between the gate and bonding pads was buried under the p^+ layer to reduce instabilities due to a parasitic channel. Moreover the surface was rounded, because a defect free and smooth surface is mechanically tough.

The feature of low output impedance leads to quick response, and therefore this enables us to observe variations in local ion concentrations within a width of only a few microns. A micro ISFET which has the ion sensitive part at the probe

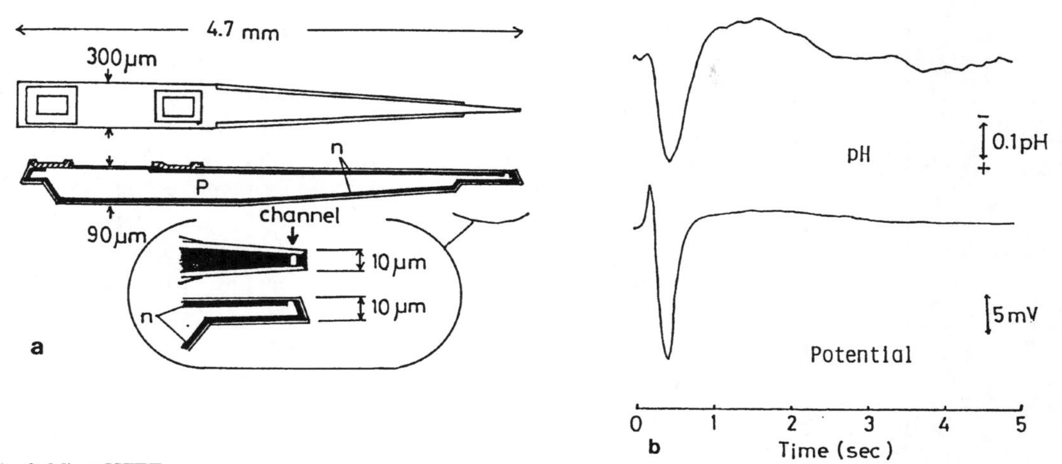

Fig. 2. Micro ISFET.
(a) Structure; (b) pH change measured by the micro ISFET and the potential measured simultaniously on a frog retina after photo stimulation.

tip has been developed to verify this. Fig. 2 (a) shows the structure of the pH sensitive micro IS-FET that has a tip size of 10 µm and a channel area of $5 \times 5\,\mu m^2$ [15]. The three-dimensional micro-machining took an important part in the fabrication process of the silicon micro probe. EPW (Ethyl-enediamine - Pyrocatechol - Water) anisotropic etching and CF_4 plasma etching were used to process the top and the bottom of the wafer respectively. The measured pH sensitivity of the micro ISFET was about 48 mV/pH.

An example of a biological application of the micro ISFET (30 µm tip size) is shown in Fig. 2 (b). The pH change measured by the micro ISFET and the potential curve measured simultaneously from a frog retina after photo stimulation were observed. The quick pH response within 1 second as seen in the figure demonstrates the usefulness of the micro ISFET.

The material of the ion sensing layer determines the ion selectivity of the ISFETs. Both inorganic and organic materials can be used. Si_3N_4, Al_2O_3 and Ta_2O_5 indicated excellent pH sensitive characteristics.

MAS ($M_2O - Al_2O_3 - SiO_2$) glass, where M corresponds to an alkalication as Na^+, K^+ or Li^+, is known as a sensing material for sodium or potassium ions. Sodium sensitive and potassium sensitive ISFETs, which have MAS membranes as their ion sensing layers, were developed by the following two methods. One is the metal alkoxide hydrolysis method and the other is the ion implantation method.

The former was as follows [8]. A mixture of metal alkoxide solution, the contents of which correspond to the composition of the membrane, was coated on the ISFET by dipping. After sintering at 500° C, an MAS layer of about 500 Å thickness was formed. Maximum sodium to potassium ion selectivity was obtained with the LAS (Li:Al:Si = 25:25:50) glass and was about 200. On the other hand, the maximum potassium to sodium ion selectivity was obtained by the KAS (K:Al:Si = 45:15:40) glass and was about 40.

The ion implantation method is rather advantageous by virtue of its compatibility with the batch processes and the controllability. The fabrication sequence of the ion-implanted ISFET is shown in Fig. 3 and was as follows [4]. An ISFET wafer having a Si_3N_4 and SiO_2 double layer on Si substrate was prepared. A thin oxide was formed on the Si_3N_4 surface by oxidation. After this, aluminum was evaporated on it and a certain amount of sodium ions was implanted through the aluminum layer into the thin oxide layer on the Si_3N_4. During this process, aluminum was pushed into the thin oxide layer by the sodium ions. Finally, the aluminum layer was removed and the device was sin-

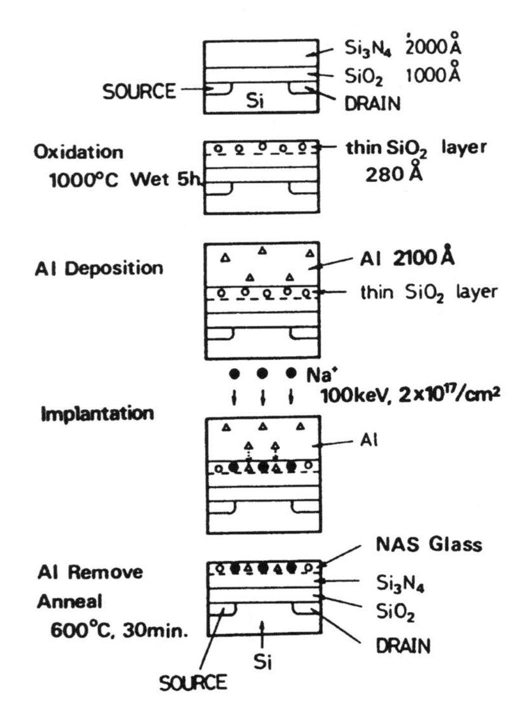

Fig. 3. Fabrication sequence of the ion implanted ISFET.

tered. Since the aluminum layer prevents the sodium ions from penetrating the bottom SiO_2 layer, the FET characteristics were not damaged. The ion selectivity could be controlled by varying the thickness of the aluminum layer and the amount of implanted ions. Both sodium sensitive and potassium sensitive FETs were obtained in this way.

SOS (Silicon on Sapphire) ISFETs shown in Fig. 4 (a) have been developed [7]. Each SOS ISFET is on a silicon island on a sapphire substrate and is therefore easily isolated from neighbouring FETs. Furthermore, it is also very well isolated from the sample solution as sapphire is a good dielectric material.

Biological molecules as urea etc. can be sensed using an immobilized enzyme membrane on an oxygen sensor or on a pH sensor. By measuring the rate of an enzyme reaction, the concentration of a specific molecule in a test solution is determined. This type of sensor is called biosensor. High selectivity can be obtained due to the specificity of an enzyme reaction. By virtue of the advantages of ISFETs, i.e., the very small size etc., ISFET type biosensors have been widely investigated. Multi-biosensors, which can detect different molecules simultaneously, have been fabricated using integrated ISFETs [3, 7].

Different deposition methods for patterning immobilized enzyme membranes of multibiosensors have been also developed. One of these was the lift off method [7], in which the wafer was first coated with a photo-polymer which is patterned to deter-

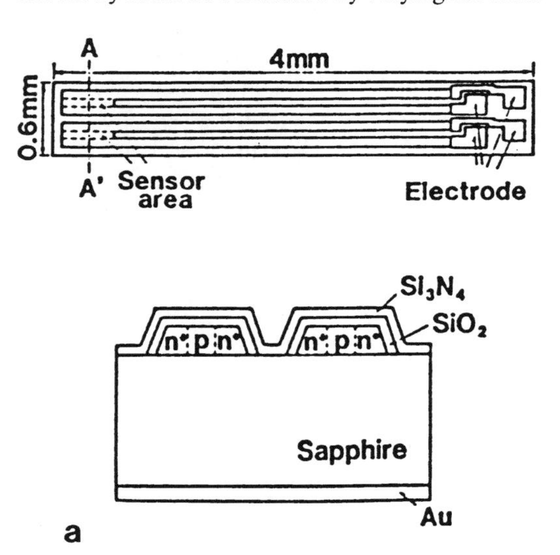

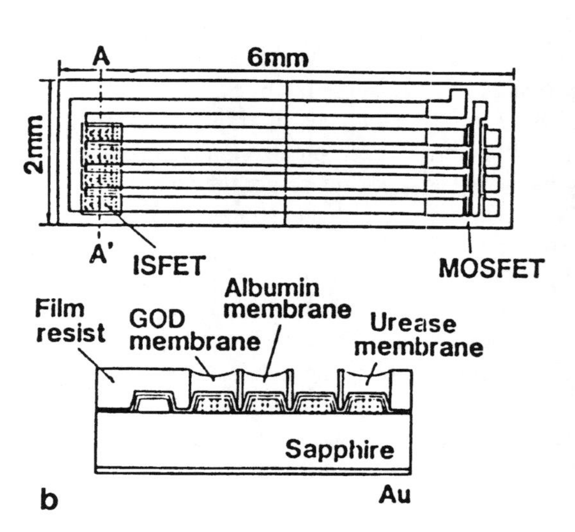

Fig. 4. SOS ISFET multibiosensor. (a) SOS ISFET; (b) Multibiosensor.

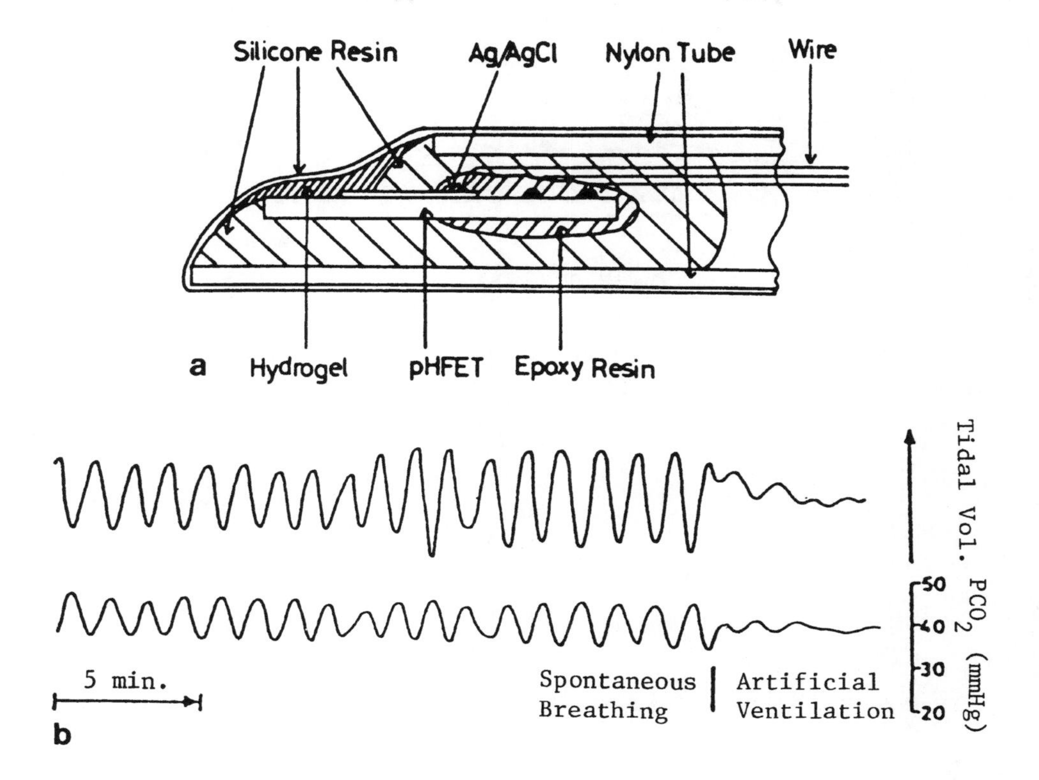

Fig. 5. Catheter-tip PCO_2 sensor. (a) Structure; (b) An example of clinical measurements of arterial PCO_2 compared with the tidal volume records.

mine the pattern of the membrane. The enzyme membrane was then spin-coated on the wafer and unwanted parts of it were lifted off by disolving the polymer in acetone in an ultrasonic bath. Another method was to use a photo-crosslinkable polymer containing an enzyme [3]. A third was the ink jet nozzle method, by which the multibiosensor shown in Fig. 4 (b) was fabricated [7]. Drops (50 μm in diameter) of enzyme solution containing albumin were emitted from an ink jet nozzle into a photopolymer micro pool, in which drops of glutaraldehyde solution were subsequently emitted by another ink jet nozzle. The number of drops can be controlled by the number of electric pulses driving the respective nozzle. This method uses only a small amount of enzyme for the membrane fabrication, making very efficient use of the often very expensive enzymes.

For the purpose of continuous blood gas monitoring in vivo, catheter-tip PCO_2 and PO_2 micro sensors have been developed [9]. Severinghaus type PCO_2 sensors have been constructed. The structure of a catheter-tip version of such a sensor is shown in Fig. 5 (a) [13]. A pH ISFET was mounted at the tip of a nylon tube of 0.8 mm diameter. A thin film Ag-AgCl reference electrode was also formed on the ISFET chip. The sensor was then coated with a poly-vinylalcohol gel containing 0.15 M NaCl and 0.15 M $NaHCO_3$ and further with a silicone rubber membrane of 50–100 μm thickness. The gel film equilibrates with the CO_2 tension in the test solution by diffusion of CO_2 across the silicone membrane. The pH of the gel, measured by the ISFET, corresponds to the CO_2 tension of the test solution.

Fig. 5 (b) is an example of clinical measurements of arterial PCO_2 compared with the tidal volume records [6]. The patient, being unconscious and

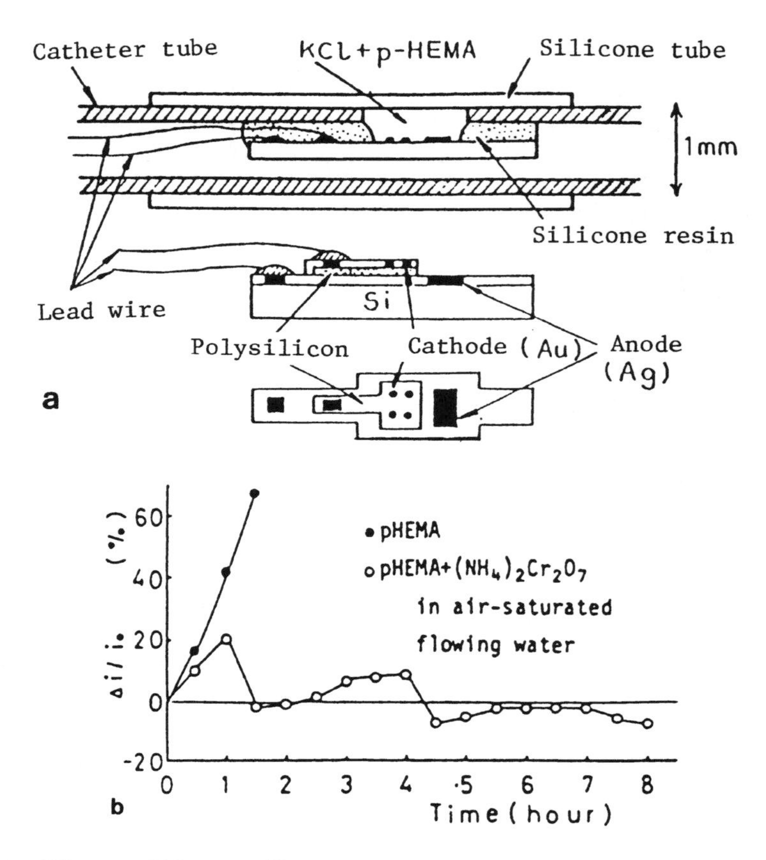

Fig. 6. Clark-type micro PO_2 sensor. (a)Structure; (b) An example of drift.

receiving treatment for a subarachnoid hemorrhage, exhibited a type of oscillatory (Cheyne-Strokes) breathing, that was abolished upon the institution of artificial ventilation.

Clark-type micro PO_2 sensors have been also developed [9]. High sensitivity, small dependence on the flow velocity, quick response and long term stability are required for PO_2 sensors. A multi cathode structure is a reasonable approach to increase the sensitivity without increasing the problems of flow velocity dependence and slow response time. Such a structure was fabricated as shown in Fig. 6 (a) by means of silicon micromachining. Clark type micro PO_2 sensors, however, have some inherent problems, namely, the dissolution of anode material (Ag) and its deposition on the cathode which increases the sensitivity and thereby causes zero drift.

This problem was reduced by filling the reservoir of the inner electrolyte with an anion exchanger which traps dissociated Ag complex ions. pHEMA (poly-2-hydroxyethyl-methacrylate) containing $(NH_4)_2Cr_2O_7$ for anion exchange sites was used for this purpose. The catheter tube was finally covered with 100 μm thick silicone rubber tube forming an oxygen permeable membrane. The silicone rubber tube, swollen in tri-chloroethylene, shrank and was fixed on the catheter tube. The experimental results in Fig. 6 (b) shows how the drift was reduced by employing the anion exchanger membrane.

Zirconia is known as a solid electrolyte through which oxygen is transported from a cathode to an anode. When the diffusion of oxygen to the cathode is obstructed, the cathode current is limited. This current is proportional to the oxygen concentration in the atmosphere. Fig. 7 shows the struc-

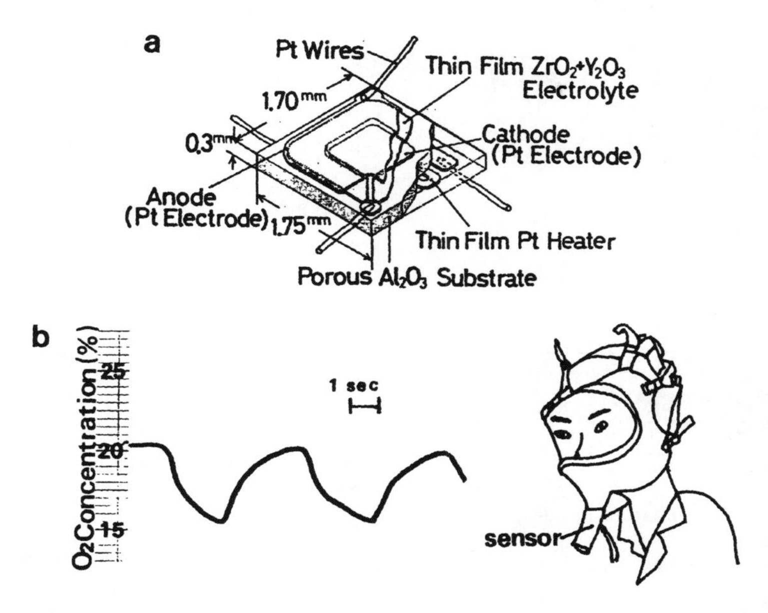

Fig. 7. Thin film limiting current type oxygen sensor. (a) Structure of the sensing element; (b) Measurement of oxygen concentration in exhalation.

ture of the sensing element of a thin film limiting current type oxygen sensor [18]. A porous Al_2O_3 substrate limits the diffusion of oxygen to the cathode. A thin film Pt heater was also integrated on the substrate. Linearity up to 70%, small size, quick response (90% response 0.6 sec), low power consumption (1W) and excellent stability make this sensor suitable for biomedical applications. One application of this limiting current type oxygen sensor was the oxygen concentration measurement in exhalation, as shown in Fig. 7 (b).

3. Physical sensors

Micro pressure sensors have been one of the most important fields in the development of physical sensors for biomedical applications, since it is almost impossible to obtain local pressure waveform with a pressure sensor of conventional size. Silicon-diaphragm micro pressure sensors have been developed for different biomedical purposes and some of them will be described below.

Fig. 8 (a) shows the structure of a catheter-tip

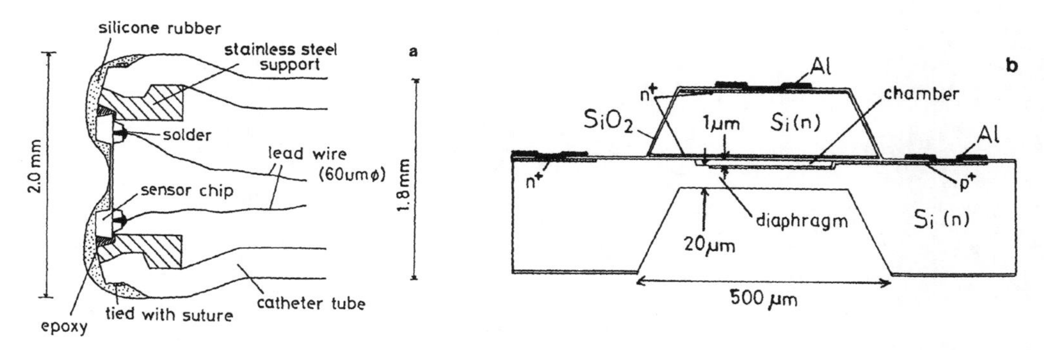

Fig. 8. Micro pressure sensors. (a) Catheter-tip piezoresistive pressure sensor; (b) Absolute type all silicon capacitive pressure sensor fabricated by a direct silicon to silicon bonding method.

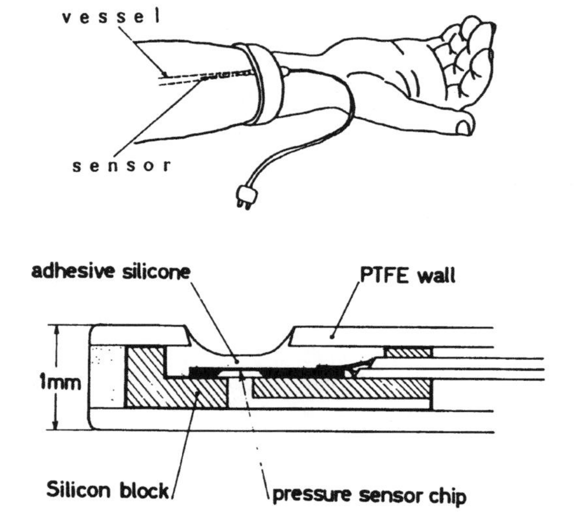

Fig. 9. Indwelling disposable pressure sensor.

piezoresistive sensor [2]. The difficulty of this kind of sensor is mainly the lead wire attachment. To reduce the assembly work and to ensure the reliability of the micro-soldering of lead wires, solder pools surrounded by polysilicon layer of 30 µm thickness were formed on the sensor chip. These pools have contact holes at their bottom and can hold lead wires in position during the soldering process.

Fig. 8 (b) is the structure of an absolute type capacitive pressure sensor [17]. This sensor can be used for biomedical implant applications. Unlike other absolute type sensors, of which built-in pressure reference vacuum chamber was fabricated by anodic bonding of silicon to pyrex glass, this sensor had its vacuum chamber between two silicon wafers. A direct silicon to silicon bonding technique was used for the fabrication [14]. By virtue of the

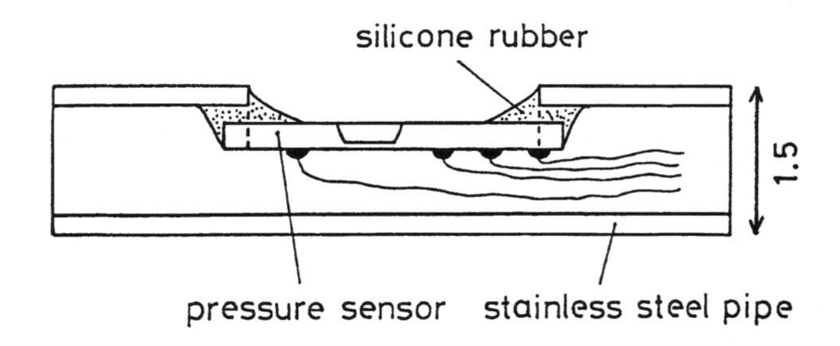

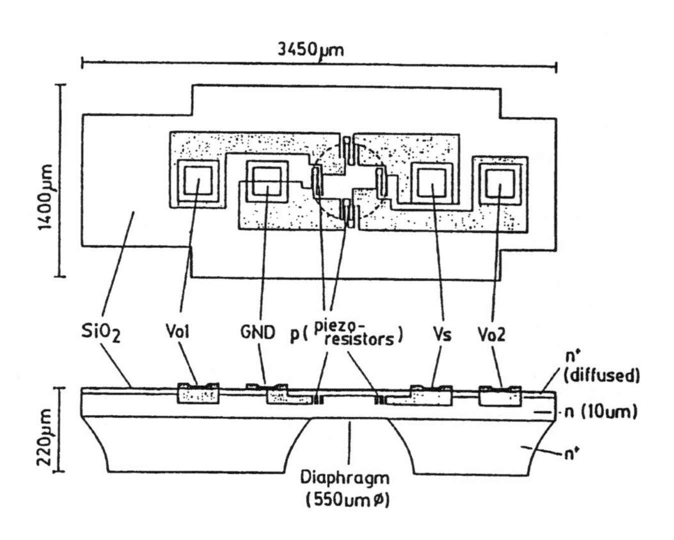

Fig. 10. Sidewall type catheter pressure sensor.

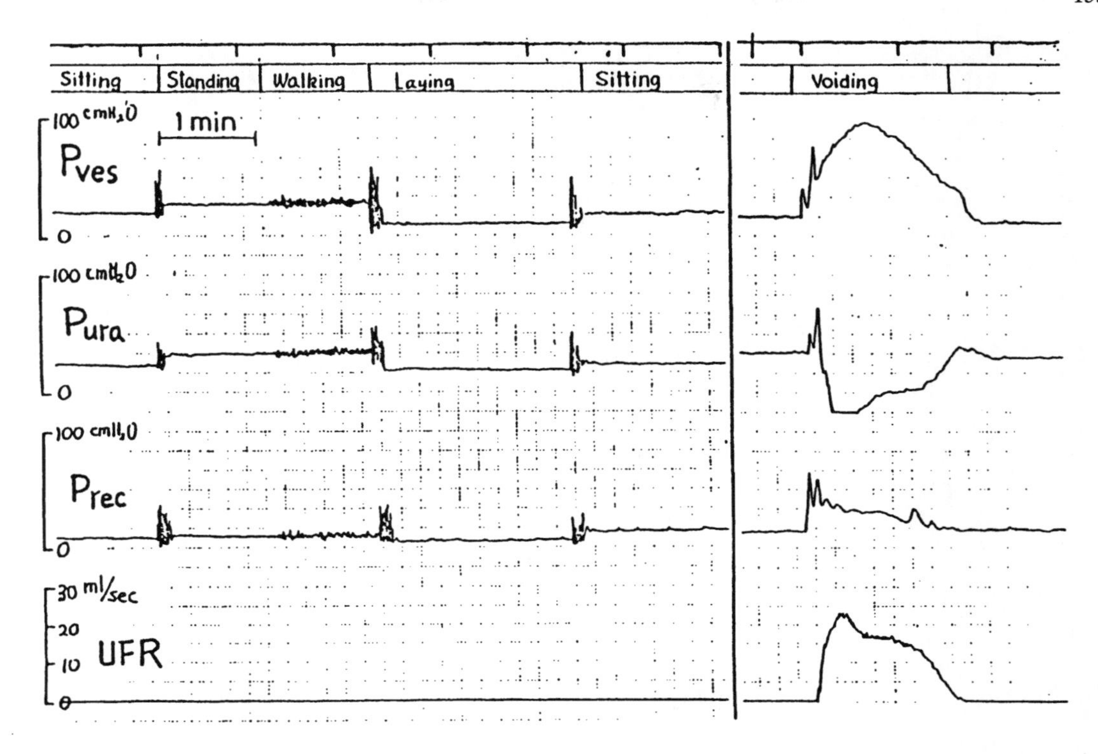

Fig. 11. A recording obtained from a clinical case showing a normal voiding pattern. The intravesical pressure (Pves) and the intraurethral pressure (Pura) were recorded simultaneously with the two-channel sensor catheter. Intrarectal pressure (Prec) and uroflow rate (UFR) were recorded simultaneously with other sensors.

thermal matching of the two elements, stress free sensor structures are available. Furthermore, the process for integration of the signal conditioning circuits on the sensor chip is allowed after making a chamber between the bonded wafers.

The fabrication of an indwelling type disposable pressure sensor has also been reported [11]. The scheme of blood pressure monitoring and the sensor structure are shown in Fig. 9. The diameter of the sensor is about 1 mm and the sensor was used continuously in a blood vessel for long term without heparine.

A sidewall type catheter sensor which is suitable for multi point pressure sensing is shown in Fig. 10 [1]. Stability of the sensor was improved with a suitable structure as follows. The problem due to the surface charge which modulates the resistance of the piezoresistor was solved by burying piezoresistors. Additionally, the problem due to the packaging stress which causes thermal disturbances was solved by using a thick supporting rim of the sensor chip and further by mounting on a stainless steel support with elastic material.

Fig. 11 shows a recording obtained from a clinical case showing a normal voiding pattern [2]. In this application, the intravesical pressure (Pves) and the intraurethral pressure (Pura) were recorded simultaneously with this two-channel sensor catheter.

4. Sensing systems

Portable or implantable multifunctional instrumentation systems have been constructed with different sensors, signal conditioning circuits and actuators.

Although implantable or catheter tip chemical sensors are very important in continuous monitoring, they are not always reliable because of the

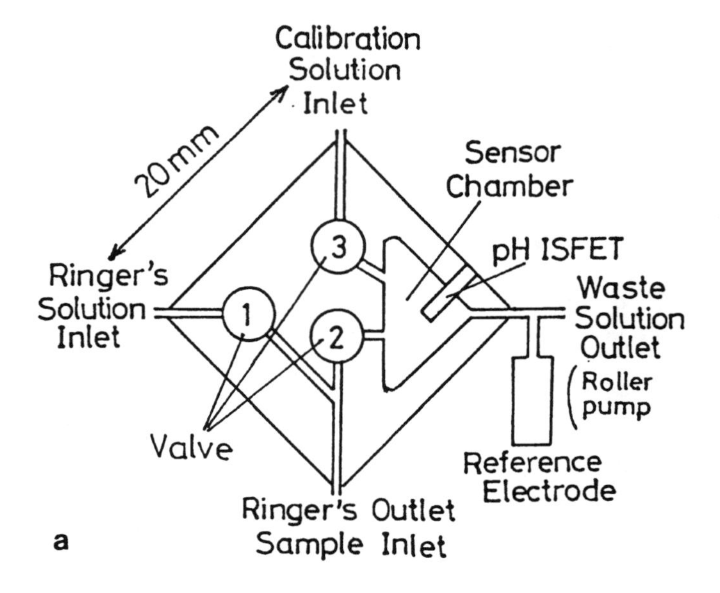

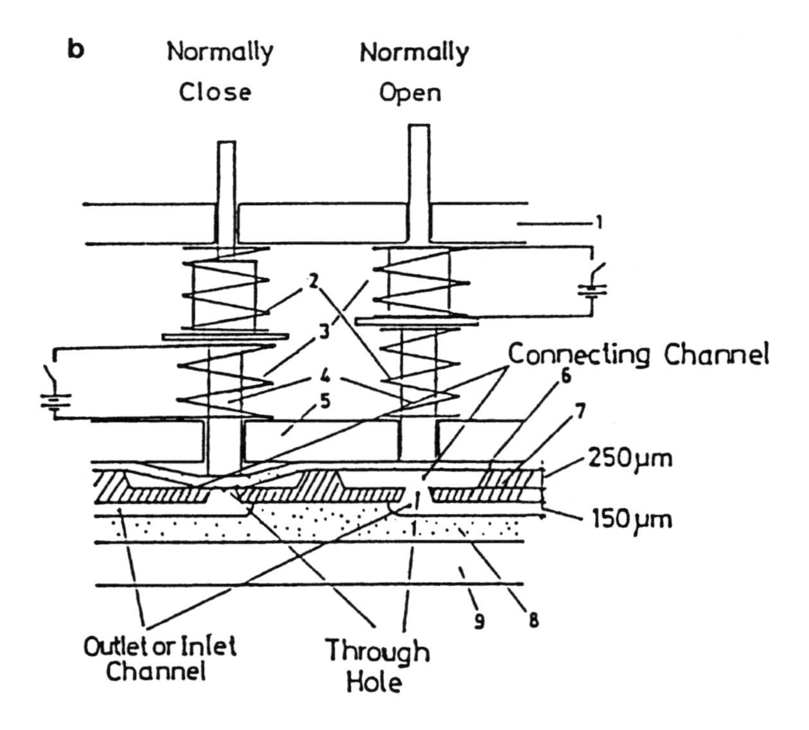

Fig. 12. Blood pH monitoring micro cell. (a) Structure of the micro cell. (b) Structure of the micro valves. 1, 5, 9: guide plate, 2: bias spring, 3: shape memory coil, 4: glass cylinder, 6: silicone rubber sheat, 7: silicon wafer, 8: glass plate.

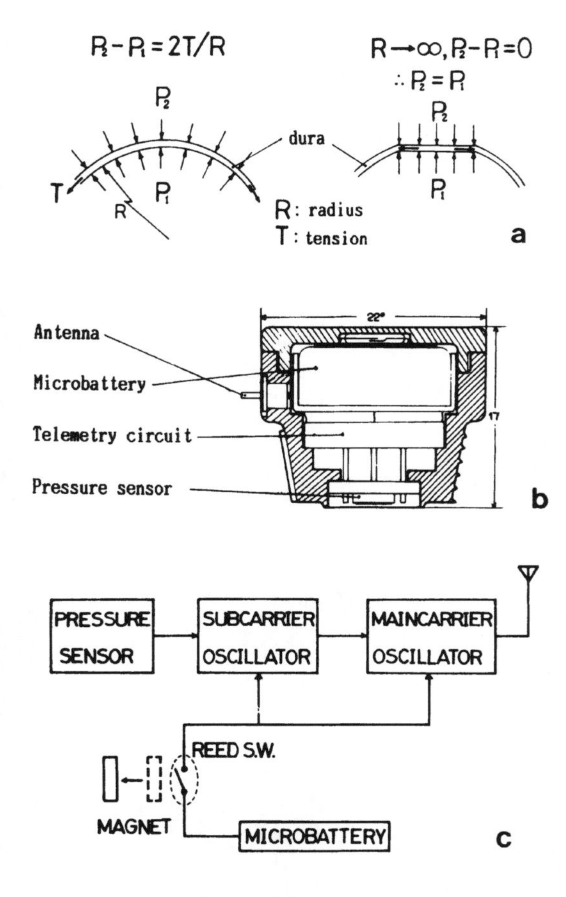

Fig. 13. Implantable telemetry system for the epidural measurement of intracranial pressure. (a) Principle of the coplanar measurement method; (b) Cross section of the telemetric intracranial pressure sensor; (c) Blockdiagram of the telemetry transmitter.

blood coagulation, the inability of in vivo calibration and so on. Intermittent blood analysis in vitro can be applied if the blood sample volume is small enough to prevent blood loss. Such a system (the micro cell) for blood pH monitoring has been developed [16]. The structure of this micro cell is shown in Fig. 12. This cell is made in a silicon wafer and the sample volume of the cell is about 5 nl. The cell has following modes:

1. Infusion of ringer solution to a vein.
2. Sampling blood from a vein to measure its pH.
3. Cleaning the sensor with ringer solution.
4. Calibration of the sensor.

Three microvalves shown in Fig. 12 are used to alter the modes. The valve actuator is composed of a shape memory alloy coil memorizing its expanded state. When actuated it is heated above the critical temperature (50° C) by passing a direct current through it whereupon it expands to its memorized shape. The response time of the valve is about 1 second. Other sensors for O_2, CO_2, etc. could be also integrated in the micro cell.

Implantable telemetry system for the epidural measurement of intracranial pressure has been developed [4]. The principle of the epidural pressure measurement by a coplanar method is shown in Fig. 13 (a). When the dura is flat, the intracranial pressure P_1 equilibrates with the external pressure P_2. An absolute pressure sensor was assembled with a telemetry transmitter as shown in Fig. 13 (b). The block diagram of the telemetry transmitter is shown in Fig. 13 (c). An external magnet is used to connect the internal battery through a reed switch when the measurement is carried out. After an operation, the telemetric sensor system is implanted and works for 3 to 4 weeks monitoring the intracranial pressure of a patient.

Fig. 14 shows an implantable multi sensor telemetry system on a custom CMOS IC chip [12]. One sensor at a time is selected according to a request from the external circuit and its signal is transmitted from the implantable circuit. To save battery power, the power switch of the implantable circuit is controlled by the external circuit. A pulse powered command receiver is included on the chip for this purpose. This chip consists of four separate chips.

Another telemetering system using custom integrated circuits has been developed for optical biotelemetry [10].

5. Conclusion

Recent research activities on solid state micro sensors and on sensing systems in Japan are presented in this review. Basic problems of biomedical micro sensors are also discussed.

The development of micro sensors depends on the fabrication facilities. Establishment of sensor

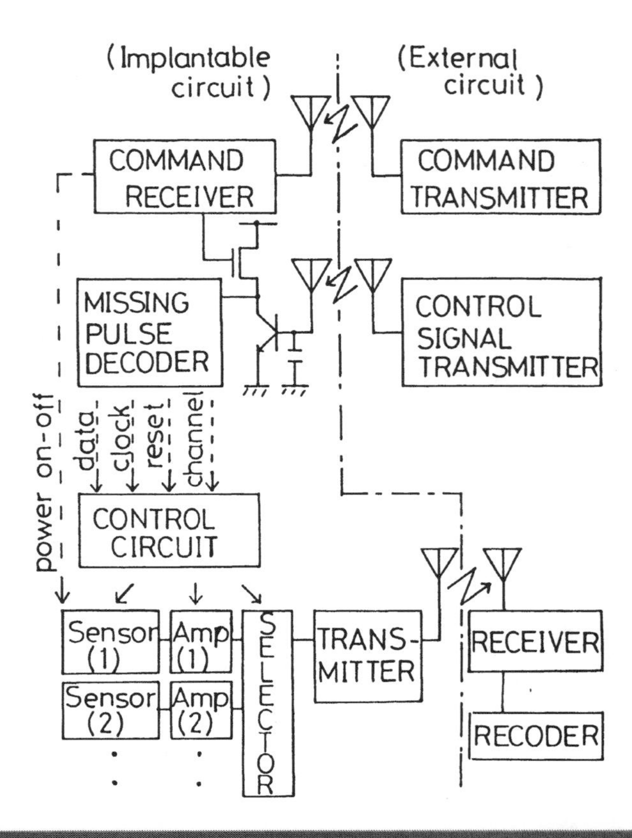

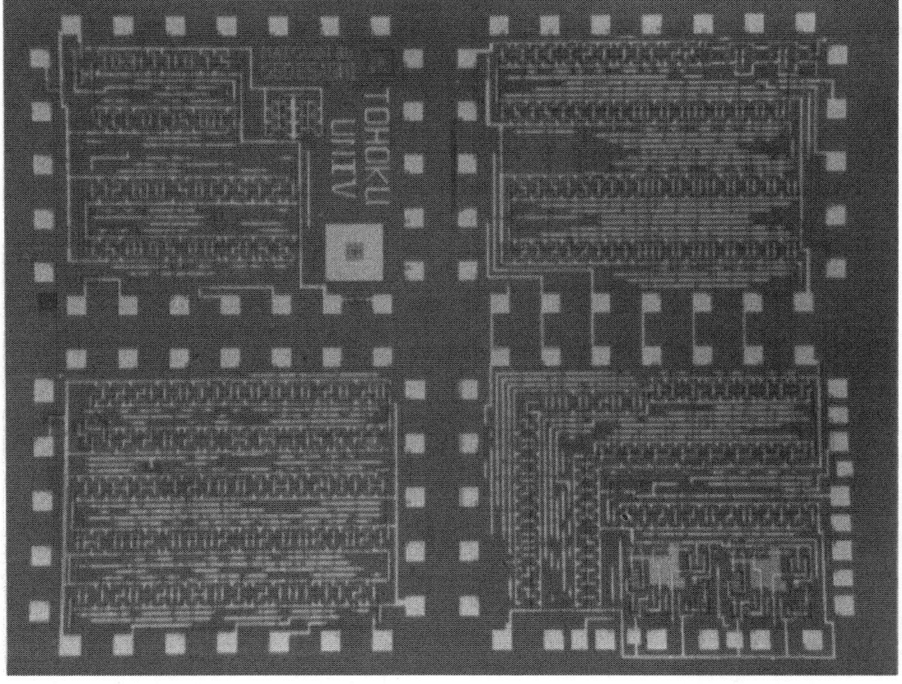

Fig. 14 **Implantable multisensor telemetry system.** (a) Blockdiagram; (b) Photomicrograph of the CMOS IC chip.

laboratories which have semiconductor processing facilities are desired for further development of micro sensors.

Acknowledgment

The authors express appreciation to Mr. Fredrik Enquist for English correction of this paper.

References

1. Esashi M, Komatsu H, Matsuo T: Biomedical pressure sensor using buried piezoresistors. Sensors and Actuators 4: 537–544, 1983.
2. Esashi M, Komatsu H, Matsuo T, Takahashi M, Takishima T, Imabayashi K, Ozawa H: Fabrication of catheter-tip and sidewall miniature pressure sensors. IEEE Trans on Electron Devices ED–29: 57–63, 1982.
3. Hanazato Y, Nakako M, Maeda M, Shiono S: Application of watersoluble photocrosslinkable polymer to enzyme membrane for FET-biosensor. Proc of the 2nd Int Meeting on Chemical Sensors: 576–579, 1986.
4. Ikeyama A, Maeda S, Nagai H, Furuse M, Igarashi I, Inagaki H, Kitano T: Epidural measurement of intracranial pressure by a newly-developed pressure transducer. Neurologia Medico-chirurgica 17: 1–7, 1977.
5. Ito T, Inagaki H, Igarashi I, Kitano T: ISFETs for Na^+ and K^+ (2nd Rep.) ISFETs using ion implanted membranes. Proc of the 25th Conf Japan Soc ME & BE: 357, 1986.
6. Kohama A, Nakamura Y, Nakamura M, Yano M, Shibatani K: Continuous monitoring of arterial and tissue PCO_2 with sensors based on the pH-ISFET. Crit Care Med 12: 940–942, 1984.
7. Kuriyama T, Nakamoto S, Kawana Y, Kimura J: New fabrication methods of enzyme immobilized membrane for ENFET. Proc of the 2nd Int Meeting on Chemical Sensors: 568–571, 1986.
8. Matsuo T, Esashi M: Methods of ISFET Fabrication. Sensors and Actuators 1: 77–96, 1981.
9. Matsuo T, Esashi M, Shibatani K: Catheter-tip PCO_2 and PO_2 sensors. Proc of the Symp on Biosensors: 33–34, 1984.
10. Nakamura T, Usui S, Ishida M: Optical bio-telemetry by singlechip V/F converter. Proc of the 25th Conf Japan Soc ME & BE: 114, 1986.
11. Nakashima A, Inagaki H, Igarashi I, Kitano T, Okino H: Indwelling miniature blood pressure sensor (3rd Rep.) application. Proc of the 25th Conf Japan Soc ME & BE: 499, 1986.
12. Seo H, Esashi M, Matsuo T: Fabrication of biotelemetry system by CMOS custom IC. Digest of S 61 Tohoku Joint Meeting on Electricity in Japan: 240, 1986.
13. Shimada K, Yano M, Shibatani K, Komoto Y, Esashi M, Matsuo T: Application of catheter-tip ISFET for continuous in vivo measurement. Med & Biol Eng & Comput 18: 741–745, 1980.
14. Shimbo M, Furukawa K, Tanzawa K, Fukuda K: Direct bonding of silicon wafers. Digest of 33rd Meeting on Applied Physics Japan: 525–526, 1986.
15. Shoji S, Esashi M, Matsuo T: Micro ISFET of 10 μm tip size. Proc of the 1st Int Meeting on Chemical Sensors: 473–478, 1983.
16. Shoji S, Esashi M, Matsuo T: Blood pH monitoring micro cell using micro valves. Proc of the 2nd Int Meeting on Chemical Sensors: 550–553, 1986.
17. Shoji S, Nisase T, Esashi M, Matsuo T: Fabrication of pressure sensor by silicon direct bonding. Digest of S 61 Tohoku Joint Meeting on Electricity in Japan: 227, 1986.
18. Takahashi H, Saji K, Kondo H, Takeuchi T, Igarashi I: Influence of gas composition on the characteristics of limiting current-type oxygen sensor. Proc of the 5th Sensor Symposium: 133–137, 1985.

Address for reprints:
M. Esashi
Department of Electronic Engineering
Tohoku University
Aza Aoba Aramaki Sendai 980, Japan

Medical Progress through Technology 12: 159–170 (1987)

Electrical measurement of fluid distribution in legs and arms

Hiroshi Kanai, Makoto Haeno & Katsuyuki Sakamoto
Dept. of Electrical Engineering, Sophia University, 7-1 Kioi-cho, Chiyoda-ku, Tokyo 102, Japan

Key words: intra-cellular fluid, extra-cellular fluid, frequency characteristics, artificial dialysis, tissue impedance

Summary

Intra- and extra-cellular fluid distribution is very important to know the physiological and clinical state of living subjects. However, it is quite difficult to measure the distribution in vivo. Electrical impedance of living tissue is mainly affected by extra-cellular fluid at an applied frequency lower than the β-dispersion frequency, and is affected by both extra- and intra-cellular fluid at higher applied frequencies than that.

In this paper, we discuss the problems of measurement of intra- and extra-cellular fluid distribution in living tissues by means of electrical impedance. The intra- and extra-cellular fluid distribution is related to some physiological parameters, such as blood circulation, metabolism of tissues, and the electrolytic concentration of intra- and extra-cellular fluids. Therefore, the information about the distribution of fluids in tissues is quite useful for the diagnosis of various diseases, the monitoring of seriously ill patients, and in medical treatments such as artificial dialysis. We discuss the method of measurement and the results of experiments.

1. Introduction

Electrical properties of living tissues have been studied both theoretically and experimentally by many researchers [3, 4, 8, 9].

The frequency characteristics of the electrical properties of living tissues show that there are three kinds of frequency dispersion, called α, β, and γ dispersions, due to the three different mechanisms of relaxation [6, 9]. β dispersion is well known as a structural relaxation and occurs at radio frequencies between 10 kHz and 10 MHz. This frequency range was used in the impedance method for various clinical diagnosis, such as the measurement of edema and so on [1, 10]. In this paper, the β dispersion phenomenon is used for the measurement of extra- and intra-cellular fluid distribution. Fig. 1 shows a schematic arrangement of tissue cells. The resistivity of the cell membrane is much higher than that of the extra- and intra-cellular fluids. The capacitance of the cell membrane is quite large, between 1 μF/cm^2 and 10 μF/cm^2, because the thickness of the membrane is very small. When a low frequency voltage is applied to the tissue shown in Fig. 1, current flows mainly through the extra-cellular fluid as shown by the solid lines because the impedance of the membrane is very large at low frequencies. Therefore, information about the extra-cellular fluid can be obtained from the measured results at low frequencies. At higher frequencies, current flows through the extra- and intra-cellular fluids as shown by the broken lines in Fig. 1. From the measured results at both low and high applied frequencies, information about the intra-cellular fluid can be obtained. The measured impedance is mainly affected by the resistivity and volume of each fluid and by the geometrical shape of the cells. It is very difficult to obtain separate information about the resistivity and the volume of each fluid. However, the measured ratio of extra-

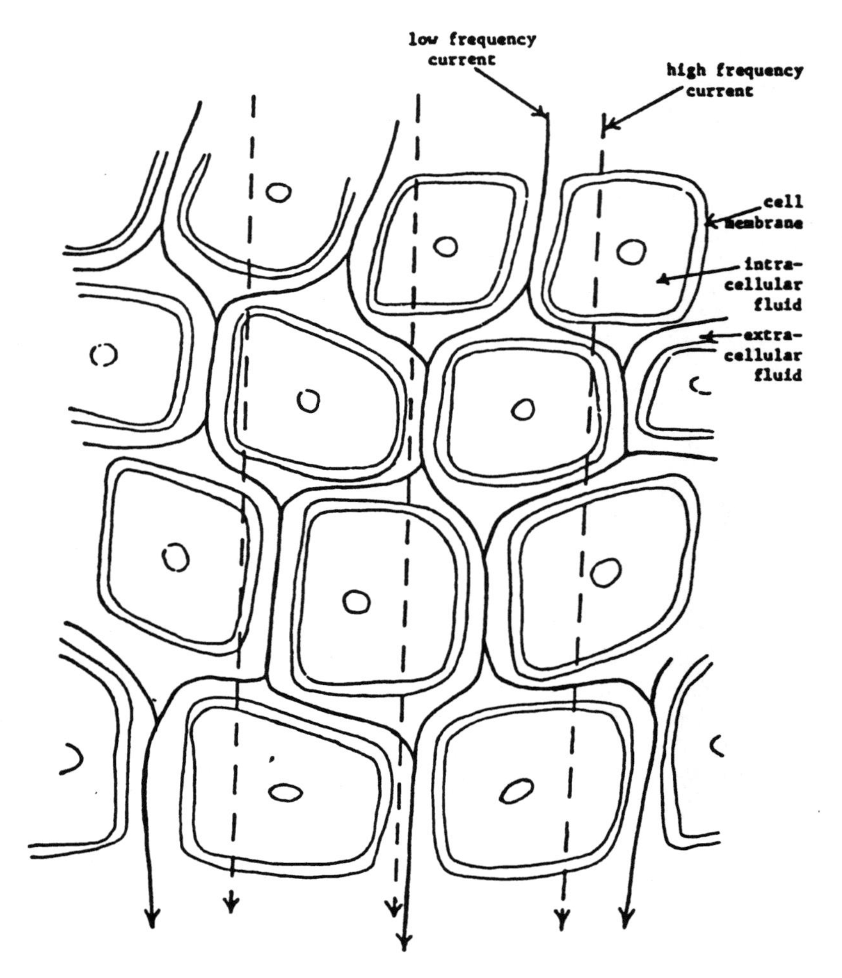

Fig. 1. Schematic diagram of tissues and current flow.

cellular resistance to intra-cellular resistance gives us the approximate value of fluid distribution, because the resistivity of the fluids usually does not change much. The change of extra- and intra-cellular fluid resistance is also very useful for monitoring the condition of a seriously ill patient, monitoring artificial dialysis, the estimation of athletic ability, and the activity of the circulatory system.

We proposed a new method for the measurement of intra- and extra-fluids distribution by means of electrical impedance [5, 6, 7]. In this paper the method is briefly shown and some clinical applications of the measured results are discussed.

2. Method

An equivalent electrical circuit for a cell embedded in tissue is derived from Fig. 1 and is shown in Fig. 2 (a). R_e is the extra-cellular fluid resistance, C_e is the parallel capacitance of the extra-cellular fluid. R_m, C_m, R_i, and C_i are the resistance and capacitance of the two layers of cell membrane and the resistance and capacitance of the intra-cellular fluid, respectively. This equivalent circuit shown in Fig. 2 (a) can be reduced to the more simplified form shown in Fig. 2 (b) in the frequency range 1–500 kHz. The admittance locus of this simplified circuit is a semi-

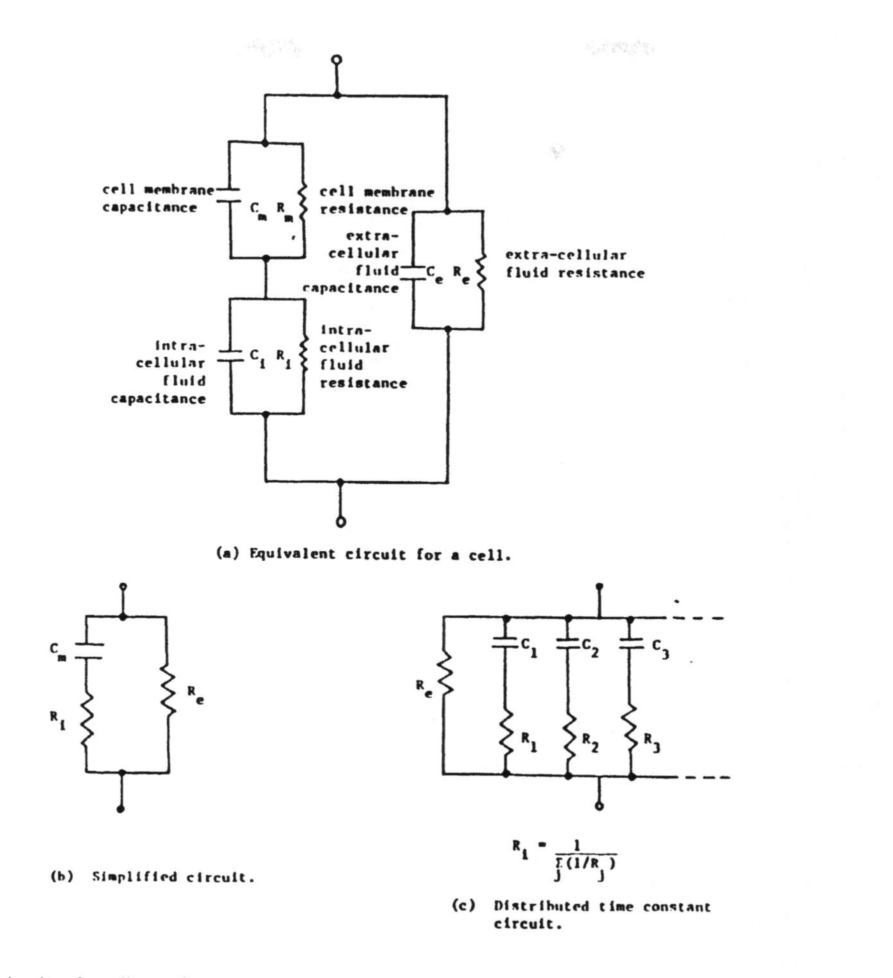

Fig. 2. Equivalent circuits of a cell or a tissue.

circle and is shown by the solid line in Fig. 3. This phenomenon results from the series circuit of membrane capacitance C_m and intra-cellular fluid resistance R_i and is therefore called structural relaxation or β dispersion. The time constant of structural relaxation T_0 is C_mR_i and the characteristic frequency of β dispersion f_0 is $1/2\pi T_0$. The characteristic frequency of most muscle tissue is about 50 kHz and that of blood is about 2 MHz. Measurement admittance loci are usually not semicircular but are only part of a semicircle with the center below the real axis. A typical measurement locus is shown by the broken line in Fig. 3. This result suggests to us that the values of the time constant C_mR_i for all the cells are not the same but distributed. The distribution function of the time constant should be a normal distribution function because the sizes of cells are statistically distributed. The admittance loci of the normal distributed time constant circuit are not exactly part of a semicircle but are similar to one. The distribution function, which forms an admittance locus which is a part of a semi-circle, is well known as the Cole-Cole distribution function. The Cole-Cole distribution function for the time constant is easily calculated from the radius and the angle θ of the measured admittance locus (Fig. 3) [2, 6, 9]. Therefore, the real equivalent circuit for the tissues should be represented by a distributed time constant circuit as shown in Fig. 2 (c). The admittance Y of this Cole-Cole distributed circuit is derived as:

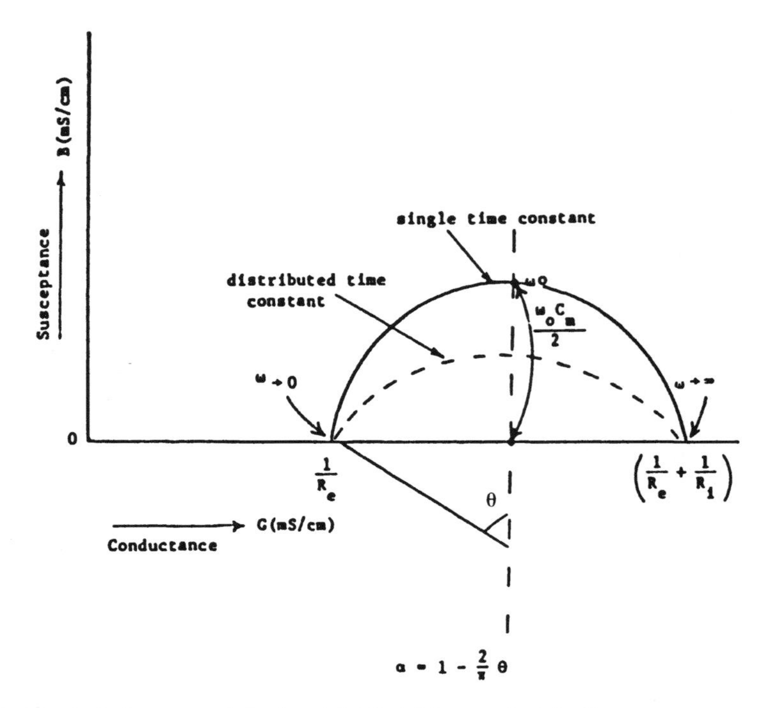

Fig. 3. Admittance loci for single time constant circuit and distributed time constant circuit.

$$Y = \frac{1}{R_e} + \frac{1}{R_i} - \frac{1/R_i}{1+(j\omega T_0)^{1-\alpha}} =$$

$$\frac{1}{R_e} + \frac{1}{R_i} - \frac{1}{R_i}\int_0^\infty \frac{f(T)}{1+j\omega T}\,dt \qquad (1)$$

where f(T) is the Cole-Cole distribution function and

$$f(T) = \frac{1}{2\pi}\,\frac{\sin\alpha\pi}{\cosh\,[(1-\alpha)\log T/T_0] - \cos\alpha\pi} \qquad (2)$$

and T_0 is the average value of the distributed time constant. In this paper, the Cole-Cole distribution function is used for the analysis of the measured results instead of the normal distribution function because of its simplicity in the calculation of various parameters. From the measured results, the coordinates of the center and the radius of the circular admittance locus are calculated by the least square curve fitting method. The entire admittance locus is then obtained. From this calculated admittance locus, the parameters α, T_0, R_e, and R_i are easily obtained as shown in Fig. 3. For the discussion of the results, the simplified circuit shown in Fig. 2(b) is used instead of the distributed time constant circuit shown in Fig. 2(c). C_m in Fig. 2(b) is obtained by the equation $T_0 = R_iC_m$, and is different from the real capacitance.

3. Experimental arrangement

β dispersion frequency of most muscle tissues is between 30 kHz and 80 kHz. Therefore, it is desirable to vary the applied frequency used for measurement from 1 kHz to 1 MHz. At applied frequencies higher than 200 kHz, the accurate measurement of the electrical properties of living human subjects is very difficult because of stray capactances. The applied frequency is varied from 1 kHz to 500 kHz in our experiment. Fig. 4 shows a block diagram of our experimental arrangement. The four-electrode method is used in this experiment to reduce the effects of electrode impedance, skin impedance, and spread impedance. One of the two current electrodes is put on the lower thigh,

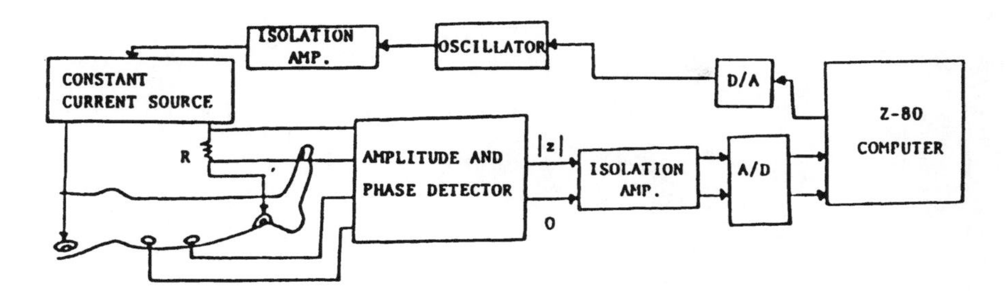

Fig. 4. Block diagram of experimental arrangement.

and the other on the ankle of the subjects for the measurement of legs and on the arm and on the wrist for the measurement of arms. Two detecting electrodes are put on the measurement portions of the subjects 10 cm apart from each other. A constant current source supplies a constant current of 100 μA to the current electrodes. This circuit is floated from ground to prevent electric shock hazard. The potential difference between two detecting electrodes is amplified and measured by an amplitude detector and phase detector. The detecting circuits are also floated from ground for safety. All input and output leads are shielded by the shield wire whose potential is kept at the same potential as the inner wire to reduce the effect of stray capacitances. The outputs of the amplitude detector and phase detector are connected to a microcomputer. An output of the microcomputer is also connected to the constant current source and automatically changes the frequency stepwise. The computer extrapolates the admittance represented by Eqs (1) and (2) in the frequency range from 1 kHz to 500 kHz and then calculates R_e, R_i, C_m, T_0 and α. In this paper, only R_e and R_i are used for discussion. Much useful information should be derived from C_m, T_0, and α and will be discussed elsewhere.

The common mode noise rejection ratio mainly depends on the impedance of the detecting electrodes. To reduce the electrode impedance of the

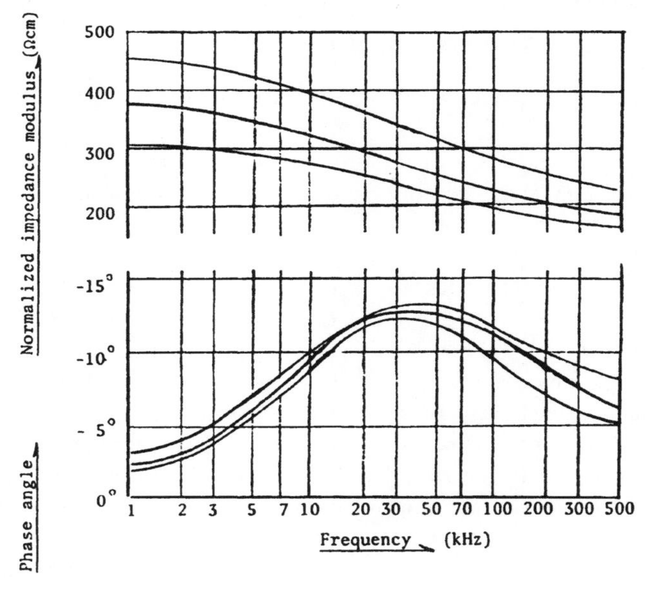

Fig. 5. Frequency characteristics of some human legs.

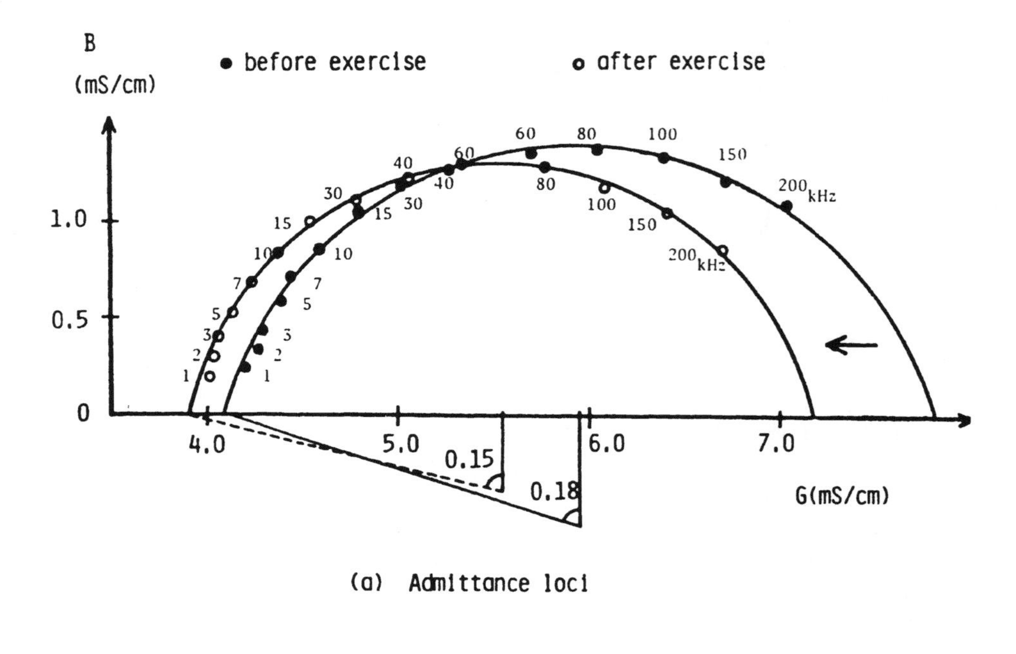

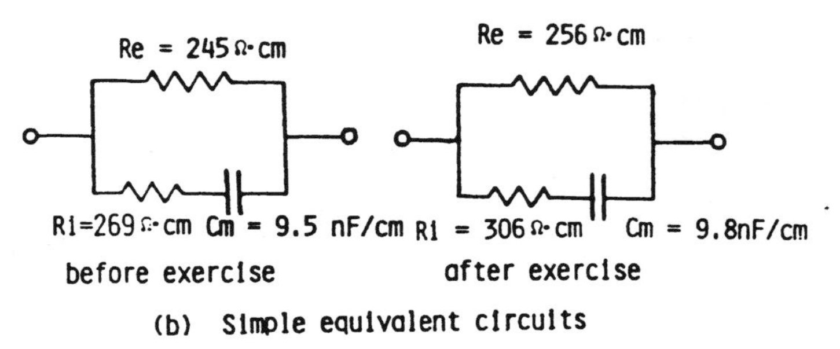

Fig. 6. Admittance loci and simple equivalent circuits for a trained subject: the change due to ergometer exercise.

detecting electrodes, Karaya gum electrodes of 1 cm diameter are used together with electrolytic gel. The constant current electrodes are band electrodes of 0.8 cm width or Karaya gum electrodes of 3 cm diameter.

The measurement error is less than 2% for the amplitude and 1 degree for the phase angle. All measurement is done within 5 seconds. Resistivity and hematocrit values of blood sampled from a patient are measured by a capillary tube measurement cell of 1 mm inner diameter and 70 mm length.

4. Results and discussion

Fig. 5 shows some typical measured results of impedance in human legs. The upper diagram shows the frequency characteristics of the impedance modulus, normalized with respect to the diameter of each leg and the distance between the two detecting electrodes. The lower diagram shows the frequency characteristics of the phase angle. At low frequencies, the resistivities of most men's legs are between 250 and 450 Ω · cm. The resistivity decreases with increase of applied frequency. At 200 kHz, the resistivities of most men's legs are between 180 and 250 Ω · cm. The phase angle is

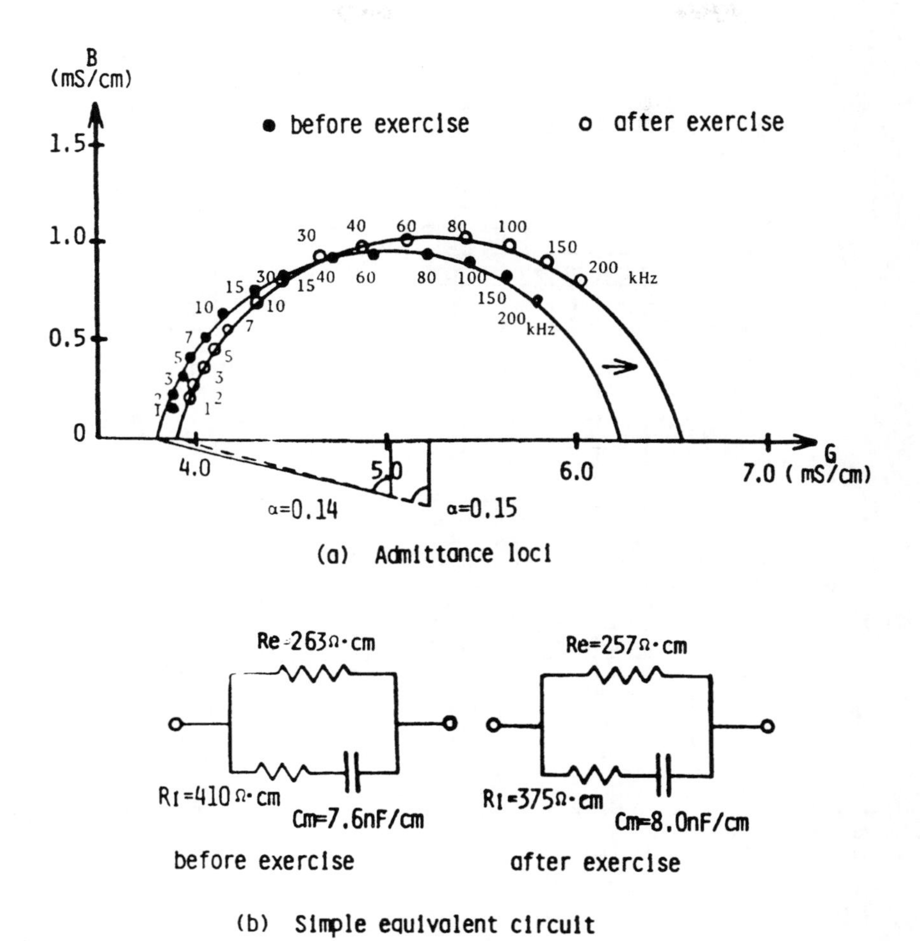

Fig. 7. Admittance loci and simple equivalent circuits for an untrained subject: the change due to ergometer exercise.

maximum at a frequency slightly lower than the characteristic frequency of β dispersion. From the lower diagram, it can be seen that the characteristic frequency of β dispersion is about 50 kHz for human legs and that the maximum phase angle is about −13 degrees. From these measurement results, admittance loci and simple equivalent circuits were calculated.

These values are used to calculate the extra- and intra-cellular fluid resistivities R_e and R_i. For simplicity, it is better to use the equivalent circuit shown in Fig. 2 (b). Average calculated values of R_e and R_i are 400 Ω · cm and 380 Ω · cm, respectively.

It is very important to know how the frequency characteristics are affected by the condition of human legs. The changes in the frequency characteristics of human legs as a result of exercises like running or swimming were measured for several subjects. A result obtained on a well-trained athlete is shown in Fig. 6. The open circles show the results obtained after ergometer exercise and the closed circles those before exercise. The body weight of this human subject reduced from 56.0 kg to 55.2 kg as a result of the exercise. The resistivity slightly increases due to the exercise. The characteristic frequency of β dispersion also increases slightly. The calculated values of R_e, R_i, and C_m are shown in Fig. 6 (b). R_i and R_e are increased by 12% and 5% as a results of exercise. This increase is reasonable since the weight decreases by the exercise. A result obtained on an untrained subject is

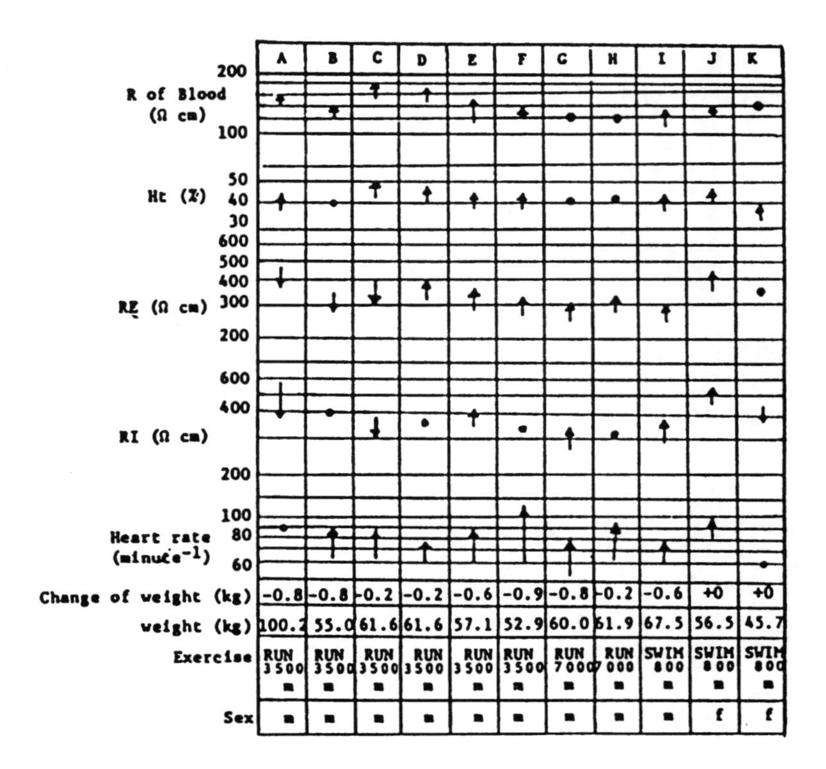

Fig. 8. Changes of various values in 11 subjects (A-K) due to running or swimming exercise. Arrows show the value and direction of the changes. Closed circle means no change.

shown in Fig. 7. R_e does not change much (1% decrease), but R_i decreases by 9% as a result of exercise. This phenomenon is not understood well. However, it is very interesting that the intra-cellular fluid of the untrained subject increases in spite of the decrease of body weight as a result of exercise. This phenomenon might be used as a measure of athletic ability of subjects, and also used for the monitoring of patients because the change of intra-cellular fluid depends on metabolic and recovery abilities of the patients.

The changes in the frequency characteristics of human arms due to exercises like running and swimming were also measured. The changes for both trained and untrained subjects are similar. R_e of arms does not change much but R_i remarkably increases by ergometer exercise. From these results, it might be concluded that the fluid distribution in a body is changed by exercise and that the fluid in the arms moves into the legs as a result of exercise. Detailed discussion will be published elsewhere.

R_e and R_i are affected not only by the fluid volume but also by the resistivity of the fluid. To discuss the effect of the resistivity of fluid, we also measured resistivity of whole blood and plasma, hematocrit value, heart rate, body weight and body weight change before and after exercise. Some of the results are shown in Fig. 8.

Subjects A, B, C, and D were untrained males. Subjects E, F, G, H, and I were well-trained male athletes. Subjects J and K were well-trained female athletes. Exercise consisted of 3,500 m running, 7,000 m running, or 800 m swimming. Changes of body weight are less than 1 kg. The resistivity of blood and the hematocrit value increases by the exercise. These results are reasonable because the volume of plasma decreases due to exercise with the decrease of body weight. The resistivity of plasma does not change measurably. The resistivity

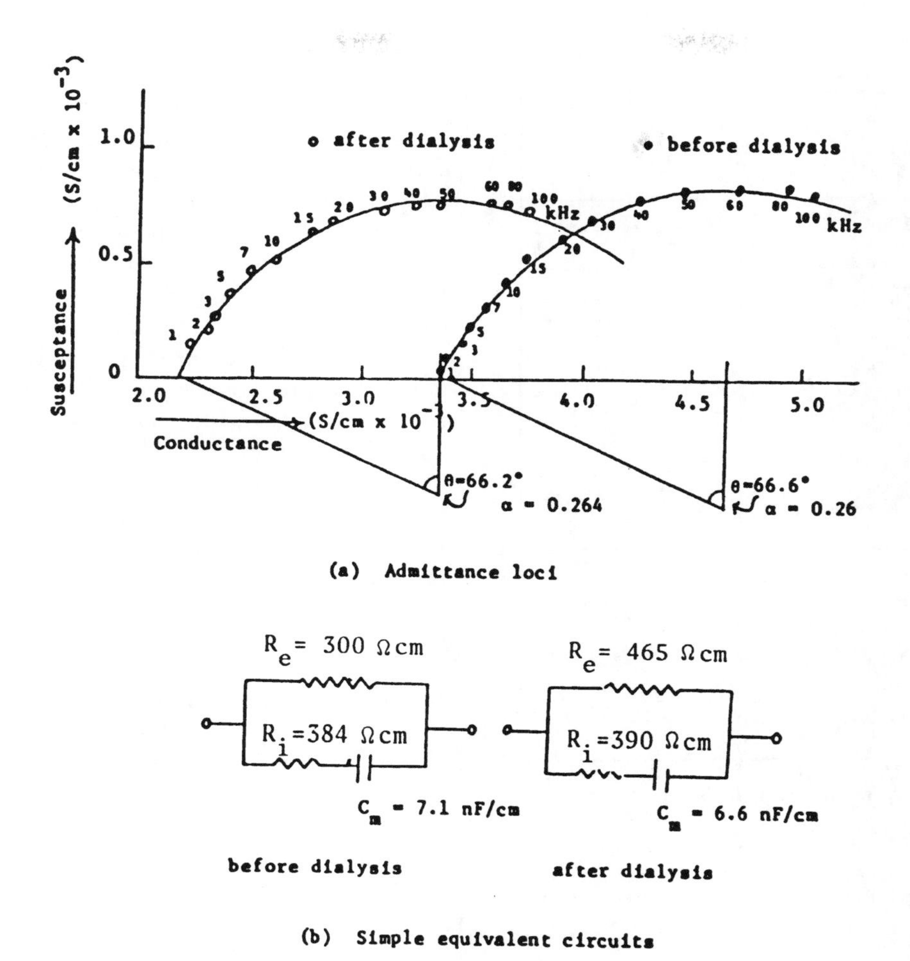

Fig. 9. Admittance loci and simple equivalent circuits for a patient before and after artificial dialysis.

of extra-cellular fluid decreases remarkably for the untrained subjects even though the resistivity of blood increases and the body weight decreases. However, R_e for the well-trained athletes usually increases by exercise as shown in Fig. 6. This difference may be caused by the difference in metabolic and recovery rates of individuals. The recovery rate mainly depends on the ability of the circulatory system. Therefore, this phenomenon can be used for the diagnosis of circulatory diseases and also for the investigation of athletic ability. The resistivity R_i of intra-cellular fluid shows similar results. The change of R_i might depend on the biophysical characteristics of the cell membrane. The decrease of R_e and R_i is due to the increase of fluid volume. Total fluid volume decreases by exercise. Therefore, the fluid volume of some parts of the body must decrease remarkably. As mentioned above, measured results show that the resistivity of human arms usually increases by exercise.

Artificial dialysis causes a great volume change of body fluid. Therefore, the resistivity of tissues also changes greatly by artificial dialysis. The frequency characteristics of the resistivity of a patient's legs are measured before and after dialysis. One of the results is shown in Fig. 9. The body weight of this patient was 64.5 kg before dialysis and reduced by 1.4 kg after dialysis. The resistivity increases 50% due to artificial dialysis at low frequencies and 40% at high frequencies. The re-

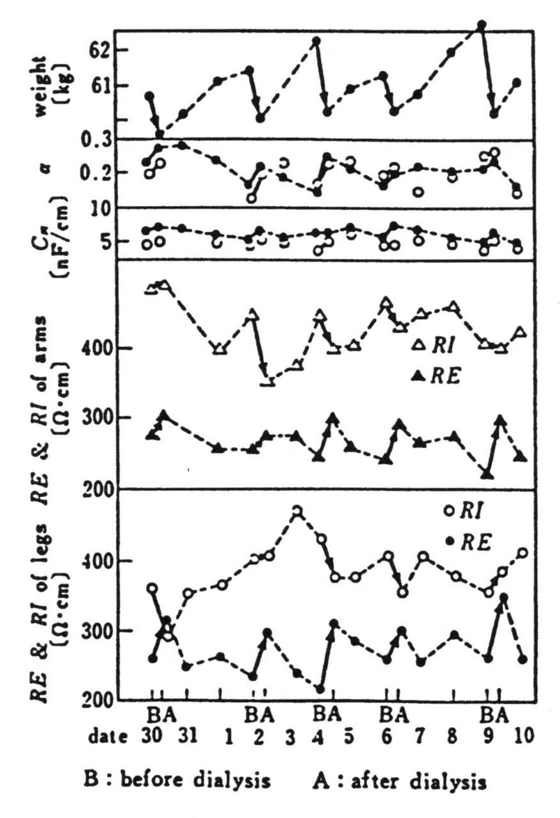

Fig. 10. Changes of various values of a patient as a result of artificial dialysis.

sistivity before dialysis is much smaller than the values for normal subjects and the resistivity after dialysis is a little higher. The phase angle before dialysis is also much lower than for normal subjects. After dialysis, the phase angle is almost equal to the normal value; however, the characteristic frequency is much lower than the normal value.

R_e increases remarkably by the artificial dialysis. On the contrary, R_i does not change much in this case and sometimes remarkably decreases as a result of artificial dialysis. These results show that the body water is mainly extracted from extra-cellular fluid by artificial dialysis and that the intra-cellular fluid volume increases by dialysis even when the total body water decreases. Fig. 10 shows the change of R_i and R_e of both a leg and an arm of a patient in a series of artificial dialysises. R_es of both the leg and the arm increase after dialysis. On the contrary, R_is of the leg and the arm sometimes do not change and sometimes decrease. This phenomenon is caused by low sodium concentration in dialysate which is used for regular artificia dialysis and is in agreement with physiological knowledge. Therefore, it is supposed that the intra-cellular fluid volume must be decreased by high sodium concentration dialysis. The change of R_e and R_i of patient leg due to low and high sodium concentration dialysis are shown in Fg. 11. The upper diagram in Fig. 11 shows the change of R_e and R_i by series treatments of high sodium (153 m Eq/1) and low sodium (136 m Eq/1) concentration dialysis. At first, the patient was treated by high sodium dialysate for 2 hours, and then by low sodium dialysate for 4 hours. R_e increases remarkably by both high and low sodium dialysis. R_i slightly increases or does not change by high sodium concentration dialysis. On the contrary, R_i usually decreases by low sodium concentration dialysis. For comparison, a result obtained by only low sodium concentration dialysis is shown in lower diagram in Fig. 11. Detailed discussion will be shown elsewhere.

5. Conclusions

The frequency characteristics of the electrical properties of human legs and arms can be measured with sufficient accuracy within a few seconds. From these results, the equivalent resistivity R_e of extra-cellular fluid, the equivalent resistivity R_i of intra-cellular fluid, the characteristic frequency of β dispersion, the equivalent capacitance C_m of cell membrane, and the extra- and intra-cellular fluid distribution can be calculated. The electrical characteristics of human legs and arms are represented by a simple equivalent circuit which consists of R_e, R_i, and C_m. These values give us approximate information about the extra- and intra-cellular fluid volumes and their distribution.

The effects of exercise on the values of R_e and R_i are discussed in this paper. The effects of artificial dialysis are also discussed.

It is concluded that R_e and R_i are very useful for the monitoring of artificial dialysis and the estimation of athletic ability, and we can also get more

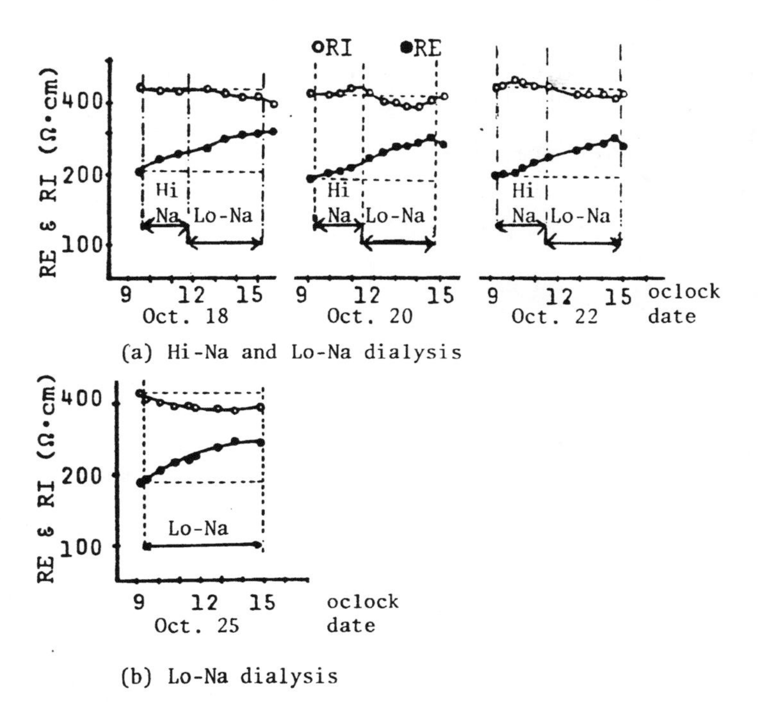

Fig. 11 Change of R_e (closed circle) and R_i (open circle) by high sodium (Hi-Na) and low sodium (Lo-Na) dialysis.

information from the measured results, such as the equivalent membrane capacitance, the characteristic frequency of β dispersion, and the Cole-Cole distribution function. These might be very useful for various clinical purposes. R_e, R_i, and other parameters are quite useful for the measurement of edema, the estimation of metabolic and recovery abilities, the diagnosis of various circulatory diseases, and the monitoring of seriously ill patients. These clinical applications will be discussed elsewhere.

Acknowledgement

We are very grateful to Mr. T. Higashiizumi, Yokogawa Electric Work, Tokyo, Japan, and Mr. M. Tanishima, Nihon Koden Ltd., for their valuable assistance in these experiments. We are also very grateful to Prof. K. Nakayama for his valuable discussion. A part of this work was supported by Suzuken Memorial Foundation.

References

1. Ackman JJ, et al.: Complex bioelectric impedance measurement for the detection of pulmonary edema. Digest of the 11th ICMBE, Ottawa, Canada, 1976, pp 288–289.
2. Cole KS, Cole RH: Dispersion and adsorption in dielectrics. J Chem Rev 9: 341–352, 1941.
3. Geddes LA, Baker LE: The specific resistance of biological material. Medical and Biological Engineering 5: 271–293, 1967.
4. Guy AW, et al.: Therapeutic applications of electromagnetic power. Proc IEEE 62: 55–75, 1974.
5. Haeno M, Sakamoto K, Kanai H: Estimation of fluid distribution by impedance method. Japanese Journal of Medical Electronics and Biological Engineering 23: 354–360, 1985.
6. Kanai H, Sakamoto K, Haeno M: Electrical measurement of fluid distribution in human legs: Estimation of extra- and intra-cellular fluid volume J. of Microwave Power 18: 233–243, 1983.
7. Sakamoto K, Higashiizumi T, Kanai H: Frequency characteristics of the electrical impedance of legs. Japanese Journal of Medical Electronics and Biological Engineering 17: 264–270, 1979.
8. Schwan HP: Electrical properties of tissue and cell suspension. In: Lawrence JH, Tobias CA (eds) Advances in bio-

logical and medical physics, Vol. V. New York, Academic Press, 1957, pp 147–224.
9. Schwan HP: Alternating current spectroscopy of biological substances. Proc IRE 10: 1845–1855, 1959.
10. Tender BT: Automatic recording of biological impedances. J Med Eng Technol 2: 70–75, 1978.

Address for offprints:
Hiroshi Kanai
Dept. of Electrical Engineering
Sophia University
7-1 Kioi-cho, Chiyoda-ku
Tokyo 102, Japan

Medical Progress through Technology 12: 171–183 (1987)

Measurement of electrical bio-impedance and its applications

Yoshitake Yamamoto & Tatsuma Yamamoto
Department of Electrical Engineering, Okayama University, Okayama, Japan

Key words: bio-impedance, skin impedance, applications of bio-impedance

Summary

This paper describes: 1) the measurement method of electrical bio-impedance; 2) presentations of models of bio-impedance and their applications to some impedance analyses; 3) the analyses of steady state and dynamical state of electrical properties of the skin; and 4) the applications of bio-impedance. The applications include: 1) the influence of skin impedance to biological potential measurement; 2) skin moisturization measurement using skin admittance; and 3) gait analysis using lower leg electrical impedance.

1. Introduction

There are many sorts of electrical bio-impedance from very low value impedance such as tested in the blood and liver to very high value such as found in skin and teeth [6]. The frequency ranges which are of interest are also over a wide area from direct current to the MHz range. Bio-impedance cannot be explained in only a few words. The research of bio-impedance was started over one hundred years ago and now there are plenty of reports on the results of numerous studies.

Discussed in this paper are the results of our research on bio-impedance, mainly skin impedance and its applications. However, the Proceedings of Fifth International Conference on Electrical Bio-impedance in 1981 (Tokyo) [4] include reports of many instances of other bio-impedance works in Japan. Furthermore, many interesting research projects have been performed as follows; impedance of flowing blood [5], bacterial test by electrical impedance [2], measurement of electrical resistivity of articular cartilage [1] and measurement of electrical bio-impedance in breast tumors [3].

2. Measuring methods of electrical bio-impedance

2.1 Measurement device [14]

Bio-impedance changes due to various factors inside and outside the body and also according to time. We must rapidly measure bio-impedance under constant conditions for obtaining the most reliable data. Because of this, the measurement system shown in Fig. 1 which is constructed of a synchronous rectifier with a phase sensitive detector has been proposed. It can be utilized to measure automatically and continuously the real part (resistive component) and the imaginary part (reactive component) of the impedance. A sine wave voltage from a generator is converted by a voltage to a current convertor into a sine wave current of constant amplitude to be delivered to the impedance Z. The terminal voltage of Z is applied to two multipliers M_1 and M_2. The voltage from the generator is also applied to M_1 directly and M_2, with an equivalent amplitude, after phase shifts of 90 degrees. The outputs of M_1 and M_2 pass through each lowpass filter and, as a result, the output from M_1 becomes proportional to a resistance Rs while that from M_2 is proportional to a reactance Xs. Using this system, the impedance at an expected one

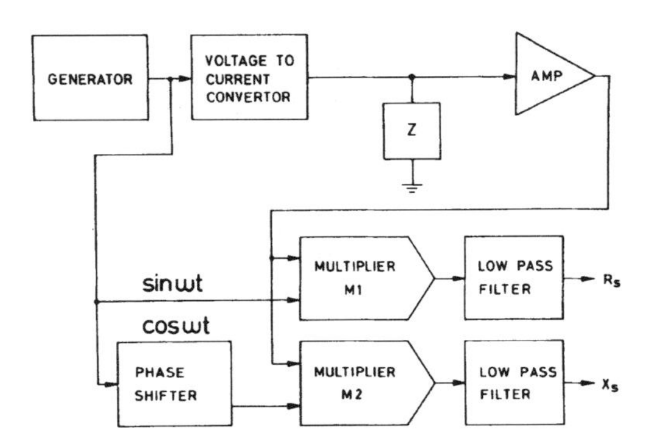

Fig. 1. Continuous impedance measurement device.

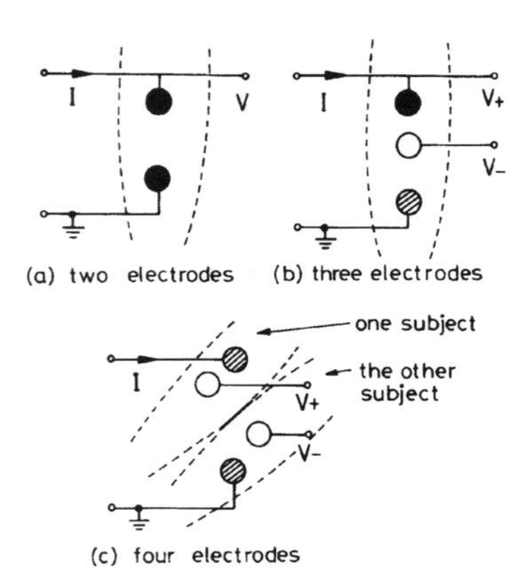

Fig. 2. Construction of electrode system in impedance measurement by constant current method. ● equals electrode of current and potential, ◍ equals current electrode and ○ equals potential electrode.

frequency can be obtained instantaneously and continuously.

If the measurement frequencies are set up subsequently, the frequency characteristics of bio-impedance can be easily obtained. In the study on bio-impedance of time variation, it is necessary to be able to measure simultaneously the impedance for one point on the skin at some different frequencies and to measure the impedance simultaneously for some different points at one frequency. For this purpose, a dynamic measurement device was developed which was constituted of an n channel measurement employing a time multiplex. It is possible to analyze the bio-impedance variously by developing these devices.

2.2 Two, three and four electrodes

An impedance is decided by the ratio of subject voltage and current. Then, an electrode system must be constructed for measuring an impedance. In the two electrode method (Fig. 2a) the potential difference between the two electrodes is picked up and the impedance between these two electrodes can be measured. In this case, if one electrode is made a large size, i.e. indifferent electrode, the impedance of the side of this large electrode can be ignored and only the impedance of the side of the other electrode can be detected. If a third electrode, i.e. potential electrode is added as shown in Fig. 2b, only a single side impedance can be measured. This three electrode system is very useful because the electrode of large size is not necessary.

The construction in Fig. 2c is for a four electrode method which ignores the impedance of current electrode portions and can measure the impedance of the central portion between two potential electrodes. In Fig. 2c, the skin impedance in case of contact of skin with skin can be measured.

2.3 Telemetry

It is necessary to be able to measure bio-impedance in a state of no restriction on subject's free actions during a long period of time. It can be accomplished only by applying a wireless telemetry. Therefore, the telemetry system with a transmitter portion as shown in Fig. 3 was designed and constructed, by means of PWM/FM, to obtain the skin impedance of 20 Hz [16]. Its dimensions are 46 × 46 × 40 mm and it weighs 60 grams including batteries. It enables continuous operation of about 30 hours. In the modulation portion, the resistive and reactive components of skin impedance are measured by synchronous rectifier the same as Fig. 1.

3. Analysis of bio-impedance using models

3.1 Cole-Cole dispersion system and its parallel equivalent circuit

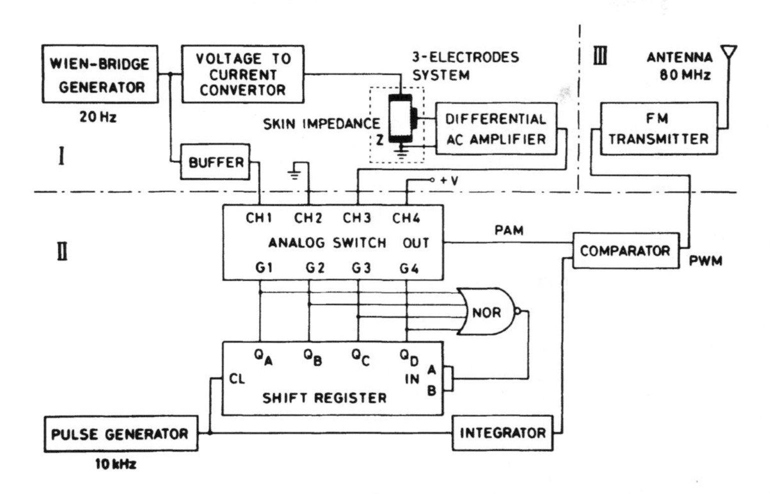

Fig. 3. Block diagram of transmitter in telemetry system. The part of I is an impedance measurement circuit, II is a digital circuit for modulations PAM (puls amplitude modulation) and PWM (puls width modulation) and III is an FM (frequency modulation) transmitter.

The vector locus of bio-impedance such as skin, tooth, muscle, etc. satisfies Cole-Cole circular arc's law as shown in Fig. 4 and can be represented by [7]

$$Z = R_s - jX_s = Z_\infty + \frac{R_2}{1 + (j\omega\tau_m)^\beta} \tag{1}$$

where $Z_\infty = \lim_{\omega\to\infty} Z$, $Z_0 = \lim_{\omega\to 0} Z$.

And $R_2 = Z_0 - Z_\infty$ is a resistive component based on ionic conduction, $\tau_m (f_m = 1/2\pi\tau_m)$ is the central relaxation time representing relaxation phenomenon, β (≤ 1) is a parameter representing the degree of deviation from Debye type ($\beta = 1$) and ω is an angular frequency. And then, this equation can be expressed by the parallel equivalent circuit in Fig. 5a [9] and parameters of the circuit are given by

$$\frac{1}{Z - Z_\infty} = \frac{1 + (j\omega\tau_m)^\beta}{R_2} \tag{2}$$

$$= G_2 + g_p + j\omega C_p \tag{2}$$

$$G_2 = 1/R_2, \; G_\infty = 1/Z_\infty \tag{3}$$

$$g_p = \omega^\beta g_0, \; C_p = \omega^{\beta-1} C_0$$

$$g_0 = G_2 \tau_m^\beta \cos\frac{\beta\pi}{2} \tag{4}$$

$$C_0 = G_2 \tau_m^\beta \sin\frac{\beta\pi}{2}$$

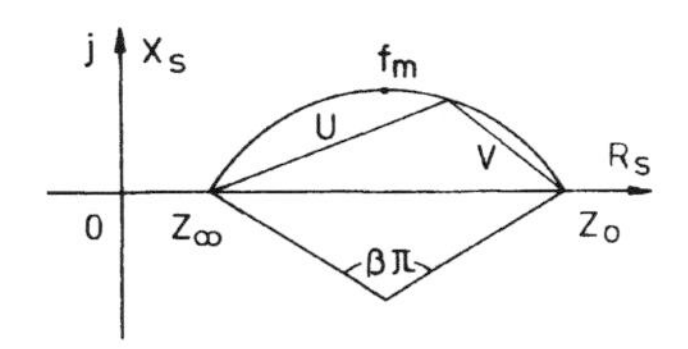

Fig. 4. Vector locus of bio-impedance Z=Rs−jXs. f_m is the characteristic frequency.

g_p and c_p are respectively conductance and capacitance based on polarization. In the skin, $Z_\infty = 0.0$. Fig 5a is a circuit in the case that the extinct cells, such as skin, tooth, bone, are dominant over the value of impedance. Fig. 5b is also the equivalent circuit satisfying Cole-Cole arc's law [11]. This is a circuit for blood or muscular tissues which contain

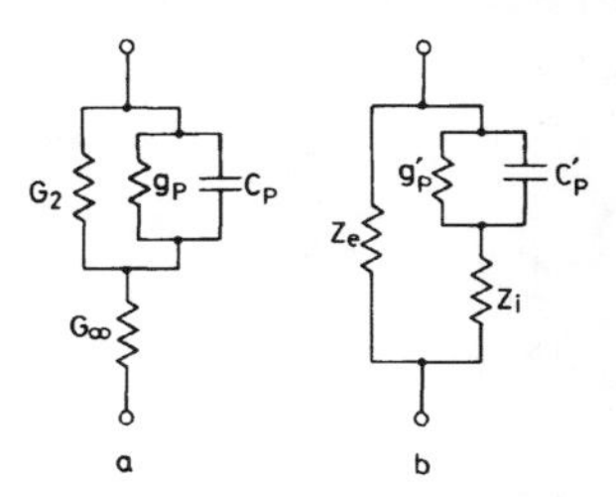

Fig. 5. Equivalent circuits of bio-impedance of satisfying Cole-Cole arc's law.

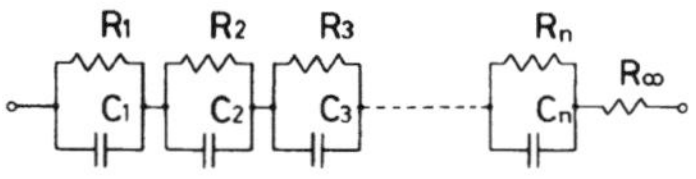

Fig. 6. Equivalent circuit of discretely distributed type for bio-impedance.

living cells. Resistors Ze and Zi of ionic conduction are resistances of the outer and inner cellular solution respectively. Where, $Z_0 = Ze$, $Z_\infty = ZeZi/(Ze + Zi)$, and the polarization impedance is given by $Zp' = (Ze + Zi)/(j\omega\tau_m)^\beta = 1/g_p' + j\omega C_p')$.

3.2 Approximation of Cole-Cole circular arc with distributed relaxation time and its equivalent circuit

The construction of an equivalent circuit with fixed elements for bio-impedance satisfying the Cole-Cole circular arc's law is explained. The Cole-Cole dispersion system having continuously distributed relaxation times can be simulated by the system of some discrete relaxation times, and approximate equation is assumed as follows [12]:

$$Z(\omega) = Z_\infty + \sum_{i=1}^{n} \frac{R_i}{1 + j\omega C_i R_i} \tag{5}$$

Equation (5) can be explained by the equivalent circuit in Fig. 6 ($R_\infty = Z_\infty$). The optimum circuit elements were obtained with $\beta = 0.5$–0.9 for the cases $n = 3, 5, 7$. Some approximate arcs are shown in Fig. 7. The equivalent circuit simulates in good agreement with skin impedance over the wide frequency range. It is useful to simulate the skin impedance in the case, for example, of signal distortion caused by skin impedance appearing in electrocardiography.

3.3 Non-linear bio-impedance

The impedance can be described by Eq. (1) in the case that the frequency vector locus of bio-impedance obeys the circular arc's law in Fig. 4. But, its decision must be done carefully by Cole and Cole's method. If U and V are evaluated for each mea-

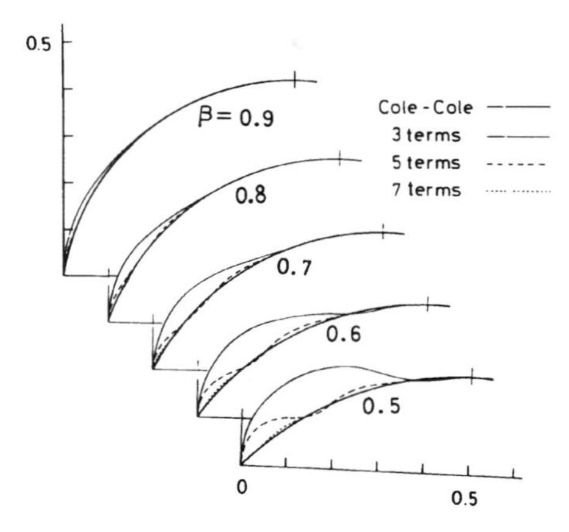

Fig. 7. Cole-Cole circular arcs and approximate arcs of 3, 5 and 7 terms. Expressions of arc are normalized. It is possible to approximate with a small number of terms when β of arc is large.

surement value, the ratio V/U is described using a new parameter α as follows:

$$V/U = (\omega\tau_m)^\alpha \tag{6}$$

If parameter α (≤1) equals β of the circular arc, the impedance is described by a linear Equation (1). However, when $\alpha \neq \beta$, the impedance is non-linear and is described by the following Equation [10].

$$Z(\omega) = Z_\infty + \frac{Z_0 - Z_\infty}{1 + j^\beta(\omega\tau_m)^\alpha} \tag{7}$$

Vector loci of Eq. (1) and Eq. (7) have the same form, but locations on the circular arc for each frequency are mutually shifted according to the two equations. The parameters of equivalent circuit for Eq. (7) are given by

$$\begin{aligned} g_p &= \omega^\beta g_0, Cp = \omega^{\beta-1} C_0 \\ g_0 &= G_2\, \tau_m^\alpha \cos\frac{\beta\pi}{2} \\ C_0 &= G_2 \tau_m^\alpha \sin\frac{\beta\pi}{2} \end{aligned} \tag{8}$$

Non-linear bio-impedance is explained again in Section 4.3.

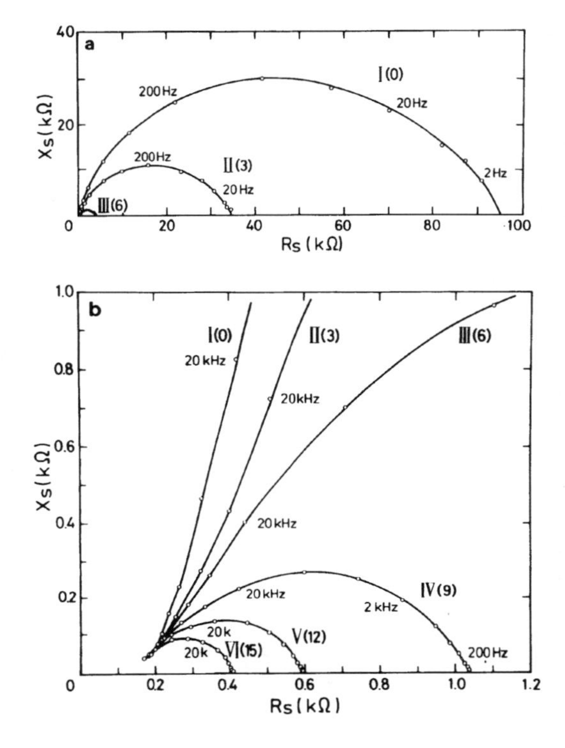

Fig. 8. Skin impedance loci due to succesive strippings. A figure in the parentheses shows the number of the stripping. Two Ag-AgCl electrodes of 9 mm diameter were placed with Beckman electrode paste on the ventral side of forearm with a distance of 50 mm.

4. Characteristics of skin impedance

4.1 Laminate structure of epidermal stratum corneum

The skin impedance mainly consists of the impedance of the stratum corneum. Then, it is important for the understanding of the skin impedance that the formative mechanism of the stratum corneum impedance be analyzed [7, 8]. The removal of the stratum corneum was carried out stepwise by cellulose-tape stripping. A stabilization time of about 30 minutes after applying the electrode was allowed before measurements were taken. The skin impedances for each time are shown in Fig. 8. Considering these results, the characteristics on skin impedance, resistivity and dielectric constant are made clear in view of the laminate structure of epidermal stratum corneum. The frequency characteristics of the average resistivity and dielectric constant, and effective resistivity ϱ (x) and dielectric constant ε (x) at every point of the stratum corneum are evaluated. ϱ (x) decreases exponentially in the form of $\varrho(x) = \varrho_0\, e^{-ax}$ and ε (x) increases nearly exponentially in the form of $\varepsilon(x) = \varepsilon_0\, e^{bx}$, x is the distance towards the deeper tissues from the surface, and a>0, b>0. The frequency dispersion of skin impedance originates in the relaxations due to the inhomogeneous structure from the cellular level appearing in ϱ (x), ε (x) and due to the laminate structure from the morphological standpoint appearing in the impedance equation. Namely, the skin impedance equation which simultaneously estimates two types of relaxation by the complex dielectric constant and integral operation is given by:

$$Z(\omega) = Z_\infty + \int_0^d \frac{\varrho(\varkappa)}{1 + j\omega\varepsilon(\varkappa)\varrho(\varkappa)} d\varkappa/S \qquad (9)$$

where Z_∞ is the impedance of the deep tissues, d is the thickness of the stratum corneum. S is the area of electrode. Equation (9) can be transformed in the style of Eq. (1) under the some conditions [8].

4.2 Time variation and dispersion

The impedance of living tissues is kept at about constant level because of homeostasis. However, the skin impedance has very large variations with time and dispersion because of the existence of an extinct laminate cellular structure. Although there are many types of time variation, the variation with time due to osmosis of paste which is caused just after applying the electrode to the skin, is appearing generally and is shown in Fig. 9. These impedances always satisfy the Cole-Cole arc's law. Impedance parameters, Z_0 and R_2 decrease, characteristic frequency f_m increases and β decreases only a little in the course of time.

Next, the dispersions are explained [13]. The frequency characteristics and correlations of the skin impedance were measured on the forearm and ankle of several subjects 1 minute after the appli-

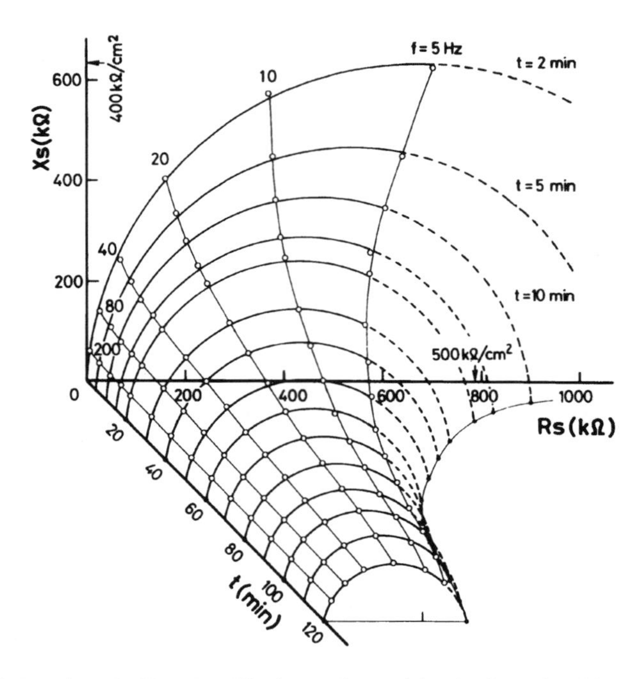

Fig. 9. Time course of skin impedance loci from 2 to 120 minutes after applying the electrodes with paste to the forearm. The electrodes used are the same as Fig. 8.

cation of the electrodes. Then, R_2, C_0 and f_m were evaluated from Eqs (1)–(4). These results are shown in Fig. 10 and Fig. 11. The distribution ranges of R_2 and C_0 are different from each other, i.e. about 200 times for R_2 and 10 times for C_0, but both parameters obey the logarithmic normal distribution. R_2-f_m have a high correlation ($r = -0.97$), and R_2-C_0 and f_m-C_0 have a low correlation (-0.20 and -0.02), respectively. These correlations can be presupposed to some degree by Eq. (4).

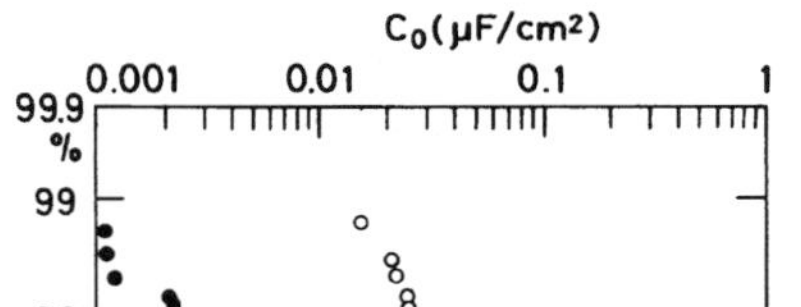

Fig. 10. Log normal cumulative probability plots of the parameters R_2 (●) and C_0 (○). Beckman electrode and paste are used. The values of parameters are converted to per area of $1\,cm^2$.

4.3 Non-linear characteristics

The vector loci of skin impedance for several current values are shown in Fig. 12 [10]. Skin impedance has a marked dependency on the current, but all frequency points fall onto a circular arc. Furthermore, the current dependencies of parameters in various cases on the human forearm and on rabbit skin have been obtained. From those results the non-linearity classification of the skin impedance has been made as shown in Table 1. The relationship between α and β for some experimental values of forearm skin impedance are shown in Fig. 13. Generally nonlinearity becomes distinguished when measurement current value is larger and measurement frequency is lower. Impedance analysis can not be applied in the case of the sub-

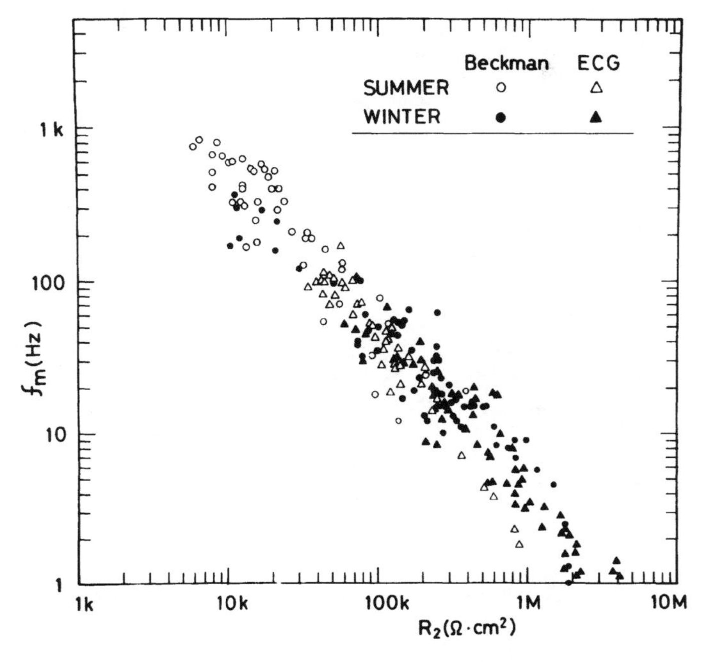

Fig. 11. Correlation between skin impedance parameter f_m and R_2. The experiments were carried out in summer using Beckman electrode and paste: ○ and ECG plate electrode and 0.9% saline: △, and in winter using Beckman electrode and paste: ● and ECG plate electrode and 0.9% saline: ▲.

division in Table 1, and the analysis by voltage-current Lissajous figure must be done, because the degree of non-linearity is too large to apply a impedance concept into their signals.

5. Applications of bio-impedance

5.1 Application to measuring bio-electrical potential

In the early state of the development of electrocardiography (ECG) and electroencephalography

Table 1. Classification of non-linearities.

	Subdivision			
	I	II	III	IV
Linearity	← linear →	←	non-linear	→
Frequency	high ←			→ low
Current	small ←			→ large
Shape of voltage wave	←	sine wave →	← almost sine wave →	← distortion wave →
α, β	←	α = β →	← α ≠ β →	
Current dependency	← independent →	←	dependent	→
Method of analysis	←	impedance	→	← Lissajous figure →

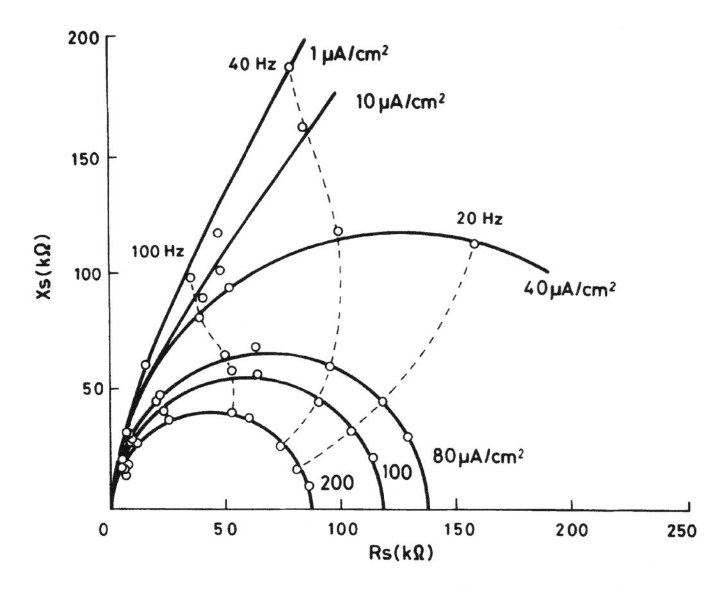

Fig. 12. Current dependency of skin impedance vector loci. These results were measured with several current values after stabilization of osmosis of paste.

(EEG), the influences of the polarization impedance of an electrode to these wave forms were very large. The various contrivances for reducing the influence of the polarization impedance have been conducted. Nowadays, the influence of the polarization impedance became quite small with the development of an electronic amplifier. However, the accuracy required for the waveforms is progressively increasing. The skin impedance causes distortion to the wave form more than in case of the polarization impedance, but the skin impedance has not been fully treated up to date. It is necessary to grasp precisely the situation of the waveform distortion by the skin impedance. Then, the problem due to the skin impedance are examined by using the equivalent circuit of skin impedance, shown in Fig. 6, from a point of view as the interface for a biomeasurement amplifier. The wave form distortions caused by the skin impedance are obtained and examined according to the characteristics of skin impedance [15].

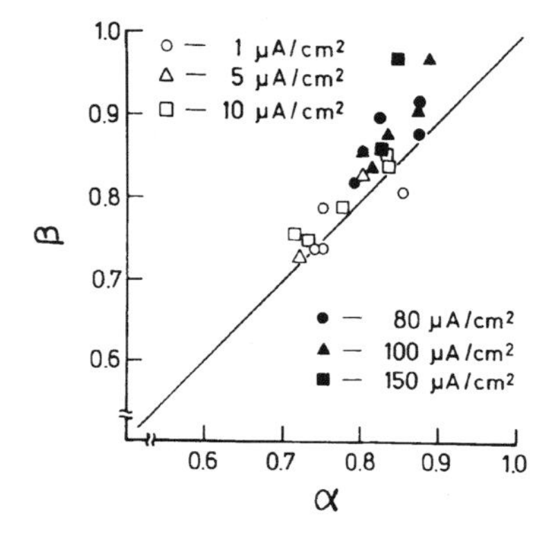

Fig. 13. Relationship between α and β of arcs measured at various current value.

5.2 Applications of skin impedance to skin sciences

(i) Performance evaluation of drugs and cosmetics [17]. Skin impedance fluctuates considerably due to various factors, both internal and external conditions of the body, and, consequently, various biological measurements are possible by utilizing skin impedance changes. One of the basic problems in this field is the variation in skin impedance caused by other factors besides the factor of interest. It is necessary to remove as many meaningless changes as possible by defining conditions such as the environment etc. and simultaneously handling by statistical treatment the changes and variances which

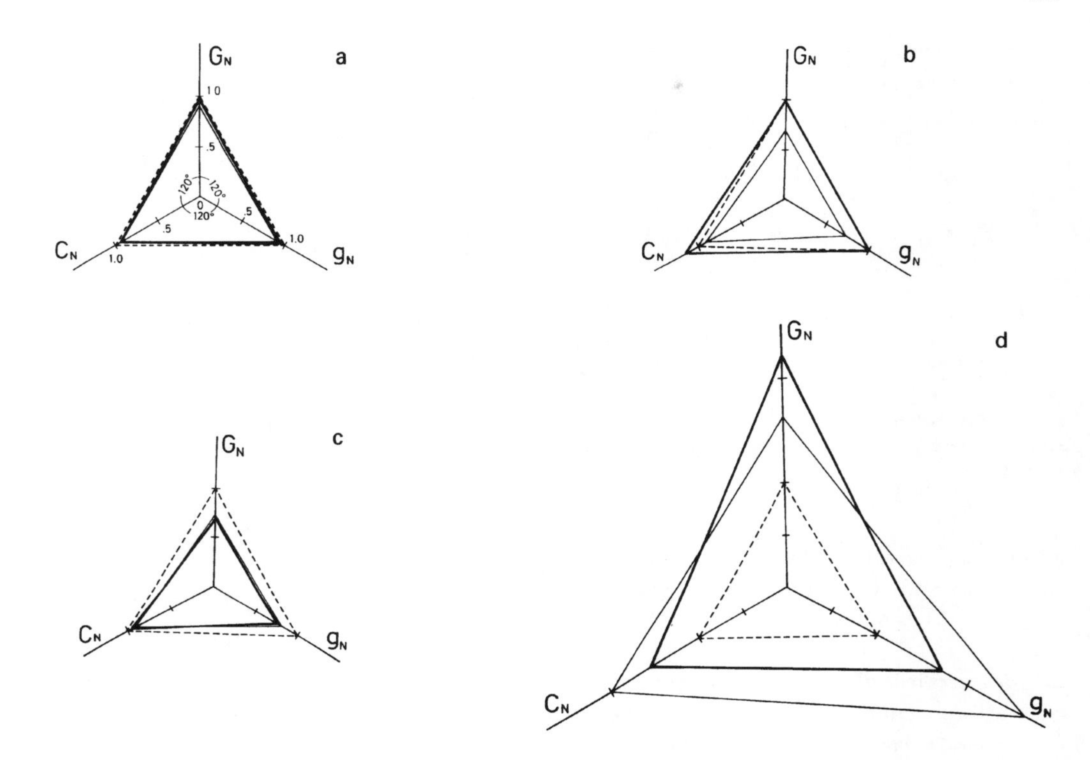

Fig. 14. Rate of change triangles. Broken line is before treatment, fine solid line is 30 minutes after treatment and heavy solid line is 3 hours after treatment. (a) is no treatment and shows identity of skin impedance under controlled condition; (b) O/W cream; (c) W/O cream; (d) PCA-Na (DL-2-pyrrolidone-5-carboxylic acid).

cannot be eliminated. It is then important to produce a stable reference impedance (reference level) which is unaffected by the factor of interest; then it will be possible to pick out change which is due only to the factor in question.

A method for setting a reference level based on the identity of the skin impedance in place of the well-known bilateralism of human skin impedance, which has been considered up to date as the basis for removing factors other than the factor of interest, has been proposed. The experiments which previously required a large number of subjects for a long time can be carried out within a short time with only a few subjects, e.g. three, in the present study. As the rate of change of impedance was expressed as the triangle shown next, this assists the intuitive understanding of the electrical properties of the skin before and after treatment and makes performance evaluation easy.

The effects on skin impedance 30 minutes after applying the sample and three hours after the first application were measured, when the three kinds of samples of saponified O/W cream, nonionic W/O cream, and PCA-Na (50% aqueous solution) were applied on the arms and the results are shown in Fig. 14. This is a triangular expression of the rate of change (called the rate of change triangle) indicated particularly in the plane: for example, C_N, g_N, and G_N components of the figure indicate the rate of change of three impedance parameters which are expressed by C_0, g_0, and G_2, respectively. It was found that a difference in the type of cosmetic characterizes the differences in the rate of change triangles. It is believed that these results suggest the possibility of the application of skin impedance measurements in a practical sense to the effects of drugs and cosmetics on the skin; i.e. to the performance evaluation.

Problems which must be resolved in the future are: clarification of the physical and chemical

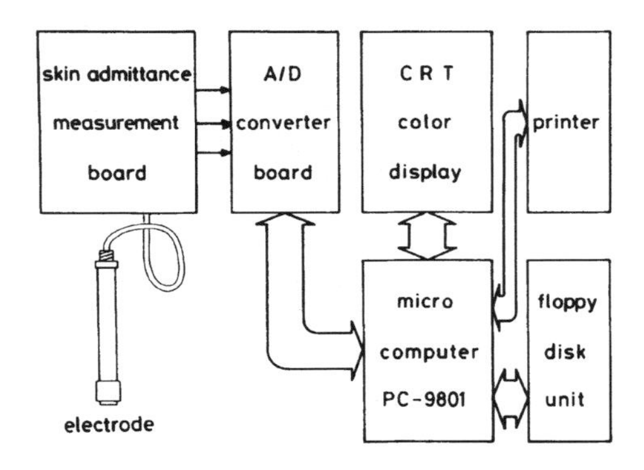

Fig. 15. Block diagram of the skin admittance measuring system. Skin admittance was measured as absolute value of admittance at 100kHz.

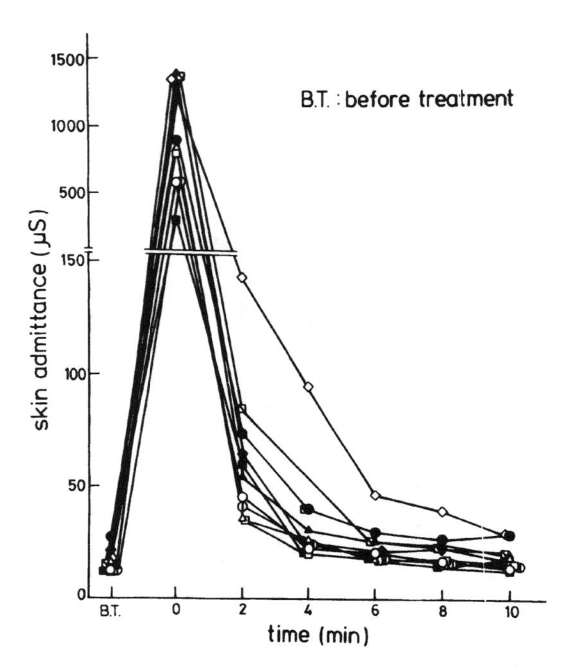

Fig. 16. Changes of skin admittance during the process of dehydration. BT: before treatment.

meanings of the rate of change in these impedance parameters and clarification of its significance in respect to drugs or cosmetics.

(ii) Measurement of skin moisturization [20]. The electrical resistance in impedance of the skin at a low frequency has been used as the index of moisturization in some methods. However, ions rather than water in the skin largely influence the result, leaving problems in its general use. These problems are discussed based on experimental observation, and the conditions required for the measurement of skin admittance to estimate skin moisturization are made clear. The influence of ions upon the admittance was found to be much smaller in a frequency range higher than about 10 kHz in comparison with the influence in the lower frequency ranges. The admittance becomes too large when the frequency is extremely high. Therefore, a frequency of about 100 kHz is appropriate. Since the admittance is largely changed by the contact pressure for a dry electrode, the pressure should be adjustable. The appropriate pressure was found to be about 100 gcm^{-2}. As far as variations in observed admittance values are concerned, the larger the surface area of a measuring electrode, the smaller the variation. However, taking the size of an indifferent electrode into account, we recommend a diameter of about 5 mm for a measuring electrode in practice. Skin admittance is primarily determined by the relative permitivity, the resistivity and the thickness of the stratum corneum and by the contact ratio between a dry electrode and stratum corneum. Among these, the contact ratio predominantly determines the change of the admittance. The moisturization measurement utilizing skin admittance is based on the change of the contact ratio induced by differing the skin moisturization. Based on the observations and considerations stated above, an instrument for the measurement of skin admittance was constructed. Fig. 15 is the block diagram of this system. With this system measuring procedures were automatic, therefore, the experimental conditions were almost constantly arranged and variations in observed data were reduced and the reliability of the result was improved. The ventral side of the forearm of each of several subjects was dipped into 42° C warm water for 5 min, then wiped off with gauze, and the time course of changes in the skin admittance was measured. The result obtained is shown in Fig. 16. The skin admittance was markedly increased by hydration and decreased with the progress of dehydration. Thus it could be confirmed that the skin admittance is strongly correlated with the water content of skin.

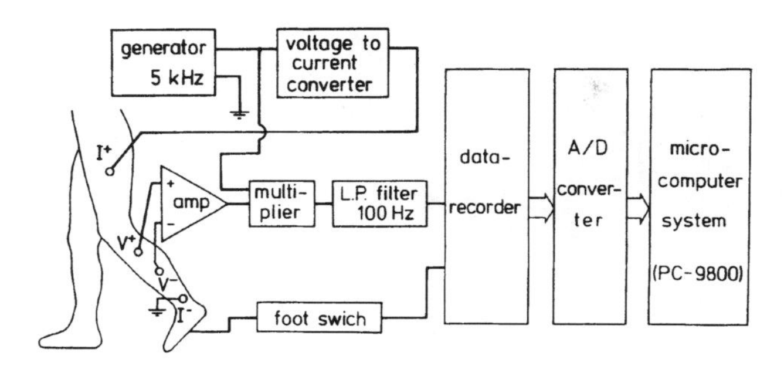

Fig. 17. Block diagram of measuring system of lower leg electrical impedance.

The skin admittances at some portions of the human body of three normal subjects were measured five times and the results are shown in Table 2. The admittances are greatly different with various body portions. The skin moisturizations are less in an upper limb, in a lower limb, and middle of the face, and more in the palm and on the sole because of continuous psychological perspiration.

5.3 Gait analysis using lower leg impedance

Gait analysis using lower leg electrical impedance for clinical application is being proposed, because lower leg electrical impedance varies with walk [18, 19]. The measuring method is constituted by a four electrode technique of a current with constant amplitude as shown in Fig. 17 and Ag-AgCl skin electrodes of 10 mm dia. were used. Lower leg impedance Z varies with the positions of electrodes applied on a lower leg. Therefore, positions are decided in view of similar figures. That is, electrodes are attached on a leg, their distances have constant ratios corresponding to the length of the lower leg. Obtained signals are input to a data recorder and 10 bits AD converter and they are stored in a microcomputer. Data processing are carried out as follows: (i) division of gait cycle; (ii) superimposed display; (iii) normalization; (iv) averaging; (v) fast Fourier transform analysis.

In static condition, Z is dominated by the magnitude of an ankle angle θ and the magnitude of the moment M of the ankle acting as the foot force, and is not influenced very much by the knee angle, the moment acting on the knee and so on. Fig. 18 is the waveform of Z (absolute value) in the case that the subject was at first standing straight, then started a normal gait for about 30 meters, and was again standing. Z is varing periodically with gait. Z during gait can be characterized by two phases, one being the impedance pattern $\triangle Z$ of its variation and the other, its mean impedance level $\overline{Z}$. Thus, $Z = \overline{Z} + \triangle Z$. As a result of deliberate discussions, the pattern $\triangle Z$ is dominated by the magnitudes of

Table 2. Skin admittances at some portions of human body.

Site	Subject age, sex	A 23,M	B 23,M	C 41,M
forehead		30.5 ± 5.3	34.3 ± 6.8	38.2 ± 6.8
cheek		33.6 ± 3.7	25.0 ± 7.5	22.0 ± 7.4
ext. forearm		10.5 ± 0.8	14.1 ± 1.2	16.8 ± 1.1
flex. forearm		17.2 ± 1.2	18.9 ± 1.9	24.5 ± 1.8
calf		19.2 ± 2.7	12.8 ± 1.4	17.1 ± 3.2
palm		539.2 ± 55.	335.6 ± 27.	265.2 ± 90.
sole		522.2 ± 34.	321.0 ± 96.	115.2 ± 47.

(unit: μS)

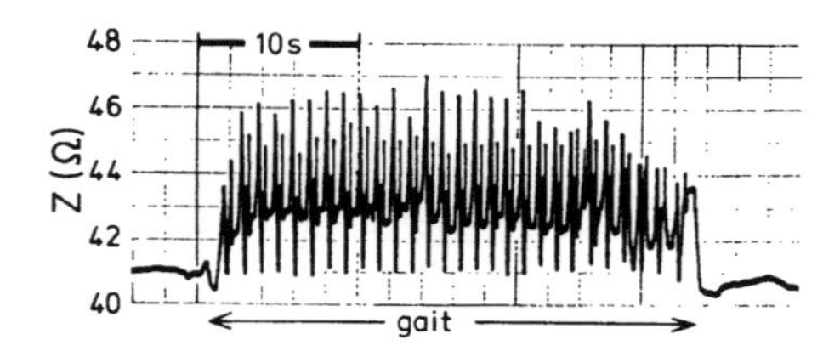

Fig. 18. Lower leg impedance during gait.

θ and M in static condition. The θ causes variation of the muscular transverse sectional area and M causes variations of blood volume (vascular transverse sectional area) and electrical conductivity of musculature. The level $\overline{Z}$ is higher than that in static condition and responds to the change of M with a fairly large time constant, because the blood volume reserved in the lower leg gradually decreases by a muscular pump action with gait. Every gait pattern has different forms of θ and M, and also has different levels and patterns of Z. These suggest that the difference appears in Z for pathological gaits.

Furthermore, information obtained from pattern and level of impedance are of all sorts such as the normality, stability and mobility of gait. The entire time of all gaits can be easily and non-restrictively measured by the impedance. Therefore, this method could be applied in rehabilitation clinics and sport training.

6. Conclusions

The fundamental studies and some applications of electrical bio-impedance for medical fields have been described. Especially this paper treated of the measurement method of electrical bio-impedance, presentations of models of bio-impedance, the analyses of steady state and dynamical state of electrical properties of the skin, and the applications of bio-impedance.

References

1. Hasegawa I, Matsuno S, Kriki S, Matsumoto G: A new measuring method of the fixed charge density of the articular cartilage measurement of electrical resistivity (in Japanese). Proceedings Conf Japan Soc Med Elect & Biol Eng 2-D-15: 302, 1982.
2. Hashimoto H, Miike H, Ebina Y, Miyaji T: An automated method for bacterial test by simultaneous measurement of electrical impedance and turbidity (in Japanese). Japan J Med Elect & Biol Eng 19: 23–29, 1981.
3. Nishimoto K, Sonoo H, Morimoto T, Inoue K, Kinouchi Y, Iritani T, Hayashi K, Bando T: In vivo measurement of electrical bioimpedance in breast tumors (in Japanese). Proceedings Conf Japan Soc Med Elect & Biol Eng M-29: 547, 1983.
4. Proceedings of Fifth International Conference on Electrical Bio-impedance, Business Center for Academic Societies Japan, Tokyo, Japan, 1981.
5. Sakamoto K, Kanai H: Electrical characteristics of flowing blood. IEEE Trans Biomed Eng BME-26: 686–695, 1979.
6. Schwan HP: Electrical properties of tissue and cell suspension. In: Lawrence LH, Tobias CA (eds) Advances in biological and medical physics. Academic Press, New York, 1957, pp 154–174.
7. Yamamoto T, Yamamoto Y: Electrical properties of the epidermal stratum corneum, Med & Biol Eng 14: 151–158, 1976.
8. Yamamoto T, Yamamoo Y: Dielectric constant and resistivity of epidermal stratum corneum. Med & Biol Eng & Comput 14: 494–500, 1976.
9. Yamamoto T, Yamamoto Y: Analysis for the change of skin impedance. Med & Biol Eng & Comput 15: 219–227, 1977.
10. Yamamoto T, Yamamoto Y: Non-linear electrical properties of skin in the low frequency range. Med & Biol Eng & Comput 19: 302–310, 1981.
11. Yamamoto T, Yamamoto Y, Mizufune E: Mathematical structure of Bio-electrical impedance obtained from linear functional point of view. Transactions of Institute of Electronics and Communication Engineers of Japan E66–6: 352–358, 1983.
12. Yamamoto Y, Yamamoto T: Construction of equivalent circuit or skin impedance (in Japanese). Japan J Med Elect & Biol Eng 14: 129–132, 1976.
13. Yamamoto Y, Yamamoto T: Dispersion and correlation of the paramters for skin impedance. Med & Biol Eng & Comput 16: 592–594, 1978.
14. Yamamoto Y, Yamamoto T: Dynamic system for the measurement of electrical skin impedance. Med & Biol Eng & Comput 17: 135–137, 1979.
15. Yamamoto Y, Yamamoto T: Influences of the skin impedance as the interface in bioelctric potential measurement: Memoirs of the School of Engineering. Okayama University 15–1: 17–28, 1980.

16. Yamamoto Y, Yamamoto T, Nishiura N: Telemetry system for measuring vector impedance of human skin. Proceeding of Fifth International Symposium on Biotelemetry. Sapporo and Kyoto, Japan, 95–98, 1980.
17. Yamamoto Y, Yamamoto T, Ohta S, Uehara T, Tahara S, Ishizuka Y: The measurement principle for evaluating the performance of drugs and cosmetics by skin impedance. Med & Biol Eng & Comput 16: 623–632, 1978.
18. Yamamoto Y, Yamamoto T, Okamoto T, Jikuya K, Hiragami F, Akashi K: Studies on lower leg electrical impedance for gait analysis (in Japanese). Japan J Med Elect & Biol Eng 22: 433–438, 1984.
19. Yamamoto Y, Yamamoto T, Okamoto T, Jikuya K, Hiragami F, Akashi K: Gait analysis using lower leg electrical impedance. XIV Intern Conf on Med & Biol Eng, VII Intern Conf on Med Physics, Espoo, Finland, 9.19: 416–417, 1985.
20. Yamamoto Y, Yamamoto T, Ozawa T: Characteristics of skin admittance for dry electrodes and the measurement of skin moisturization. Med & Biol & Comput 24: 71–77, 1986.

Address for offprints:
Yoshitake Yamamoto
Department of Electrical Engineering
Okayama University
Tsushima-Naka 3
Okayama 700, Japan

Medical Progress through Technology 12: 185–195 (1987)

Estimation of tissue parameters derived from reflected ultrasound

Tsuyoshi Shiina, Kenji Ikeda & Masao Saito
Institute of Medical Electronics, Faculty of Medicine, University of Tokyo, 7-3-1 Hongo, Bunkyo-ku, Tokyo 113, Japan

Key words: Ultrasound, attenuation, resolution improvement, adaptive filtering, tissue characterization

Abstract

We propose a method of estimating two tissue parameters, that is, the reflection coefficient and attenuation coefficient from the reflected ultrasound for the purpose of improving the resolution of ultrasonic images and obtaining information on tissue characterization. The reflection coefficient is estimated by deconvolution technique using Kalman filter taking into account the distortion of the propagating pulse due to the frequency-dependent attenuation. The attenuation is estimated by adaptive processings based upon the criterion function calculated using estimates of the reflection coefficient. Simulated signals are used to investigate the ability of this method. Additionally, actual reflected signals from soft tissues are processed by the method. The results show that the method can be applied in clinical cases.

1. Introduction

Diagnostic ultrasound imaging is now widely used as a noninvasive technique for examining the body, and the images have been enhanced to some degree during recent years, e.g. the grey scale technique and improvement of the transducer. However, the technology is based upon a rather simple idea which is used in industrial measurement and does not take into account the properties of biological tissues. As a result, the resolution of images still does not meet at the order of the wavelength, and only a part of much information on tissue characteristics contained in reflected ultrasound, i.e., only information on anatomical structures of soft tissues, is currently used. Therefore, more sophisticated signal processings are now required to improve the resolution and extract information on tissue characteristics. These problems can be commonly discussed from the point of view of estimating tissue parameters from the reflected signal. That is to say, improvement of the resolution can be carried out by correctly extracting information on the structure of tissues, which corresponds to estimating the reflection coefficient defined as the differential of acoustic impedance from the reflected signal.

On the other hand, to obtain tissue characterization information, it is necessary to estimate the acoustic parameters which determine pathology of tissue by ultrasonic signal [2, 10]. Results of many investigations show that attenuation characteristic of soft tissues increase almost linearly with frequency and the slope can be one of the most important parameters to be utilized in diagnosis. For example, cirrhotic livers produce larger attenuation than normal, whereas in diffuse infiltration of livers attenuation is lower than normal [6, 8]. The values of attenuation of infarcted regions of myocardium is larger than in the surrounding tissue because attenuation increases with the amount of collagen [9]. Thus, the attenuation coefficient is an important parameter from a diagnostic point of view. Furthermore, its estimation is also necessary, as will be shown later, for estimating the reflection coefficient.

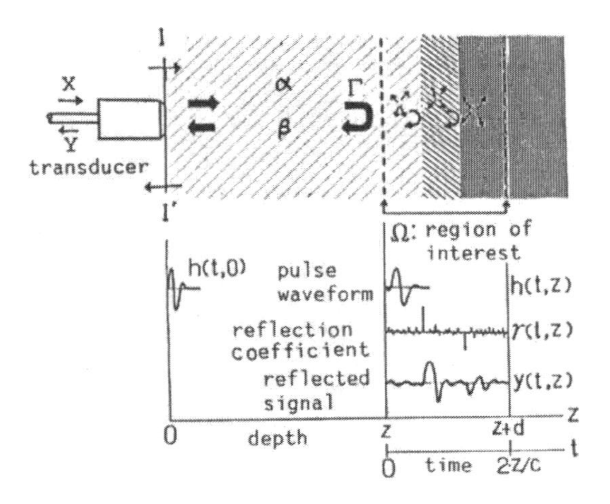

Fig. 1. Models of reflected signals in the pulse echo system.

In this paper, we describe a new method to extract two tissue parameters, i.e., reflection coefficient and attenuation coefficient from the reflected ultrasonic signals for resolution improvement and tissue characterization. This paper is organized as follows. First the model for reflected signal is given in Section 2, and tissue transfer function is described in Section 3. Next, in Section 4, we model the pulse echo system as a time-varying linear dynamic system and show that the resolution improvement and tissue characterization problem is equivalent to the parameter estimation and state identification of the system. This problem is solved by application of Kalman filtering and other adaptive processing in Section 5, 6. Finally, in Section 7, results using simulated signals and real data (pork) are presented and demonstrate the ability of this method for clinical application.

2. Models of reflected signal

Consider a region Ω which ranges from depth z to z+d along the transducer axis, i.e., the acoustic path of the propagating pulse as shown in Fig. 1. Then it is possible to select a part of the reflected signal, denoted by y(t,z), which corresponds to reflection from the region Ω. Assuming that the attenuation within the region Ω is negligible and tissues as the medium exert a linear influence on the propagating pulse, the Fourier transform of y is described as

$$Y(f,z) = X(f)I(f)I'(f)G(f,z)\Phi(f,z) \cdot \Gamma(f,z) + N(f,z) \tag{1}$$

where

X	:	electric indicent pulse
$I \cdot I'$	:	acousto-electric transfer function
G	:	radiative transfer function from transducer face to the depth z
Φ	:	two-way tissue transfer function between transducer and the region Ω
Γ	:	reflection coefficient of the region Ω
N	:	noise component

In the right side of Eq. (1), factors $X \cdot I \cdot I' \cdot G$ are dependent on only the properties of transducer and measurement system, thus letting us define

$$Ho(f,z) = X(f)I(f)I'(f)G(f,z) \tag{2}$$

Eq. (1) then becomes

$$Y(f,z) = Ho(f,z)\Phi(f,z)\Gamma(f,z) + N(f,z) \tag{3}$$

In particular, when $\Phi \cdot \Gamma$ is equal to 1 and N can be neglected, Y becomes equal to Ho. Thus, Ho is pulse waveform in the lossless and homogeneous medium and can be obtained by measuring the reflected signal from a normally-oriented plate at the depth z in the water.

The reflected signal in time domain is written as

$$y(t,z) = h(t,z) * \gamma(t,z) + n(t,z) \tag{4}$$

where

$$h(t,z) = ho(t,z) * \varphi(t,z) \tag{5}$$

and $*$ indicates convolution. y,ho,φ,γ and n are the inverse Fourier transform of Y,Ho,Φ,Γ and N respectively. Eq. (4) shows that the reflected signal from the region Ω is described as the convolution of the pulse incident on Ω and the reflection coefficient within Ω.

Next, let us discuss the reflection coefficient in particular. We have defined the basic components of the reflected signal in [13] based upon the difference in their statistical characteristics. Thus, one is the 'specular component', which is the large echo from definite interfaces whose dimensions are large compared with the wavelength, such as boundary of organs, and produces the bright outline in B-mode image. The other is the 'random component', which is the small echo from random interfaces whose dimensions are small compared with the wavelength such as liver tissue, and give a grey level background texture. The reflected signal is described as the superposition of the two components:

$$y(t,z) = y_S(t,z) + y_R(t,z) \quad (6)$$

where y_S and y_R represent the specular and random components respectively. In addition, the reflection coefficient is similarly expressed as

$$\gamma(t,z) = \gamma_S(t,z) + \gamma_R(t,z) \quad (7)$$

where γ_S and γ_R are basic components of γ corresponding to y_S and y_R respectively.

The random component can be regarded as random time-sequential signal, hence statistical parameters such as mean and variance of amplitude are significant and its power spectrum is flatter than that of the specular component. Several methods for estimating the attenuation from reflected signals have been reported [1, 5, 11]. They commonly use power spectra of reflected signals on the assumption that signals are reflected from the tissue model that is composed of random ensemble of small scatterers, which corresponds to the random component. However, actual reflected signals contain the specular component, so implementation of these methods requires averaging of power spectra over a large region, which leads to degradation of the spatial resolution. In order to reduce the averaging region, it is effective to separate the two components as pre-processing, which is discussed in detail in [13]. The method proposed here has the advantage that there is no need for such averaging since it uses the specular components for the estimation of the attenuation and reflection coefficient. On the other hand, the specular component is deterministic and directly related to the structure of tissues, thus it can be modelled as layered structure:

$$\gamma_s(t,z) = \sum_{i=1} \sigma_i \cdot \delta(t-\tau_i) \quad (8)$$

where σ_i is the reflection coefficient of i-th reflecting boundary, and τ_i is two-way propagating time corresponding to the position of i-th boundary. To improve the resolution is, in other words, truly to extract information on the tissue structure from reflected signals, and it corresponds to estimating the specular component, as mentioned above. In Section 5, we discuss the method for estimating reflection coefficient of the specular component from the reflected signal.

In the practical case, the structure of tissues is more complicated and there are various dimensions of interfaces compared with wavelength. Thus, in the real signal, the concept 'basic component' is relative, and the values of parameters to separate the two components must be set according to the purpose [13].

3. Tissue transfer function

In this section, we will discuss the tissue transfer function for ultrasonic wave propagation, Φ, in detail. Using attenuation constant α and phase constant β, the transfer function Φ is described as

$$\Phi(f,z) = \exp \{ -2 [\alpha(f \cdot \xi) + j\beta(f \cdot \xi)] \, d\xi\} \quad (9)$$

It is well known that the attenuation constant increases almost linearly with frequency for most soft tissues [1, 5]:

$$\alpha(f,z) = a(z) \cdot f \quad (10)$$

As already mentioned, recent results have shown that the slope a(z) is an indicator of disease condition of tissue. Any non-flat attenuation characteristic is accompanied by the associated phase characteristic. The correct phase characteristic is not necessary in many methods for estimating the attenuation since they use only the power spectra of the reflected signal and the phase information is discarded. On the other hand, to make a inverse filter for estimating the reflection coefficient, both magnitude and phase characteristics of the tissue transfer function must be specified. However, it is very difficult to measure the absolute phase characteristics of medium with band limited signals used in diagnostic ultrasound. Therefore, we have implemented the *minimum-phase model* for the transfer function of tissues in [12]. There can be an argument as to whether or not the biological tissue as the medium of ultrasound is minimum-phase. In visualizing the equivalent circuit for plane wave, for example, one can be convinced that the wave propagation follows the minimum-phase principle, except for the undetermined component being the term proportional to the frequency, i.e., the term representing the uniform time delay. It is well-known that the phase characteristic in the minimum-phase system is related to the attenuation characteristic by the Hilbert transformation $H[\cdot]$ as follows

$$\beta(f,z) = H[\alpha(f,z)] = \frac{2f}{\pi}\int_0^{\infty} \frac{\alpha(u,z)-\alpha(f,z)}{u^2-f^2}\,du \quad (11)$$

If one substitutes the expression for α in Eq. (10) into Eq. (11), the integral diverges. One may then assume that the attenuation far from the frequency range of interest does not affect significantly the phase within the range. From such a point of view, the attenuation is assumed to be proportional to the frequency from $1/\nu$ to ν and flat outside of this range as shown in Fig. 2.(a), where ν is a sufficiently large value. The integral in Eq. (11) then converges, giving the following phase each frequency range.

$$\beta(f) = \begin{cases} \dfrac{a\cdot f}{\pi}\left[\ln\dfrac{\nu^2-f^2}{\nu^{-2}-f^2} + \dfrac{\nu^{-1}}{f}\ln\dfrac{\nu^{-1}-f}{\nu^{-1}+f} - \dfrac{\nu}{f}\ln\dfrac{\nu-f}{\nu+f}\right], & (f<\nu^{-1}) \\ \dfrac{a\cdot f}{\pi}\left[\dfrac{\nu^{-1}-f}{f}\ln\dfrac{\nu-f^{-1}}{\nu+f^{-1}} + 2\ln\dfrac{\nu+f}{\nu^{-1}+f} - \dfrac{\nu-f}{f}\ln\dfrac{\nu-f}{\nu+f}\right], & (\nu^{-1}\le f\le\nu) \\ \dfrac{a\cdot f}{\pi}\left[\dfrac{\nu^{-1}}{f}\ln\dfrac{f-\nu^{-1}}{f+\nu^{-1}} + \ln\dfrac{f^2-\nu^2}{f^2-\nu^{-2}} - \dfrac{\nu}{f}\ln\dfrac{f-\nu}{f+\nu}\right], & (\nu<f) \end{cases} \quad (12)$$

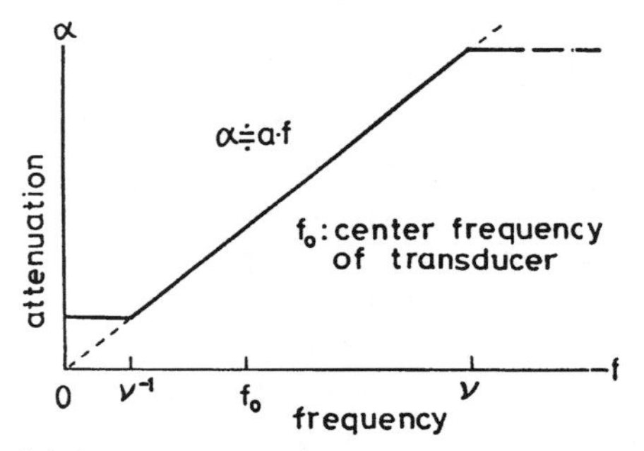

(a) A model of the attenuation characteristic

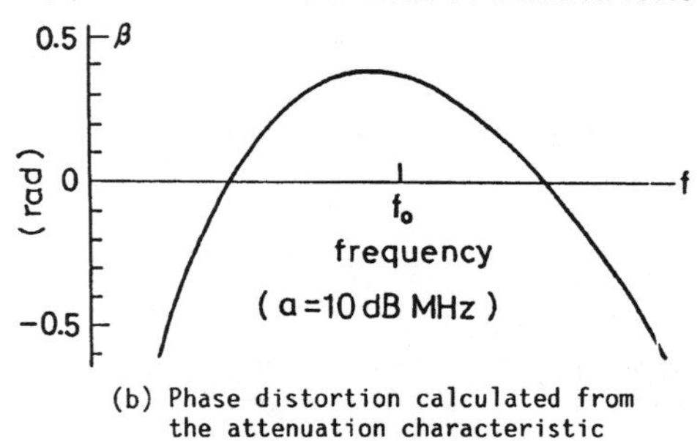

(b) Phase distortion calculated from the attenuation characteristic

Fig. 2. A model of the propagation characteristics of biological tissues.

The problem then is how the phase is affected by the choice of ν. It was shown that the curves of β are slightly convex upward and its slope with frequency is monotonously increasing as a function of ν, whereas the deviation of β from the straight-line is almost completely the same if ν is larger than a certain value [12]. Thus, the choice of ν affects only the time-delay and has little effect on the waveform distortion. As an example, the waveform distortion is calculated as shown in Fig. 3. Fig. 3(a) is the transmitted pulse waveform which is an impulse response of a resonant circuit with $Q=1$. The returned waveform calculated with the phase of Eq. (12) and the attenuation being 40 dB at the center frequency is shown in Fig. 3(b). In contrast, Fig.

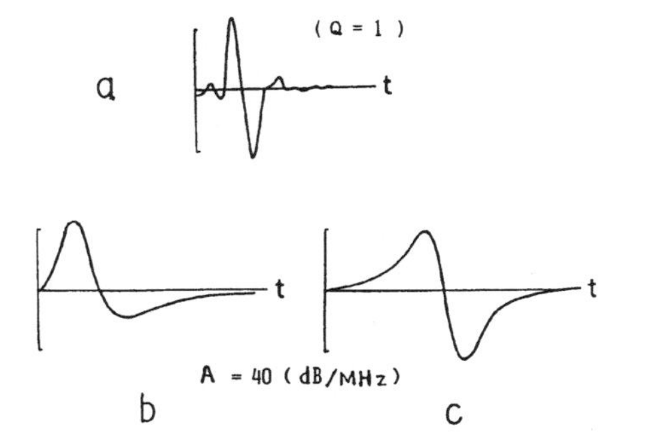

Fig. 3. Waveform distortion by frequency-dependent attenuation:(a) transmitted pulse waveform; (b) returned waveform calculated with the phase of Eq. (12); (c) returned waveform calculated without considering phase distortion.

3(c) is the waveform calculated considering only the phase incurred by the resonant characteristics and neglecting the phase of Eq. (12). Comparison of the two waveform indicates that the phase distortion due to the attenuation must be taken into account for the problem of treating the waveform.

Now we rewrite Eq. (9) as

$$\Phi(f,z) = \exp\left[-A(z)\cdot f - jB(f,z)\right] \tag{13}$$

where

$$A(z) \triangleq 2\ \ a(\xi)d\xi$$

$$B(f,z) \triangleq H[A\cdot f]$$

$$= 2\ \ \beta(f,\xi)d\xi \tag{14}$$

Thus, given the value of parameter A, which is referred to as the attenuation slope in this paper, the tissue transfer function with frequency is determined and the pulse waveform h is obtained from Eq. (5).

4. Resolution improvement and tissue characterization by parameter estimation

As mentioned in the preceding Section, the pulse waveform changes with propagation, so the convolution model described in Eq. (4) can be regarded as the time-varying system whose input is the reflection coefficient, output is the reflection signal and impulse response is the propagating pulse. The resolution improvement can be realized by estimating the specular component of the reflection coefficient, that is, estimating an input of the system. On the other hand, the estimation of the attenuation coefficient is equivalent to that of system parameter. If the pulse waveform h is given, the reflection coefficient can be estimated by deconvolution technique from the reflected signal. The pulse waveform, however, is unknown since it contains the unknown parameter A as described in Eq. (5). Thus, both pulse waveforms, i.e., the attenuation A and reflection coefficient must be estimated.

In order to estimate these two parameters, besides the relation described in Eq. (4), one more a priori knowledge or assumption about them is required. Usually, it is assumed that the reflection coefficient is random white sequence. Then, the power spectrum of propagating pulse $|H|^2$ is equivalent to that of the reflected signal $|Y|^2$ except for a noise component N. As a result, the problem of estimating the attenuation coefficient reduces to that of estimating $|H|^2$ from $|Y|^2$. These procedures are employed in several methods for estimating the attenuation, e.g., *spectral-shift* and *spectral difference method* [1, 5]. Once the attenuation is estimated, the pulse waveform h is obtained, then the reflection coefficient can be estimated by an inverse filter designed using h. However, the actual reflection coefficient is not completely random white and contains the specular component so that to apply this assumption to the reflected signal, averagings over a large region is required, which degrades the spatial resolution of estimated attenuation coefficient.

In the method proposed here, we introduce a criterion function based upon the estimates of reflection coefficient to estimate the two parameters. As shown in Fig. 4, our method consists of the esimator of the reflection coefficient and the part which calculates the criterion function and generates an estimate of the attenuation coefficient. In the following section, they will be concretely described.

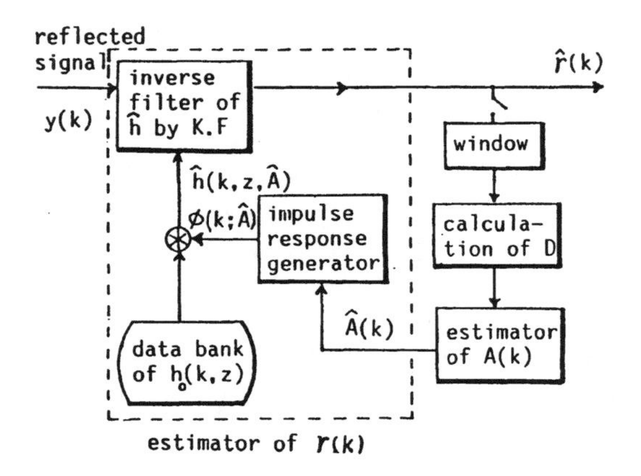

Fig. 4. Block diagram of the system to estimate the reflection coefficient and the attenuation coefficient.

5. Estimation of the reflection coefficient

A main part of the estimator of the reflection coefficient is an inverse filter whose inputs are the reflected signal and the pulse waveform h, and output is an estimate of the reflection coefficient. There may be some algorithm to constitute inverse filter. We here apply Kalman filter to the inverse filter by considering the pulse waveform as the impulse response of the time-varying system. Kalman filtering is suited to analyze a time-varying system, and has proven to be applicable to various problems such as seismic data processing and adaptive equalization for digital communication [7]. Application of Kalman filtering to the reflected signal was proposed by Kuc et al., which requires an analytical description of the pulse waveform [4]. In our approach, Kalman filter is applied more simply and directly by making use of the convolution model for reflected signals and general signal generating model for reflection coefficients [14].

In order to apply Kalman filtering, a state space representation of the system is required as follows

$$x(k) = A(k)\,x(k-1) + B(k-1)\,u(k-1) \qquad (15)$$
$$y(k) = C^T(k)\,x(k) + v(k) \qquad (16)$$

where x(k) is the $n \times 1$ state vector, A(k) is the $n \times n$ state transition matrix for n-th order system and k indicates a time domain index in the discrete form. u(k) is the $1 \times m$ input vector, y(k) is the $1 \times l$ output vector, v(k) is the $1 \times l$ measurement noise vector and B(k),C(k) are $n \times m$ and $n \times l$ matrices, respectively, where m is the order of the input vector and l is the order of output vector. C^T represents transposition of C. Eq. (15) is called the state equation of the system and Eq. (16) the observation equation. We assume that u(k) and v(k) are uncorrelated, zero mean, white noise processes:

$$\begin{aligned} &E[u(k)] = E[v(k)] = 0 \\ &E[u(k) \cdot u(j)^T] = U(k)\delta_{kj}, \text{ for all } k \\ &E[v(k) \cdot v(j)^T] = V(k)\delta_{kj} \end{aligned} \qquad (17)$$

where $E[\cdot]$ is the expectation operator and U(k) and V(k) are known diagonal matrices.

Now we formulate our problem in discrete state variable form to apply Kalman filtering as follows. At first, let us define the state vector v(k) as the set of reflection coefficients:

$$\gamma(k) \triangleq [\gamma_1(k), \gamma_2(k), \ldots, \gamma_N(k)]^T \qquad (18)$$

where

$$\begin{aligned} \gamma_i(k) &\triangleq \gamma\,((N-i)\Delta t,\, k\Delta z) \\ &= \gamma\,((N+k-i)\Delta t,\, 0) \end{aligned} \qquad (19)$$

and define the vector h as

$$h(k) \triangleq [h_1(k), h_2(k), \ldots, h_n(k)]^T \qquad (20)$$

where

$$h_i(k) \triangleq h(i\Delta t,\, k\Delta z) \qquad (21)$$

then Eq. (4) can be written in the discrete form:

$$y(k) = h^T(k) \cdot \gamma(k) + n(k) \qquad (22)$$

Eq. (22) is exactly the form of the observation equation (16).

Next, to formulate our problem in the form of state equation, we assume that reflection coefficient sequences are generated by the ARMA model as

$$\gamma_i(k) + \sum_{n=1}^{N} p_n \gamma_{i-n}(k) = w(k) + \sum_{m=1}^{M} q_m w(k-m) \quad (23)$$

This is a more general expression for multi-channel input of noise. Using Eq. (18), Eq. (23) can now be written in the form of state equation as follows

$$\gamma(k) = A(k)\gamma(k-1) + B(k)u(k-1) \quad (24)$$

where

$$u(k-1) \triangleq [w(k),\ w(k-1),\ \ldots,\ w(k-M+1)]^T \quad (25)$$

and

$$A = \begin{matrix} p_1\ p_2 \cdots p_N \\ 1 \quad\quad 0 \\ \cdots \\ 0 \quad 1\ 0 \end{matrix},\ B = \begin{matrix} 1\ q_1\ q_2 \cdots q_M \\ \\ 0 \end{matrix} \quad (26)$$

Values of coefficient p_n and q_m must be determined. It is interesting theme to estimate the optimal values of them. As a simple case, however, we here set them to $p_n = 1/N$ ($n = 1, .., N$) and $q_m = 0$ ($m = 1, .., M$), which is based upon the assumption that the value of a reflection coefficient at a particular sample time is expressed as the mean of the previous N reflection coefficients. It will be shown later that good results are obtained though this simple assumption.

After the model is formulated above, an optimal estimate of state vector, $\hat{\gamma}(k/k)$, for the given pulse waveform h(k), can be sequentially obtained by the Kalman filter equations as [3]

$$\hat{\gamma}(k/k-1) = A\hat{\gamma}(k-1/k-1) \quad (27a)$$
$$P(k/k-1) = AP(k-1/k-1)A^T + \sigma_u^2 BB^T \quad (27b)$$
$$K(k) = P(k/k-1)h(k)[h^T(k)P(k/k-1) \cdot h(k) + \sigma_n^2]^{-1} \quad (27c)$$
$$e(k) = y(k) - h^T(k)\hat{\gamma}(k/k-1) \quad (27d)$$
$$\hat{\gamma}(k/k) = \hat{\gamma}(k/k-1) + e(k)K(k) \quad (27e)$$
$$P(k/k) = [I-K(k)h^T(k)]P(k/k-1) \quad (27f)$$
$$\text{for } k = 1,2,\ldots$$

where

$$\sigma_n^2 = E[n^2],\ \sigma_u^2 = E[U^TU] \quad (27g)$$

and initial values are

$$\gamma(0/0) = 0 \quad (27h)$$
$$P(0/0) = \mu I \quad (27i)$$

where I is identity matrix, μ is a positive constant and $\hat{\gamma}(k/j)$ denotes the estimate of $\gamma(k)$ based upon measurement y(1),y(2),. . .,y(j). Finally, out of N elements of vector $\hat{\gamma}(k/k)$, $\hat{\gamma}_N(k)$ is taken as the best estimate of $\gamma(k \cdot \triangle t, 0)$. In general, many computations for matrix operations are required to carry out the discrete Kalman filtering, whereas in the above case it is possible to reduce the computational requirements by considering properties of the matrices, for example, matrix P is symmetrical and most of elements in matrix A are zero.

6. Estimation of the attenuation coefficient

In this Section, we discuss the attenuation estimator which receives estimates of reflection coefficients and produces an estimate of the attenuation coefficient that is given to the reflection coefficient estimator. As mentioned above, to estimate the two parameters from the reflected signal, it is necessary to introduce a criterion function. Based on how the shape of an estimated reflection coefficient in the case of a single reflector changes as the function of the attenuation, we here define the following criterion function:

$$D(\varepsilon) = \frac{\int_{t_1}^{t_2} Env(t)dt}{\max_{t_1 \le t \le t_2} [Env(t)]} \quad (28)$$

where

$$Env(t)\text{:envelope of } |\hat{\gamma}(t)| \quad (29)$$
$$\varepsilon \triangleq \hat{A} - A \quad (30)$$

The function D is a measure that indicates how the power of the estimated reflection coefficient is localized, in other words, how sharp each pulse composing the estimate of the reflection coefficient is. The value of the function D is positive and becomes minimum when the difference between an estimate and the true value, ε, is nearly equal to zero. Fig. 5 illustrates this situation in the case of a single reflector. Fig. 5(a) shows the function D which is calculated from the estimate, $\hat{\gamma}$, described by

$$\hat{\gamma}(t;\varepsilon) = 2\ \mathrm{Re} \int_0^{\infty} W(f) e^{-\varepsilon f - j\beta}\, e^{j2\pi ft}\, df \tag{31}$$

where W(f) is window function corresponding to the frequency band of the transducer. In Fig. 5(b) it is shown that the envelope of $|r(t;\varepsilon)|$ becomes sharper as the value of ε approaches zero, which can be understood as follows. For a simplification, assuming $\beta = 0$ and $W(f) = 0$ for $|f| > f_1$ and $W(f) = 1$ for $|f| \leq f_1$, then Eq. (31) becomes

$$\begin{aligned} r(t;\varepsilon) &= 2\mathrm{Re} \int_0^{f_1} e^{-\varepsilon f + j2\pi ft}\, df \\ &= 2\{\varepsilon\ (1 - e^{-\varepsilon f_1} \cos 2\pi f_1 t) \\ &\qquad - 2\pi t e^{-\varepsilon f_1} \sin 2\pi f_1 t\}/(4\pi^2 t^2 + \varepsilon^2) \end{aligned} \tag{32}$$

We note that for e>0 the width of Env(t) equal to ε/π is monotonously increasing as a function of ε since the term $2\varepsilon/(4\pi^2 t^2 + \varepsilon^2)$ in Eq. (32) is dominant, whereas for $\varepsilon > 0$ the terms $e^{-\varepsilon f_1}\cos 2\pi f_1 t$ and $e^{-\varepsilon f_1}\sin 2\pi f_1 t$ are dominant, thus the width of Env(t) decreases as the value of ε increases. Instead of measuring the width of Env(t) directly, the integration form is used for the function D in Eq. (28) since it is more sensitive to noise and easier to measure.

In general, when the criterion function which is convex and becomes minimum for the optimal esimate is given, the optimal value can be obtained by algorithm of adaptive processing such as the *steepest descent method.* In the practical case, however, the function D does not change smoothly due to noise and interference by adjacent pulses. Thus to detect such a value of $\hat{A}$ as that minimizes the value of D, we use the following algorithm

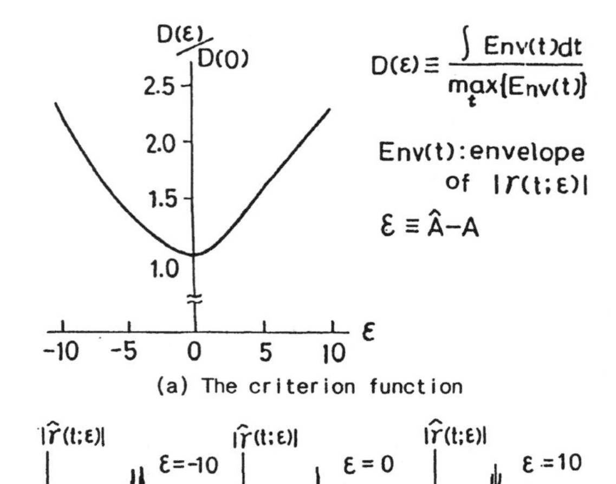

Fig. 5. The criterion function and shapes of $|\hat{\gamma}(t;e)|$ (in the case of a single reflector).

Step 1: Calculate D_i, for $i = n - L, n - L + 1, \ldots, n + L$, which indicates the values of D for A_i, where $A_i \triangleq \Delta A \cdot i$ for $i>0$ and $A_i \triangleq 0$ for $i<0$.

Step 2: Stop iteration, with $\hat{A} = A_n$ being the optimal estimate if the following condition is satisfied. Otherwise, go to Step 3.

$$D_n = \min_{n-L \leq i \leq n+L} [\ D_i\ ] \tag{33}$$

Step 3: Calculate D_{n+L+i} and return to Step 2 after increasing n by 1.

Combining the above process with the reflection coefficient estimator discussed in Section 5, the attenuation coefficient and the reflection coefficient can be estimated simultaneously. However the attenuation compared with the reflection coefficient varies slowly with depth, so in the case of estimating these parameters by sliding the region Ω, it is not always necessary to estimate the attenuation in each region. For example, it is possible to reduce computation time by means of estimating the two parameters in some regions, and operating only the reflection coefficient estimator for fixed values of the attenuation slope in other regions.

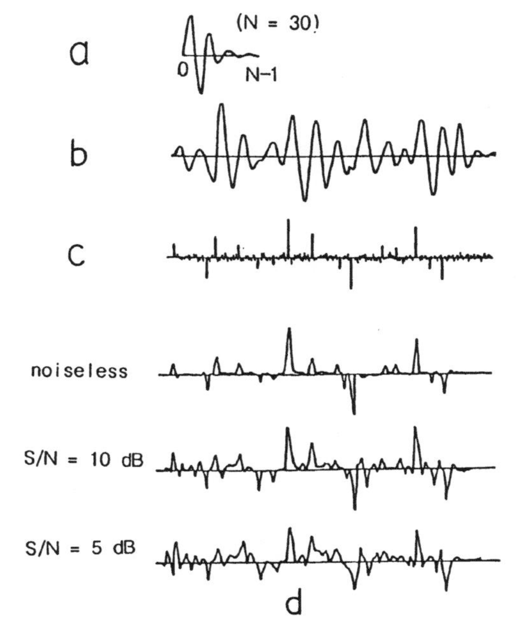

Fig. 6. Estimation of reflection coefficient by Kalman filtering: (a) pulse waveform h(k); (b) a reflected signal y(k) synthesized by (a) and (c); (c) reflection coefficient $\gamma(k)$; (d) estimated reflection coefficient $\hat{\gamma}(k)$.

7. Results of simulation and experiment

7.1 Results of simulation

To investigate the ability of the method discussed above, the synthetic echoes were generated by convolving a known pulse waveform and reflection coefficient. Fig. 6(a), (b) show the pulse waveform and the synthesized reflected signal, respectively. The pulse waveform consists of 30 sampled values. Thus the order of the system is set to $N = 30$. Fig. 6(c) is the reflection coefficient which consists of the specular component, i.e., impulse sequences whose positions conform to a Poisson distribution and amplitudes are uniformly distributed, and the random component which is a Gaussian zero-mean random sequence. To demonstrate the effect of noise on the reflection coefficient estimator, white random Gaussian noise was added to the synthetic signal of Fig. 6(b). The estimated reflection coefficients by the estimator are shown in Fig. 6(d). It can be seen that the estimator still supplies satisfying results down to a signal-to-noise ratio of 10 dB.

Next, the simulated signal containing the attenuation characteristic was used to illustrate the estimation of the attenuation slope. Fig. 7(a) is the reflected signal generated by convolving the reflection coefficient of Fig. 6(c) and the pulse waveform calculated from that of Fig. 6(a) with the attenuation slope of $A = 10$ dB/MHz. Fig. 7(b) shows the criterion function D calculated as increasing the value of $\hat{A}$ in 1 dB/MHz steps for different values of signal-to-noise ratio S/N. The values of D became minimum when $\hat{A}$ is equal to the true value (10 dB/MHz) in both cases, i.e., S/N = 20 and 50 dB. However, note that the minimum values of L requisite for detecting the optimal value of $\hat{A}$ according to the algorithm described in Eq. (33) is 3 for S/N = 50 dB, whereas it increases to 5 for S/N = 20 dB due to the larger variation of values of D. Fig. 7(c) shows estimates of the reflection coefficient $\hat{\gamma}$ for different values of $\hat{A}$. It can be seen that $\hat{\gamma}$ is most similar to γ of Fig. 6(c) and the envelope of $|\hat{\gamma}|$ most sharpens when $\hat{A}$ is equal to 10 dB/MHz.

7.2 Experimental results

The reflected signals from biological tissues were used to examine whether the proposed method can be applied to practical cases. The data were obtained with a clinically applied 3.5 MHz transducer and digitized to 10 bit accuracy, at a 20 MHz sampling rate. They were processed by the method with the order of system set to $N = 30$. Fig. 8(a) shows one of the reflected signals from a block of pork consisting of two layers, i.e., muscle and fat. Large echoes observed in Fig. 8(a) correspond to the interface between muscle and fat, and that between fat and acrylic plate used for a stand. Fig. 8(b) is an estimate of the reflection coefficient in case where only the reflection coefficient estimator was operated with the attenuation being set to $\hat{A} = 0$. Note that the width of the pulses is still broad since the attenuation characteristic has not been removed. On the other hand Fig. 8(c) shows the result of the simultaneous estimation of the attenuation and reflection coefficients. It is seen

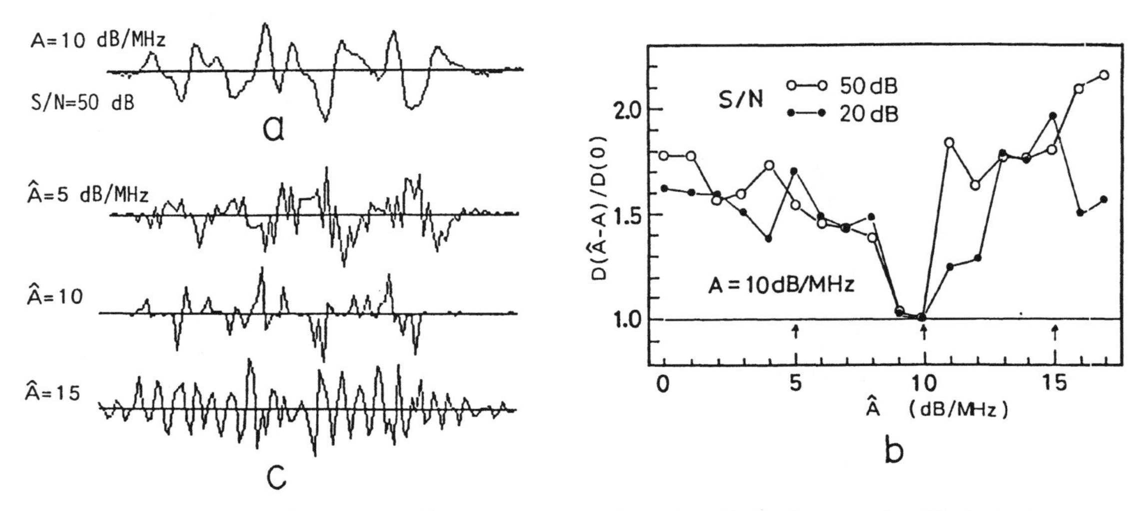

Fig. 7. Estimation of the attenuation coeficient: (a) a reflected signal synthesized considering the attenuation; (b) criterion function D; (c) estimates of the reflection coefficient for different values of Â.

that the pulse duration is compressed to less than 1/3 of that of Fig. 8(a), as a result, the resolution is improved. On the other hand the attenuation slope of the muscle layer is estimated to be 21.6 dB/MHz. To evaluate this value, it is also estimated by *spectral difference method* [5] from the random component. The result is to be 23.1 dB/MHz, which is in very good agreement with the above value. These values are different from those of live tissues since in our case the tissue sample was not so fresh and data were obtained at 24° C which is lower than body temperature.

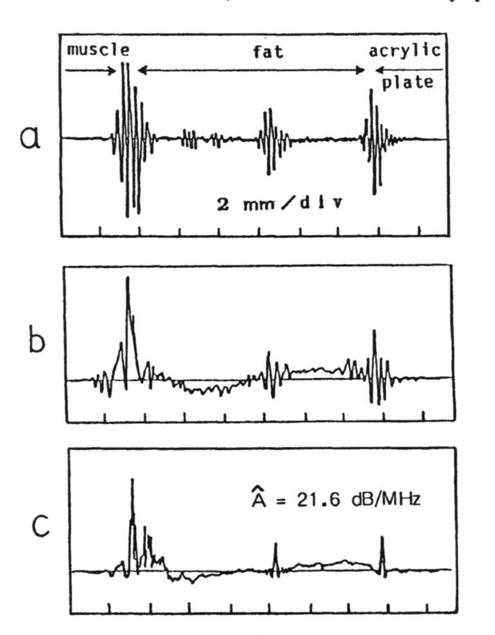

Fig. 8. Results of estimation for experimental data (pork): (a) A reflected signal; (b) estimated reflection coefficient without conpensation for attenuation; (c) estimated reflection cofficient and attenuation slope.

Furthermore, many reflected signals were similarly processed and used to construct the B-mode image as shown in Fig. 9(a). Fig. 9(b) shows a conventional B-mode image constructed by usual envelope detection of reflected signals. By comparing two images, the improvement of resolution is clear. Especially the parts corresponding to the interface between fat and acrylic plate, which is approximately equal to a plane, is indicated as a broad and blurred line in Fig. 9(b), whereas it becomes sharper in Fig. 9(a). These results verified this method is promising for implementation.

8. Conclusion

We proposed the method of extracting two tissue parameters, i.e., the reflection coefficient and attenuation coefficient from the reflected ultrasound for the purpose of improving the resolution and obtaining the information on tissue characerization.

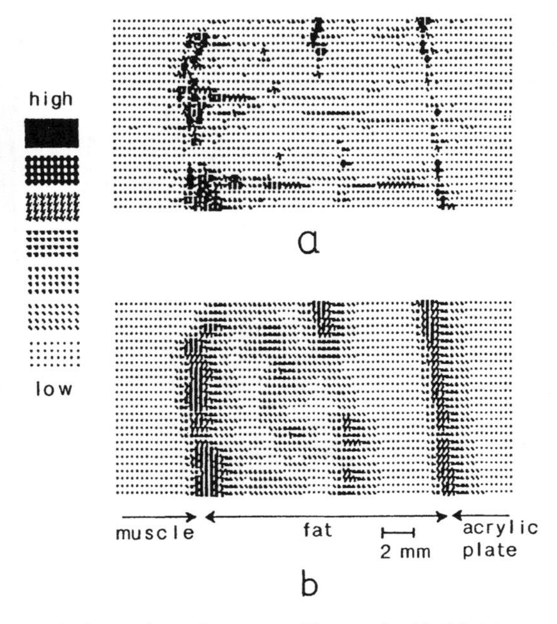

Fig. 9. Comparison of constructed images (pork): (a) A image constructed using processed data; (b) a conventional B-mode image.

First, a convolution model for reflection signals and tissue transfer function based on frequency-dependent attenuation were introduced. Next, the reflection coefficient estimator was described: the reflection coefficient is estimated by deconvolution technique using Kalman filter taking into account the distortion of the propagating pulse due to the frequency-dependent attenuation. On the other hand, the attenuation coefficient is estimated by adaptive processing based upon the criterion function calculated using estimates of the reflection coefficient.

Finally, the proposed method was examined by computer simulation and the experimental data. Results of simulation verified that this method improved the resolution and produced a good estimate of the attenuation, and experimental results showed this to be applicable in the practical case. There are some problems that are not illustrated here. For example, determining optimal values of the parameters of Kalman filter and using the random component for parameter estimating are left for future studies.

References

1. Fink M, Hottier F, Cardoso JF: Ultrasonic signal processing for in vivo attenuation measurement; short time Fourier analysis. Ultrasonic Imaging 5: 117–135, 1983.
2. Glover GH: Computerized time-of-flight ultrasonic tomography for breast examination. Ultrasound Med Biol 3: 117–127, 1977.
3. Kalman RE: A new approach to linear filtering and prediction problem. Trans ASME series DJ of Basic Eng 82: 34–45, 1960.
4. Kuc R: Application of Kalman filtering techniques to diagnostic ultrasound. Ultrasonic Imaging 1: 105–120, 1979.
5. Kuc R, Schwartz M: Estimating the acoustic attenuation coefficient slope for liver from reflected ultrasound signals. IEEE Trans Sonic & Ultrason SU-26 5: 353–362, 1979.
6. Kuc R, Taylor KJW: Variation of acoustic attenuation coefficient slope estimates for in vivo liver. Ultrasonic Med Biol 8: 403–412, 1982.
7. Lawrence RE, Kaufman H: The Kalman filter for the equalization of digital communication channel. IEEE Trans COM-19 60: 1137–1144, 1971.
8. Maklad NF, Ophir J, Balsara V: Attenuation of ultrasound liver and diffuse liverdisease in vivo. Ultrasonic Imaging 6: 117–125, 1984.
9. Mimbs JW, Yubas DE, Miller JG, Weuss AN, Sobel BE: Detection of myiocadial infarction in vivo based on altered attenuation of ultrasound. Circ Res 41, pp 192–197, 1977.
10. O'Donnel M, Miller JG: Quantitative broadband ultrasonic backscatter; an approach to nondestructive evaluation in acoustically inhomogenious materials. J Appl Phys 52: 1056–1065, 1981.
11. Ophir J, Maklad NF, Bigelow RH: Ultrasonic attenuation measurements of in vivo human muscle. Ultrasonic Imaging 4: 290–295, 1982.
12. Saito M: Basic aspects of ultrasonic signal processing. Proc of the Biological Engineering Society 6th Nordic Meeting Aberdeen, CIGI: 3, 1984.
13. Shiina T, Ikeda K, Saito M: Separation of specular and random components in ultrasonic echo. Proc of Int Symp on Noise and Clutter Rejection in Radars and Imaging Sensors, 152–157, 1984.
14. Shiina T, Ikeda K, Saito M: Analysis of reflected ultrasound by adaptive filtering; for improvement of resolution and tissue characterization. proc of 14 ICMBE and 7th ICMP, 623–624, Espoo, 1985.

Address for offprints:
Tsuyoshi Shiina
Institute of Medical Electronics
Faculty of Medicine
University of Tokyo
7-3-1 Hongo, Bunkyo-ku
Tokyo 113, Japan

Medical Progress through Technology 12: 197–211 (1987)

Recent progress of technology in obstetrics and gynecology, particularly in perinatal medicine in Japan

Kazuo Maeda
Department of Obstetrics and Gynecology, Tottori University School of Medicine, Yonago 683 Japan

Key words: perinatology, fetal heart rate, ultrasonography, computer, uterus, tissue characterisation

Introduction

There has been remarkable improvement in the perinatal mortality in Japan as noted in the reports of national statistics of the Ministry of Health and Welfare. It will be the least perinatal mortality among the countries in the world where the births are more than one million over the last 2 to 3 years. Namely, the mortality of Japan was less than 10 in 1,000 births in a year. This improvement was obtained by the change of socioeconomical condition until 1980, but the progress after that period is interpreted as the result of the efforts in the management of the mother and infant in the perinatal stage (Morio, 1985). This effort includes that of the staffs in the clinics and also the advancements of the tools in the new technologies which have been seriously studied since the 1960s. The most important modality would be the progress of fetal monitoring in labor and pregnancy in these 20 years. The external techniques include the use of fetal heart signals detected at maternal abdomen, which is the most commonly the ultrasonic Doppler fetal heart signal, and that of external tocodynamometry. This technique resulted in the monitoring of whole labor and also the diagnosis of pregnant women prior to the onset of labor with the technique of the non-stress test (NST) which is the antepartum cardiotocogram (CTG) recorded for 40 to 60 min. mainly in high-risk patients. The management with rapid delivery after the diagnosis of fetal hypoxia with the technique reduced the unexpected fetal deaths during pregnancy and in labor, and also decreased the perinatal morbidity including neonatal asphyxia, respiratory distress and the meconium aspiration syndrome. The reduction of cerebral palsy after growing-up can be expected if the fetal monitoring and the management is adequately carried out in perinatal stage. Fetal heart rate (FHR) analysis is one of the main targets of the research in order to obtain further improvement, since the main component of the fetal monitoring has been the diagnosis of FHR records. A new technique for the recording of uterine contractions is hoped for, and some trials are being carried out. Another important progress obtained in this decade is the improvement of ultrasonographic diagnosis with the real-time B-mode device which in our country mainly consists of electronic scan. The device is used not only in big hospitals but also even in most of private obstetrics clinics in our country. Fetal heart M-mode, 2 dimensional echocardiography, however, is used mostly in the hospitals where the fetal cardiologists study the fetal heart. Blood flow studies with the pulsed or CW ultrasonic Doppler device on the fetus or the mother are also still carried out in big hospitals or university laboratories. Computer processing of analog data was introduced in our field since the 1970s, and also the descriptive data analysis into the field of perinatal management. This review will deal only in the most prominent results of the recent few years.

Fetal heart rate analysis

Original fetal heart signals including fetal electrocardiogram (ECG) and phonocardiogram had been precisely analyzed and studied in order to detect fetal abnormality during labor prior to FHR monitoring in the 1960s. The results obtained were the usefulness of FHR in the diagnosis for fetal hypoxia. FHR monitoring is most frequently used in the present in fetal diagnosis for that reason. However, the basis of more correct information obtained in FHR change has been recently sought in the field of obstetrical engineering. Koyanagi (1986) reported unique mathematical analysis and the histogram on the large amount of dispersed FHR values showing the fetal CNS development in the histogram change and its variation in NTD patients.

The studies on fetal ECG and ultrasonic Doppler signals

The detecting error of fetal direct ECG in conventional fetal heart rate metering was studied with the comparison to a precise digital system, and was found to be 0.5 to 1.5 bpm, and more in the case of increased noise. From the results, the meter is suitable for LTV (long term variability) detection but may not be used for STV (short term variability) processing. Also the detection error was tested in the 1 MHz Doppler fetal heart signal in comparison to direct fetal ECG (Yagi et al., 1985a, b). Abdominal lead fetal ECG can be used in the study of fetal heart, and the QRS detecting technique has been frequently reported (Ninomiya et al., 1985, 1986). Direct lead fetal ECG was detected through a punctured maternal abdominal wall in order to obtain a clear record (Kubo et al., 1985). Tsujii et al. (1985) reported the detection of fetal heart rate between 6–9 weeks of gestation with the use of M-mode signal and autocorrelation technique. Fetal heart rate was the most accurate predictor of gestational weeks in the stage between 6–8 weeks. Fujibayashi et al. (1986) analyzed the M-mode signal of fetal heart directly by digital scan converter with FFT technique and found the heart wall signal in the fetus before 6 weeks and valve signals after 8 weeks. Maeda et al. (1981) developed a new device for the continuous recording of the systolic time intervals of the fetal heart utilizing direct fetal ECG and CW ultrasonic Doppler fetal heart signals. The technique was applied to the analysis of fetal heart action in labor (Yoneda, 1981) and during pregnancy (Nakamura, 1982). The changes were related to the FHR, but showed unique change in variable deceleration which was related to cord compression. Maeda et al. (1984) found characteristic change of PEP/VET in the cases of fetal distress in labor.

Fetal cardiac function has been studied by ultrasonic blood flowmetry with pulsed and CW ultrasound. Murakami et al. (1986) studied the pulsation in umbilical venous blood flow in the case of circulatory failure and found the high level of their pulsation ratio to be the ratio of the lowest blood flow velocity in venous blood to the highest one. The authors also found the pulsation of the blood flow profile in the inferior vena cava of a hydropic fetus (1986). Tricuspid blood flow regurgitation is now discussed in the detection of fetal heart failure.

Improvement of fetal heart rate meter with autocorrelation technique

The use of direct fetal ECG with its peak detection and trigger formation followed by interval measurement and the calculation of beat-to-beat instantaneous heart rate recording had been the standard type of old conventional FHR monitor. Recent demands to examine FHR even in nonstress tests (NST) during pregnancy with the diagnostic accuracy similar to direct fetal ECG promoted the more simple external but accurate FHR record with ultrasonic Doppler signal of the fetal heart. Real-time autocorrelation technique has matched this request. Fetal ultrasonic Doppler signal which is detected by continuous or very weak pulsed ultrasound and the real-time autocorrelation heart rate meter is capable of demonstrating almost the same LTV of FHR as obtained by fetal direct lead ECG and conventional triggering type instantaneous heart rate meters. It is very natural that other FHR patterns including the baseline, transient rise (acceleration) and fall (deceleration) are clearly recorded by the method. Although the use of this type fetal monitor has been a few years in foreign countries, Japan has widely utilized the real-time autocorrelation FHR meter in this decade. As the results: 1) all labors are monitored, since the technique is non-invasive in the case of the association of external tocodynamometry; 2) antepartum CTG is diagnosed under the same clinical accuracy as intrapartum FHR monitoring; 3) CTG examination is carried out through pregnancy, labor and delivery using single technique and uniform interpretation criteria. Full intrapartum monitoring of all labor cases and the use of NST in high-risk cases in outpatient clinics with the association of appropriate treatment of fetal hypoxia has resulted in markedly reduced perinatal mortality, decreased neonatal morbidity and significantly decreased cerebral palsy patients who were registered to the regional governmental health center, while the cesarean rate is as low as 10% or less in the affiliate hospital of the author (Tsuzaki et al., 1986). Contraction stress test (CST) has been almost discarded in our district, since fetal diagnosis is sufficient with the use of autocorrelation fetal monitors.

The improvement of external tocodynamometry

Uterine contraction is the expulsive force of the fetus in the labor, and also it is one of important factors influencing the intrapartum fetus. Therefore, the contraction curve is the reference channel of the FHR tracing in CTG. Catheter insertion and intrauterine pressure measurement had been the main technique in conventional old fetal monitoring, and modern monitoring also prepares the ability of internal measurement. However, the internal technique is as invasive to the mother as the direct ECG electrode to the fetus. External transducer of fetal monitoring has become common in our country for that reason. A guard-ring type external transducer is placed on maternal abdomen in this case. Recently, the feature of the external transducer was discussed in the study group of medical engineering in perinatal medicine of the Japan Society of Medical Electronics and Biological Engineering, and new standards for the external transducer were published (1985). The study group is also discussing the new technique for the external uterine contraction detection. There have also been presented the computer processing of the burst discharge of electrical activity of the uterine muscle, that of multiple small external transducer outputs, and the Moiré curve changes obtained at the maternal abdomen in the labor. The topogram of the electrical signal changes according to the mechanical contraction of the uterus, and the accumulation of the potentials resembles the common uterine contraction curve (Fig. 1; Takagi et al., 1986). Multiple transducer technique also presents similar results (Nakajima, 1986). The Moiré pattern is the optical method, expressing the multiple contour lines on maternal abdomen which changes along with the increase of the uterine contraction (Fig. 2; Sumimoto, 1986).

Other than the external detection technique, there are several basic studies on the action of the uterine muscle. For instance, Ikeda et al. (1984) and Kawarabayashi et al. (1986) reported their studies on the action potential of the human myometrium. They found three types of action potentials which were spike, plateau and intermediate types in the configuration, and the types were influenced by the location of the muscle or the environmental condition around the muscle cells.

Automatic analysis of FHR and its application

Automatic computer-aided analysis of FHR pattern is utilized in some computerized fetal monitoring systems (Fukuju et al., 1985; Inaba et al., 1986), signal processors (Nakajima et al., 1985) and standalone FHR analyzers in Japan. The author intended computer analysis of FHR pattern in the 1960s developing a simple FHR pattern analytic method which resulted in a unique FHR score. The score has been widely accepted in many countries. In the 1970s, the author planned to develop an automatic FHR analysis and diagnosis program utilizing HP 2100A minicomputer with the software of which main component was the FHR score. The plan was successful (Maeda et al., 1980), and the program was transplanted into a unifunctioned microcomputer system. The results were also satisfactory and

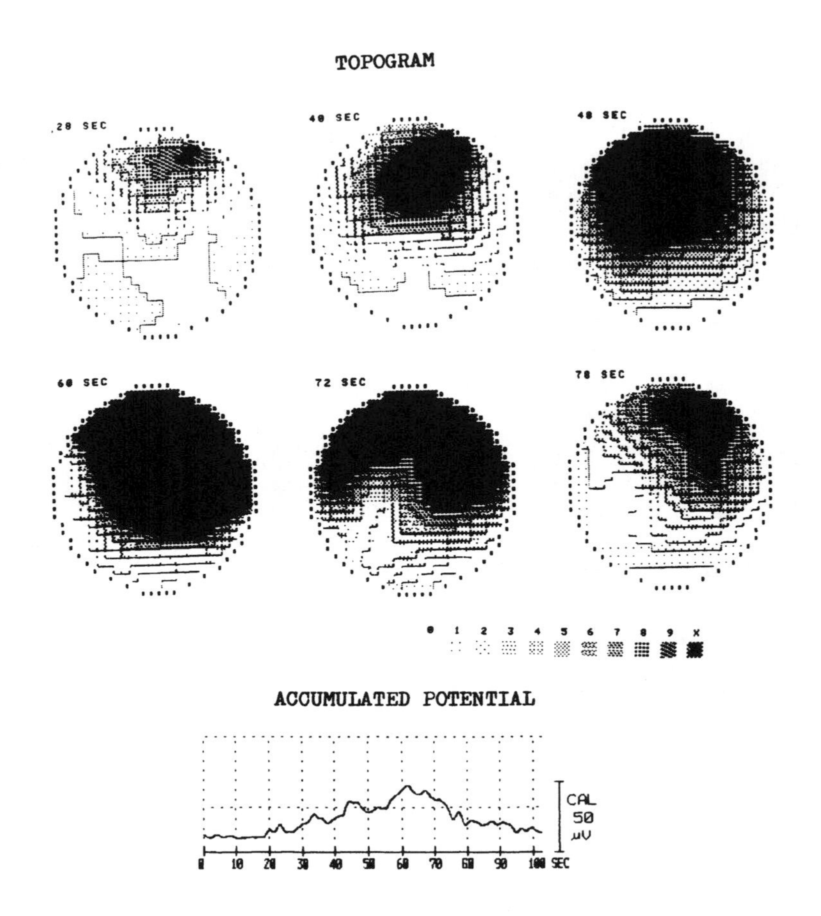

Fig. 1. The chronological changes of topograms, from left upper to right lower, which was obtained by the processing of electrical signals of the 12 points of the maternal abdomen. Accumulation of the electrical potentials forms a curve, shown at bottom, that is similar to the mechanical uterine contraction curve. (By the Courtsy of Drs. Matsuoka, Sakata, Takagi et al., Department of Obstetrics & Gynecology, Nippon University.)

coincided with the diagnosis of trained physicians (Maeda, 1981). The machine feeds a small printer which prints out the analysis parameters and also the automatic diagnosis (Fig. 3).

Wrong transducer placement or increased noise are also signaled by the printout. A remote alarm panel is also prepared. The machine is useful in clinical obstetrics, though there may be very long printout charts in a prolonged labor. Some difficulty may be present in overviewing the whole printout. Further data compression will be requested in the future in FHR data storage. For these reasons, we intended to develope the multiple simultaneous display of the automated analysis parameters on single color display including fetal distress index, FHR score, uterine contraction area, number of dips, baseline FHR, variability and lag time. The device is 'Trendgram of FHR analysis' (Fig. 4). The trendgram is easy to handle and it can analyse a long course of labor. Diagnosis is easy, and the results were compared to the states of umbilical cord arterial blood with good sensitivity and specificity (Maeda et al., 1985; Irie et al., 1985).

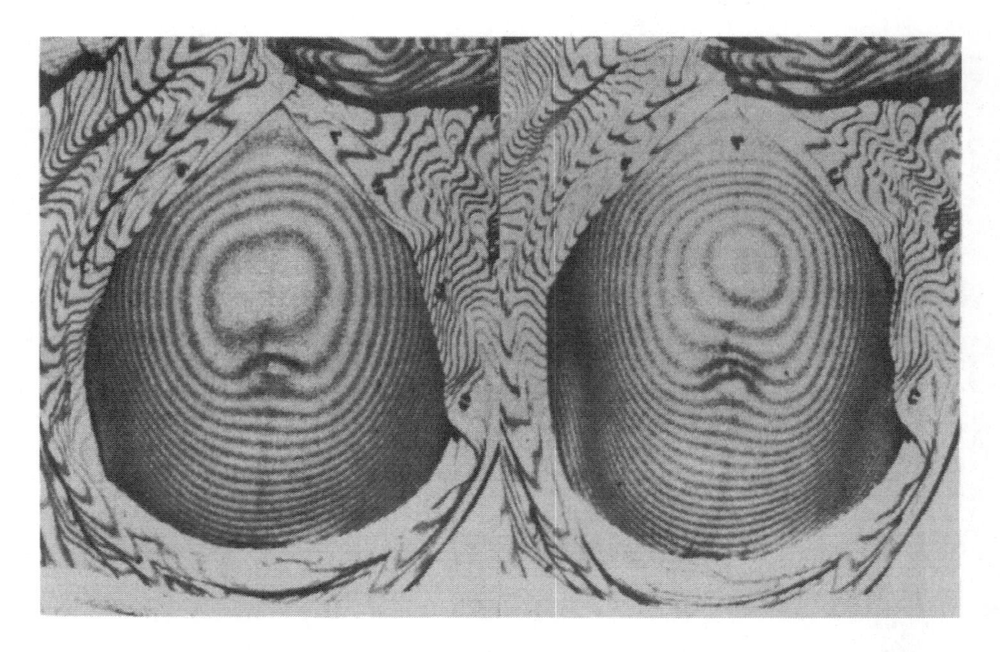

Fig. 2. Moiré effect which was produced on maternal abdomen in the labor. Left side is processed between the uterine contractions, and the right in the uterine contraction. (By the Courtsey of Dr. K. Sumimoto, Department of Obstetrics & Gynecology, Hamamatsu Medical University.)

Frequency analysis of FHR pattern

FHR curve is composed of several parameters other than the DC signal, FHR-baseline including baseline variability, acceleration and deceleration. FHR-baseline variability is discussed with the classification of LTV and STV which has been studied with many mathematical methods through computer processing. Deceleration and acceleration are usually analysed by eye, though the significance in fetal well-being is somewhat different among the two parameters. For these very complicated researches, many planned to investigate the FHR pattern using frequency analysis. Taguchi (1983) studied the FHR with FFT technique, and found the difference along with the change of fetal and neonatal resting and active states. The loss of baseline variability case, of course, showed severe loss of the high frequency component. A case of sinusoidal pattern showed the peak in the low frequency area. Kitada (1984) studied the frequency components of FHR with autocorrelation and cross correlation to the sine waves produced in the computer. The cyclic changes of FHR were observed in the cases who were in the resting state. The main frequency was between 2 and 3 cpm in these cases. Neonates showed similar results. Sugimoto et al. (1985) studied the frequency analysis of FHR with linear prediction method and found the peaks at 0.15 Hz and 0.33 Hz. Noguchi et al. (1986) also studied the frequency analysis with the method of generating function of heart-rate variability. Fukamanai et al. (1985) reported FFT analysis on LTV of FHR.

Analysis of sinusoidal FHR pattern

The sinusoidal FHR pattern (SP) is the fluctuating pattern of FHR-baseline which resembles a sine wave with the frequency usually less than 6 cycles per minute (cpm). The duration is long, and the small variation of the FHR which superimposes the sinusoidal pattern is very small, hence the pattern

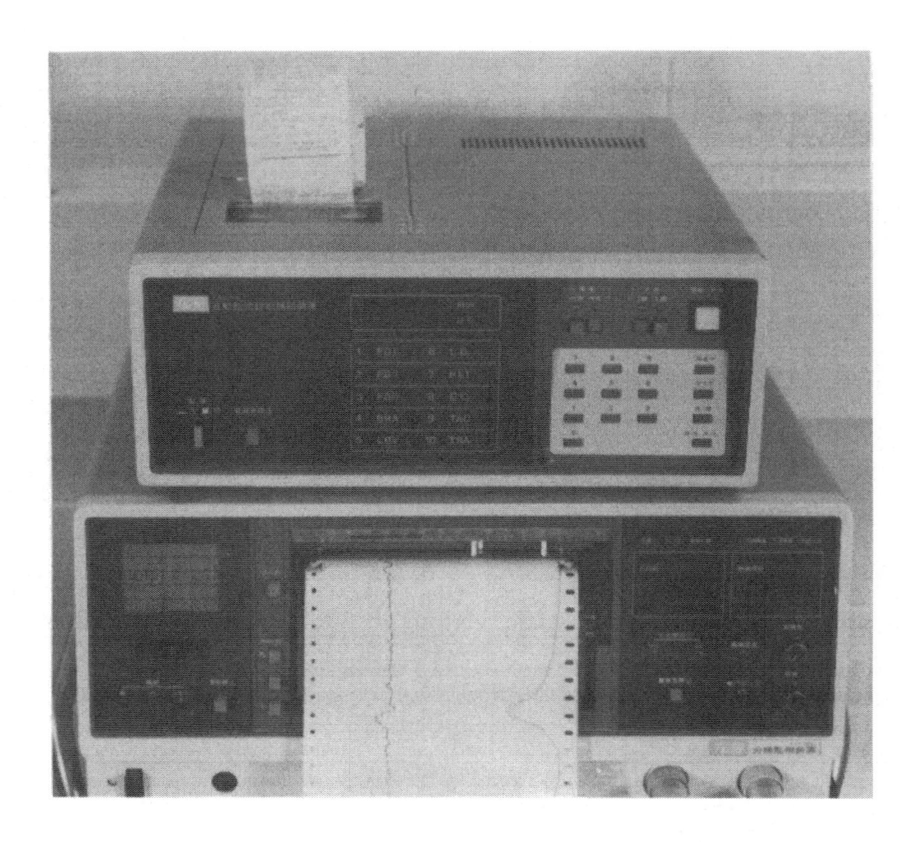

Fig. 3. The microcomputer system which incorporates the fixed automatic fetal-distress diagnosis program on PROM (upper device) and the autocorrelation fetal monitor which is connected to the microcomputer system (lower one).

seems smooth. The pattern is reported to appear in the cases of fetal anemia and hypoxia. Usually SP is an ominous sign for the fetus, and fetal distress or fetal death frequently occurs after its appearance. However, correct definition of the pattern is still uncommon due to its rare occurrence. Maeda et al. (1983) reported a tentative definition of the pattern in a very common way, namely, the pattern will be: 1) sine wave like CTG with the frequency less than 6 cpm; 2) the largest amplitude of SP is 10 bpm or more; 3) it lasts 10 minutes or longer; 4) frequency and amplitude of the waves are regular; and 5) the smaller variability superimposed on the SP is minimum, hence it looks very smooth. Although the cause of the pattern is discussed in many reports, we wanted to collect many of them in order to classify and define it from its characteristic wave form. Many CTG charts which were thought to be the SP were collected by a member of the Committee on Medical Engineering of the Japan Society of Obstetrics and Gynecology, analysed and are ready to be reported in detail in the very near future. The author (1984) intended to express the feature of the pattern with single parameter, and developed the sinusoidal pattern index (SPI) which was composed of the statistic values on its cyclicity and amplitude. Namely, the SPI is 1000 divided by square root of the sum of the square of the coefficients of variation of the intervals between the waves and that of every amplitude. SPI is expected to be 20 or more in the case of true SP. Although an on-line computer program which can be applied to the output of a fetal monitor was developed, a more convenient program which can analyze already recorded SP on the CTG was also prepared and utilized in the SP registration to the Com-

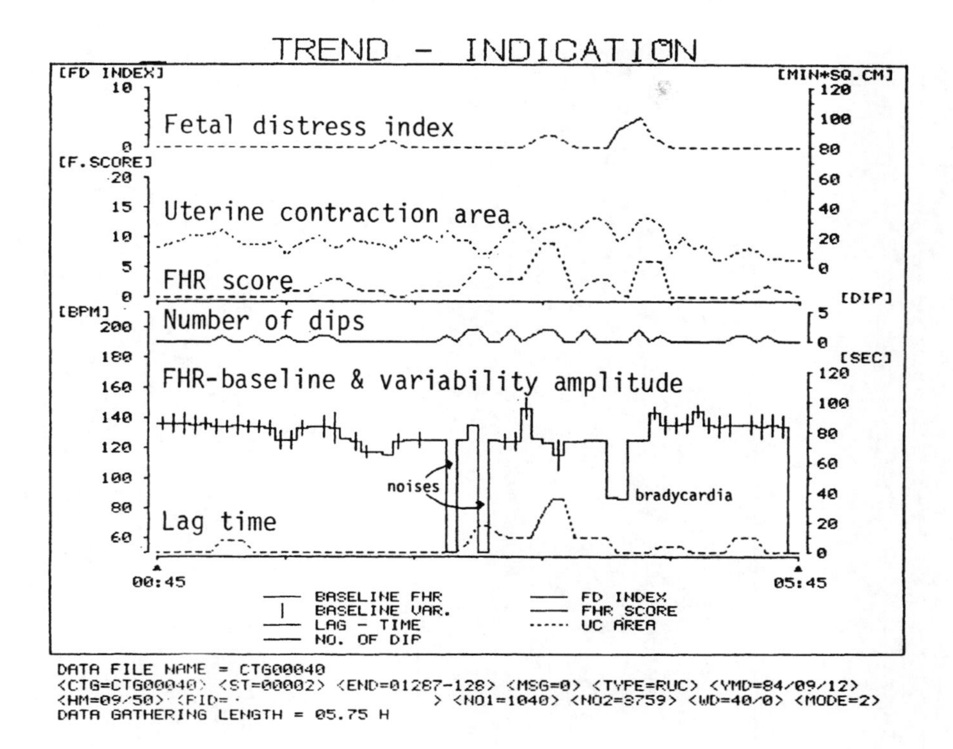

Fig. 4. A hard copy of the display of the trendgram of automated FHR analysis which was done by the automated fetal-distress diagnosis program.

mittee. Ominous SP will be a very slow, large one with large SPI and lasting for a long time span in rather early pregnancy. Details will be reported by the Committee.

Fetal gas monitoring in the labor

Shimizu et al. (1985) equipped a reflectance spectrophotometer with an optical fiber cable and microcomputer. They analyzed oxygen saturation of hemoglobin at the presenting part of the fetus in labor with the technique. Okane et al. (1985, 1986) estimated fetal arterial pO_2 and $tcPCO_2$ with transcutaneous electrodes which were attached to fetal head during labor. Continuous monitoring of fetal PO_2 and PCO_2 was carried out with the method.

Objective recording of fetal movement (fetal actocardiogram)

Maeda (1984) developed a new device for objective and continuous record of fetal gross movements in utero with ultrasonic Doppler technique (Fig. 5). The device places its transducer on the fetal back at the detection of fetal heart at the same time, and records the fetal rotating motion as the spikes on CTG chart simultaneously with FHR. The movement can be recorded from 11 weeks of pregnancy. However, the cluster of the spikes, which is called fetal movement (FM) burst, appears usually after 23 weeks. The FM burst associates FHR acceleration in the cases after about 32 weeks (Fig. 6). However, a smaller transient FHR rise than 15 bpm is observed before the stage of pregnancy, and therefore, the fetal well-being is diagnosed from a more early stage than by the conventional criteria that utilized the acceleration which is 15 bpm or

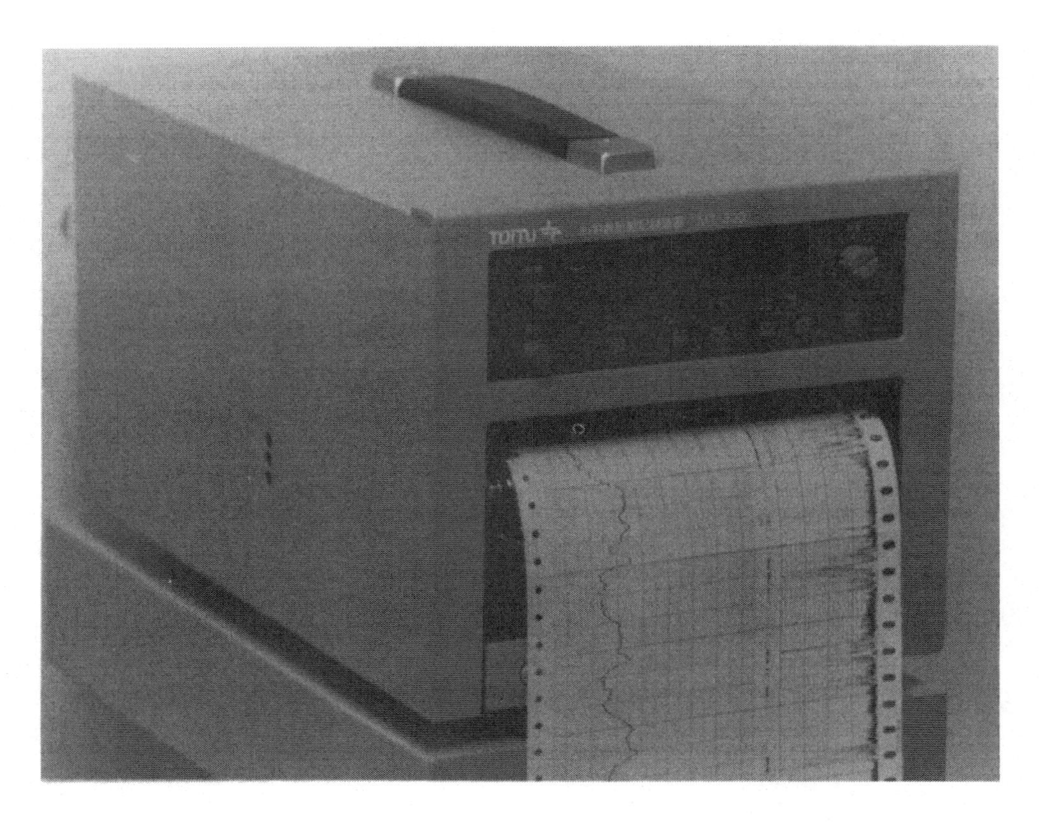

Fig. 5. Fetal actocardiograph. The principle is to detect fetal movement and fetal heart beat simultaneously with ultrasonic Doppler technique.

higher in the amplitude. The association of FHR with FM burst may indicate the will of the fetus to move, hence the technique will be capable to study fetal behavior. Actually, fetal resting and active stages are differentiated in the observation of the frequency of FM burst, namely, frequent FM bursts are observed during fetal active state, while very decreased or no FM burst is noted in the resting state that lasts for about 40 or less minutes. Imminent fetal distress (fetal hypoxia) case showed the loss of FHR acceleration in spite of frequent FM bursts (Fig. 7). The decrease of the transient FHR rise was the most sensitive sign to latent fetal distress. Fetal hiccup was also recorded with the device occasionally, though the action seemed to be a normal physiological phenomenon of the fetus (Ohta, 1985). Computer processing of FM signal is being investigated.

Neonatal monitoring

Monitoring of newborn infants, particularly premature babies, is the most important to detect neonatal abnormality immediately on its occurrence in order to obtain perfect management of pathological newborn infants. The common fetal monitor is composed of heart rate display which is detected by ECG signal and that of the rate of respiration which is detected by an impedance method which utilizes the electrodes of ECG for the heart rate. The $tcPO_2$ and $tcPCO_2$ measurements are common in modern neonatal monitoring, and the techniques clearly improved the oxygenating status of the premature newborn infants, and are indispensable in the present NICU. Other physiological phenomena are combined if necessary. The body temperature measurement is com-

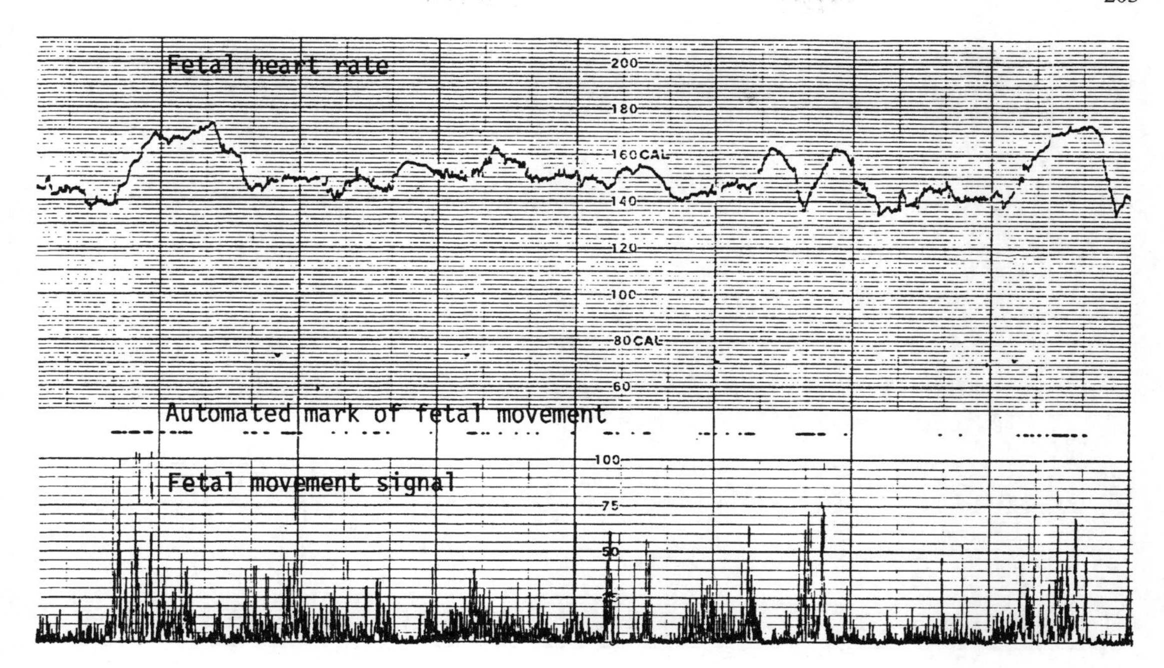

Fig. 6. Frequent FHR accelerations associate with the FM bursts in late stage of pregnancy. The finding shows normal state and fetal well-being.

mon. Neonatal blood pressure is measured by direct and indirect methods, though non-invasive technique is preferable in long time span monitoring. Electroencephalogram, brain pressure, intracranial blood flow measurement etc. are added to usual monitoring technique. Ultrasonogram of neonatal head is indispensable to monitor or manage intracranial hemorrhage including intraventricular hemorrhage (IVH) and subependymal hemorrhage (SEH). The physical parameters which are utilized in neonatal monitoring are stored in computer memory, and utilized in further study work. Since the duration of neonatal monitoring is, however, too long to fully memorize in computer, the technique of data compression and the most appropriate sampling technique are discussed in the study group on medical engineering in perinatal medicine of the Japan Society of Medical Electronics and Biological Engineering. In the medical engineering of neonatal stage, Kobayashi et al. (1986) reported the indirect measurement of neonatal arterial pressure, Inaba et al. (1985) the analysis of autocorrelation function for neonatal heart beats. The crying voice of the newborn was studied by Hashimoto et al. (1985) and Kobayashi et al. (1986), resulting in the differentiation of the demand of the newborn. The relation between mother's voice and neonatal movement was investigated by Watanabe et al. (1986), and significant relation between the two phenomena was confirmed. Neonatal respiration was monitored by sensing with airborne ultrasound by Nakagawa et al. (1986). Nakano et al. also reported the use of radio-wave in the sensing.

Computer processing of perinatal information in the management

Microcomputer and personal computer is utilized in the processing of perinatal information (Kanzaki et al., 1985; Minoura et al., 1985). Obstetrical data base construction is one of the problems in the perinatal computer system (Irie & Imai, 1986). Local area network (LAN) is utilized in the communication between several parts of perinatal cen-

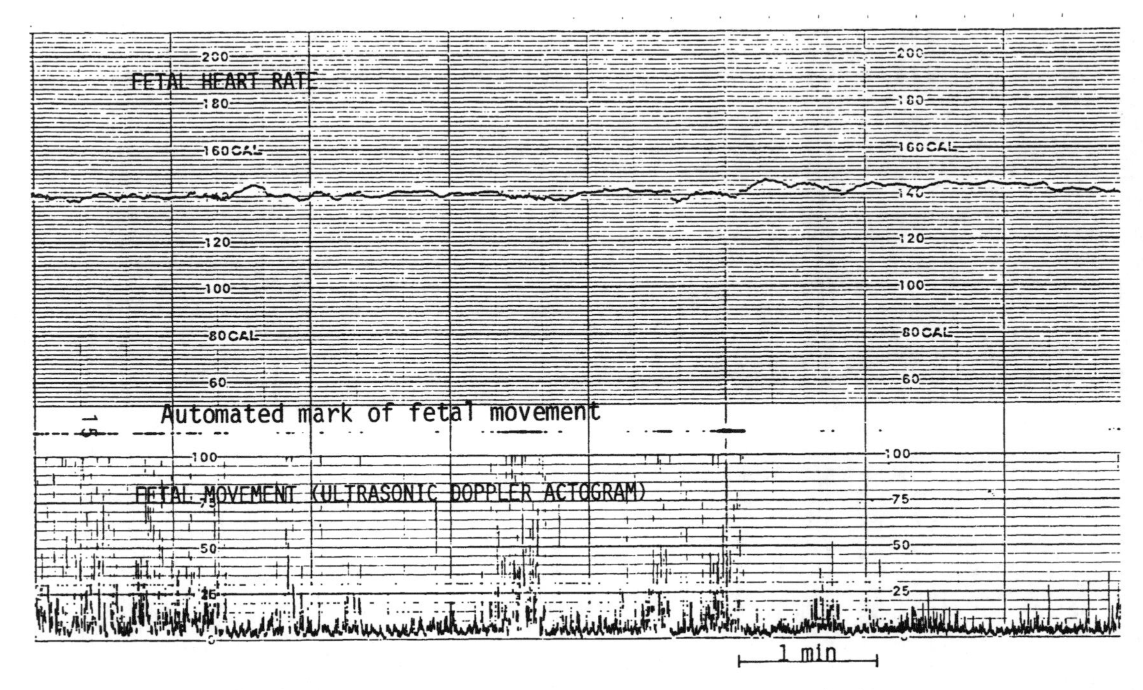

Fig. 7. EPH gestosis and IUGR in 36 weeks of pregnancy. No FHR acceleration is observed in spite of frequent FM bursts. Latent fetal distress is clearly diagnosed from the change. Fetal distress sign appeared a few days after the record, and cesarean section was carried out.

ters, as well as in the relation to large computer center or nation-wide communication (Nakahara et al., 1986). Maeda, Takeda & Yamamoto (1984) developed 'PERINATE' database in the Osaka University computer center with the support of the Ministry of Education, and enabled the communication among the study group through the N-1 nation-wide computer network. Artificial intelligence is one of the modern technologies in perinatal computer application (Minoura et al., 1985, 1986). Ultrasonographic image data are stored in computer memory, and utilized for clinical purposes (Ishiguro et al., 1985; Ogawa et al., 1985; Nishi et al., 1985). The author programmed pocket computers with several equations in perinatal medicine, for instance, gestational weeks estimation from CRL, BPD and FFL, fetal weight estimation, dystocia index, CPD index, several statistical equations (Maeda, 1984), and utilized them clinical practice and investigation.

Ultrasonography in perinatal medicine

As mentioned beforehand, perinatal medicine has been revolutionized after introduction of real-time B-mode technique in the visualization of the fetus, placenta, umbilical cord and other intrauterine structures. Estimation of correct gestational weeks, early recognition of the fetus, observation and diagnosis of fetal growth, diagnosis of fetal life, fetal anatomy and its function, fetal behavior, detection of fetal anomaly, diagnosis of fetal diseases, placental location, hydatidiform mole diagnosis, and many other morphological and functional examinations of the gestation depend on real-time ultrasonography, M-mode test, and ultrasonic blood flowmetry or other ultrasound technique. From this view point, ultrasound safety had been investigated in the study group supported by the Ministry of Health and Welfare of the government for 5 years in CW and 3 years in pulsed ultrasound. As the results, threshold intensity of CW and pulsed ultrasound were confirmed. Based on the facts, Japan Industrial Standard (JIS) limited the ultrasound intensity of obstetric Doppler fetal heart detectors and that of compound scanners. JIS draft of the electronic scanner also limits the intensity at the level similar to the compound scanner. The group work had been done mainly by the investigation of obstetric researchers under the support of engineering specialists (Maeda et al., 1986). Therefore, ultrasonic diagnostic equipment was established in safety in our country. Medical use of electronic scan device is not limited in the screening of the pregnancy (the Committee on Medical Engineering, 1986). Clinical and investigational works of ultrasonography in perinatal medicine are too many to list in this review article. Recent works report the measurements of fetal liver, adrenals or other organs (Hata et al., 1985; Murao et al., 1986). Among the works of fetal behavior, the complex of fetal action is the target in the present, and Inoue et al. (1985) reported the movement complex of fetal eye ball, urination and the onset of fetal active state. Ultrasonically guided puncture or other procedure in the body including the amniotic cavity and fetus is common in the recent ultrasonographic study, and has produced many clinical benefits.

Fetal and maternal blood flowmetries with pulsed and CW ultrasound

Pulsed Doppler fetal blood flowmetry was initiated in the measurement of blood flow volume in several fetal arteries (Maeda, Utsu & Chiba, 1984), and in the maternal pelvic artery (Ishihara, 1985). Utsu et al. measured not only the flow in the arteries but also the flow in fetal trachea which was associated with fetal breathing movement. Many researchers have studied blood flow in many instances in flow volume. However, the inconsistency of the flow volume was evaluated by the investigators, and the flow profile that is the wave form of the flow velocity pattern has become the target of investigation in the present. Maeda, Ishihara & Takeuchi (1986) reported the increase of resistance index and pulsatility index in the maternal pelvic artery and in the umbilical artery in severe EPH gestosis patients. Hata et al. (1984) reported the fetal intracardiac blood flow and its regurgitation. Kanzaki et al. (1985) investigated venous blood flow of fetal inferior vena cava, and found the characteristic change of flow profile in several abnormalities of fetal heart rhythm. Recently, fetal heart failure is estimated from the venous flow profile and tricuspid regurgitation (Tsuzaki et al., 1986). Tsuzaki (1985) also studied the flow in the placental pore, that may be the intervillous space of the placenta, and found the increased resistance index in the case of EPH gestosis. Recently, 2-dimensional Doppler color flow mapping has been reported valuable mainly in the diagnosis of structural abnormalities of fetal cardiovascular system.

Fetal cardiology

Most of congenital fetal heart anomalies have been diagnosed by the structural changes of fetal heart and large vessels in the B-mode ultrasonograms. Fetal cardiac dimensions were measured by Hata et al. (1986) with M-mode echocardiography (Fig. 8). Fetal cardiac transverse diameter (FCTD), left ventricular stroke volume (LVSV), left ventricular cardiac output (LVCO), total stroke volume (SV), and right ventricular cardiac output (RVCO) were measured and estimated. The changes in the cases of SFD and fetal heart failure was studied. This field of fetal cardiology is one of the most promising investigations in the present and will be in the future, not only in ultrasonography but also in many divisions of medical engineering.

Tissue characterization in prenatal medicine

Tissue character is a very unique field of investigation in biological ultrasound. A-mode image signal and also radiofrequency ultrasound are the materials in tissue characterization. Placental aging, the maturation of fetal organs seem to be investigated by the technique of tissue characterization, but it will not be easy to adopt the common technique of tissue characterization to these organs, because

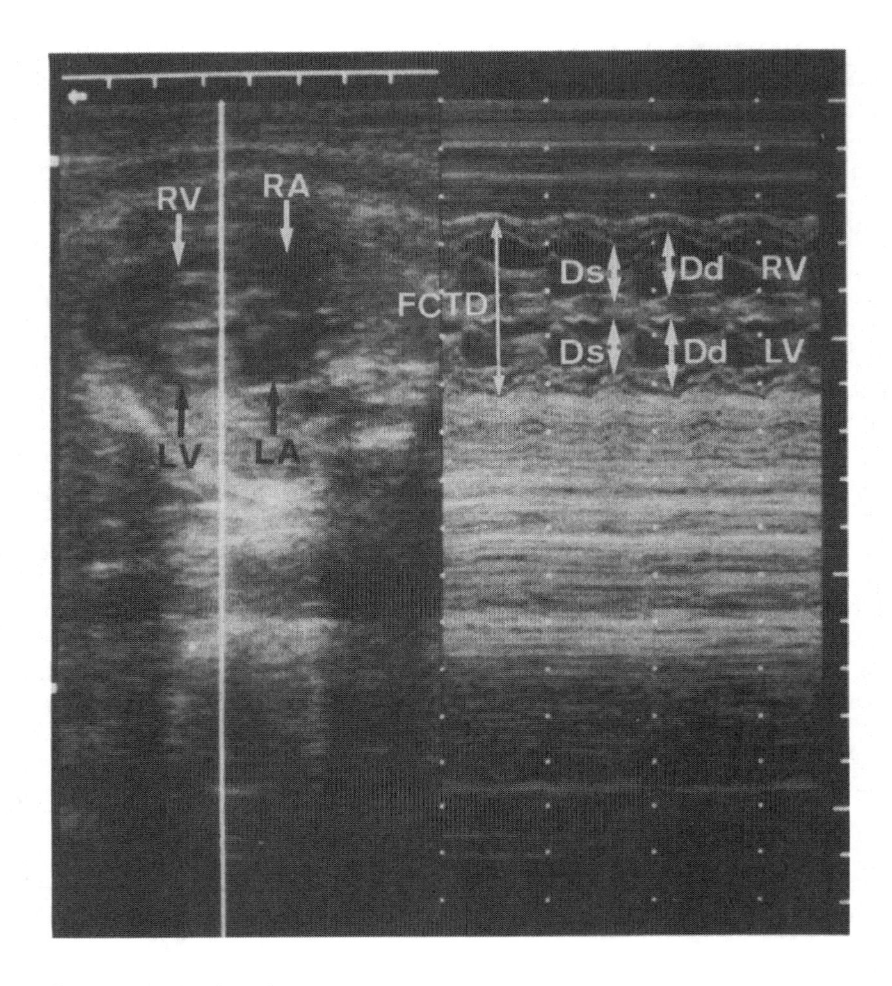

Fig. 8. Real-time-directed M-mode echocardiogram on four-chamber view. ra = right atrium; rv = right ventricle; tv = tricuspid valve; la = left atrium; lv = left ventricle; mv = mitral valve; FCTD = fetal cardiac transverse diameter; Dd = diastolic dimension; Ds = systolic dimension. (By the Courtsy of Dr. T. Hata, Dept. Obstetrics & Gynecology, Shimane Medical University.)

homogeneous distribution of the composed material is needed in the tissue characterization, but the structural characteristics are the compromising factor for the tissue characterization.

Sakao (1984) investigated the reflectivity of normal uterine muscle and fibromyoma with manual processing method, and found the difference of the reflectivities between the two materials in in vitro experiments. Research on placenta reported the aging of this organ, classifying into 3 or 4 or 5 grades according to the increase of brightness and inhomogeneosity. It seems easy to find the difference between the grades, and in fact, there have been the difference of histographic parameters of the placenta among the grades of placental aging (Maeda et al., 1986). However, in single placenta, the parameter values, for instance, the mean and SD of the gray-scale, varies according the shift of the region of interest (ROI). Therefore, a single value can not be obtained in the case of aged placenta, but can be in young and homogeneous placenta. Picker reported the increase of brightness of the lung tissue on ultrasonogram if compared to that of the liver. Although the finding contains many artefacts, the test on the fetal lung will be interesting. Liver will be one of the tissues which can be tested by ultrasound histogram in comparison to some standard tissue, if such standard is present in fetal body. In the examination of the tissue with radiofrequency ultrasonic signal, the frequency dependent attenuation coefficient was calculated by using the spectral difference method. Myomatous tissue was tested with this method, and the attenuation was obtained. Similar work has already been reported by Masaoka et al. (1986). Tissue characterization will be promising in the future, since the technique is completely different from ultrasonography.

References

1. Fujibayashi H, Ohkawa T, Yagi K, Hogaki M, Okada K, Takeuchi Y: Automatous differentiation of valve and wall signal from early embryonal heart. JJME 24 (Supp): 102, 1986.
2. Fukamanai K, Hashimoto T, Furuya H, Ebara Y: Studies on characteristic of wave form of FHR long term variability by fast Fourier transform analysis. JJME 23 (Supp): 295, 1985.
3. Fukuju M, Akatsuka T, Nagamine T, Kubo T: An intelligent fetal monitoring system. JJME 23 (Supp): 300, 1985.
4. Hashimoto T, Fukamanai K, Furuya H, Ebara Y: Computer analysis on neonatal cries. JJME 23 (Supp): 315, 1985.
5. Hata K, Hata T, Aoki S, Murao F, Kitao M: Ultrasonic identification of in utero fetal adrenal gland. Jap J Med Ultras 12 (Supp): 113–114, 1985.
6. Hata T, Hata K, Kitao M: Fetal intracardiac blood-flow patterns assessed by pulsed Doppler and B-mode ultrasound. J Cardiovasc Ultrasonog 3: 101–106, 1984.
7. Hata T, Hata K, Kitao M: Fetal cardiac function and outcome determined echocardiographically. J Cardiovasc Ultrasonog 5: 19–23, 1986.
8. Ikeda M, Kawarabayashi T, Sugimori H, Nakano H: The pattern of spontaneous contraction and the effect of Mg^{++} and Terbutaline on pregnant human myometrium. Acta Obstet Gynaec Jpn 36: 377–383, 1984.
9. Inaba J, Shigematsu S, Iwasaki M, Kubo T, Iwasaki H, Akatsuka T: Analysis of autocorrelation function for neonatal heart beats using digital data recorder. JJME 23 (Supp): 297, 1985.
10. Inaba J, Okane M, Shigematsu S, Kubo T, Iwasaki H: An intelligent fetal monitoring system. JJME 24 (Supp): 105, 1986.
11. Inoue M, Hara H, Nakahara H, Hori E, Shin T, Koyanagi T, Nakano H: Relation between eye movement and micturition of fetus assessed by real-time ultrasound. Jap J Med Ultras 12 (Supp): 123–124, 1985.
12. Irie T, Sawazumi K, Tatsumura M, Maeda K: The relationship among the umbilical cord arterial blood pH, BE, HCO_3-, the automated analysis of fetal heart rate and trendgram. JJME 23 (Supp): 302, 1985.
13. Irie M, Imai S: Construction of obstetric database based on interactive input at origination point. JJME 24 (Supp): 106, 1986.
14. Ishigura M, Fukuma H, Umayabayashi M, Yuki J, Inokuchi K, Yang R, Higashidate N, Morohashi T, Sakamoto S: An on-line digitalised image transmission system used ultrasonic tomograph and computer. JJME 23 (Supp): 309, 1985.
15. Ishihara K: Measurement of blood flow in maternal pelvic artery and umbilical cord artery with the ultrasonic pulsed Doppler flow method. Acta Obstet Gynaec Jpn 37: 2335–2345, 1985.
16. Kanzaki T, Murakami M, Sasaki K, Sakakibara S, Utsu S, Chiba Y, Hasegawa T: The management of perinatal informations by microcomputer system. JJME 23 (Supp): 306, 1985.
17. Kanzaki T, Murakami M, Sasaki S, Utsu M, Chiba Y, Hasegawa T: The monitoring of hemodynamic changes during fetal therapy for arrhythmias by pulsed Doppler ultrasound. Jpn J Med Ultras (Proc 46 meeting): 265–266, 1985.
18. Kawarabayashi T, Ikeda M, Sugimori H, Nakano H: Spontaneous electrical activity and effects of noradrenaline on pregnant human myometrium recorded by the single sucrose-gap method. Acta Physiol Hungarica 67: 71–82, 1986.
19. Kitada F: Studies on periodic changes of fetal and neonatal heart rate. Acta Obstet Gynaec Jpn 36: 2147–2154, 1984.
20. Kobayashi H, Shimazu H, Ito H, Yamakoshi K: Indirect measurement of arterial pressure in newborn babies and infants. JJME 24 (Supp): 477, 1986.
21. Kobayashi K, Oda T, Murooka H: Characteristic pattern in time series of crying vocal in early infant. JJME 24 (Supp): 107, 1986.
22. Koyanagi T: Development of mechanismus regulating heart rates in human fetuses analyzed by factor analysis. Asia-Oceania J Obstet Gynaec 12: 155–165, 1986.
23. Kubo T, Shigematsu S, Inaba J, Koresawa N, Iwasaki H, Akatsuka T: Fetal ECG derived directly through maternal abdominal wall. JJME 23 (Supp): 316, 1985.
24. Maeda K, Arima T, Tatsumura M, Nagazawa T: Computer-aided fetal heart rate analysis and automatic fetal-distress diagnosis during labor and pregnancy utilized external technique in fetal monitoring. MEDINFO 80, Part 1, pp 1214–1218, 1980.
25. Maeda K, Tatsumura M, Yoneda T, Nakamura Y: Fetal mechanocardiography recorded with the processing of ultrasonic Doppler fetal heart valve signals. Jpn J Med Ultras 8: 159–165, 1981.
26. Maeda K: Computerized automatic diagnosis of fetal distress with use of external monitoring technique. Computer-

diagnostik in Geburtsmedizin 2. Symp. pp 28–49, 1981.
27. Maeda K, Ito K: Studies on the sinusoidal pattern of fetal heart rate diagnosed by new tentative criteria. Acta Obstet Gynaec Jpn 35: 1923–1930, 1983.
28. Maeda K, Utsu M, Chiba Y: Advances in CW and pulsed ultrasonic Doppler techniques in the studies of fetal heart, circulation, fetal action and breathing. In: Kurjak A, Kossoff G (eds) Recent advances in ultrasound diagnosis 4. Excerpta Medica, Amsterdam, 1984, pp 78–97.
29. Maeda K, Ito K: Studies on fluctuating CTG with the sinusoidal pattern index. Obstetric and Gynecologic Treatment 49: 497–501, 1984.
30. Maeda K: Studies on new ultrasonic Doppler fetal actograph and continuous recording of fetal movement. Acta Obstet Gynaec Jpn 36: 280–288, 1984.
31. Maeda K, Iwamoto K, Miyamoto N, Tsuzaki T, Takeuchi K: Pocket computer assisted estimations of fetal age and fetal weight. In: Kurjak A, Kossoff G (eds) Recent advances in ultrasound diagnosis 4. Excerpta Medica, Amsterdam, 1984, pp 160–173.
32. Maeda K: Report of the study group supported by the Ministry of Education 'the study on the data processing of the fetus in perinatal stage', 1984.
33. Maeda K, Tatsumura M, Takeuchi K, Oota M, Minagawa Y, Irie T: Modern technology and the fetus. In: Kurjak A (ed) The fetus as a patient. Excerpta Medica, Amsterdam, 1985, pp 284–299.
34. Maeda K, Murao F, Yoshiga T, Yamauchi C, Tsuzaki T: Experimental studies on the suppression of cultured cell growth curves after the irradiation of CW and pulsed ultrasound. IEEE Transactions on Ultrasonics, ferroelectrics and frequency control. UFFC-33: 186–193, 1986.
35. Maeda K, Ide M: The limitation of ultrasound intensity of diagnostic devices in the Japanese Industrial Standards. IEEE Transactions. UFFC-33: 241–244, 1986.
36. Maeda K, Ishihara K, Takeuchi Y: Studies on pulsed ultrasonic flowmetry, ultrasonic color Doppler technique and the evaluation of continuous wave ultrasonic Doppler flow metry. In: Kurjak A, Kossoff G (eds) Recent advances in ultrasound diagnosis 5. Excerpta Medica, Amsterdam, 1986, pp 189–200.
37. Maeda K, Sakao A, Mio Y, Kikukawa A, Akaiwa A, Kihaile PE: The Quantification of ultrasonic B-mode images with the trials of tissue characterization in obstetrics and gynecology. In: Kurjak A, Kossoff G (eds) Recent advances in ultrasound diagnosis 5. Excerpta Medica, Amsterdam, 1986, pp 215–222.
38. Minoura S, Fujii K, Kaihara S, Koyama T: Perinatal care consultation system by using MECS-AI. JJME 23 (Supp): 308, 1985.
39. Minoura S, Wagatsuma T, Fujii K, Kaihara S, Koyama T: Consultation system for the ultrasound diagnosis of ovarian tumor by using MECS-AI. JJME 24 (Supp): 112, 1986.
40. Morio S: Quantitative relationship between infant mortality and social factors. Yonago Acta medica 28: 8–37, 1985.
41. Murakami M, Matsui Y, Okudaira Y, Kanzaki T, Utsu M, Chiba Y: A study of the pulsation in the umbilical venous blood flow. JJME 24 (Supp): 474, 1986.
42. Murao F, Takamori H, Hata K, Hirayama K, Hata T, Yamamoto K, Kitao M: Measurement of fetal liver sizes by ultrasound. Jap J Med Ultras 13 (Supp): 133–134, 1986.
43. Nakagawa M, Yagi K, Ohkawa T, Hogaki M, Arai K, Takeuchi Y: Remote sensing of neonatal heart beat and respiration with the use of airborne ultrasound. Acta Obstet Gynaec 38 (Supp): 195, 1986.
44. Nakahara H, Koyanagi T, Nakano H: Application of LAN on the basis of micro-computer system in obstetric practice. JJME 24 (Supp): 70, 1986.
45. Nakajima Y, Inokuchi K, Amemiya T, Inou Y, Morohashi T, Sakamoto S, Kawakami J, Takahashi R, Moroe T, Ohta I, Kosugi M: Fetal information processing system. JJME 23 (Supp): 307, 1985.
46. Nakajima Y: New technique of uterine contraction evaluation with multiple transducer technique. 30th meeting of the study group on medical engineering in perinatal medicine. 1986.
47. Nakamura Y: Studies on the systolic time intervals obtained by ultrasonic Doppler mechanocardiograph and the triggering with abdominal lead FECG during pregnancy. Jpn J Med Ultras 9: 29–35, 1982.
48. Ninomiya S, Yano F, Nishimura J: Fetal R wave detection and its application. JJME 23 (Supp): 317, 1985, 24 (Supp): 104, 1986.
49. Nishi M, Masaoka H, Kohchi T, Ukita N, Kirai T, Yuhara A, Fujita T, Jukumoto S, Akamatsu N, Sekiba K, Tsubota N: Ultrasound measurement and computer aided diagnosis in obstetrics. JJME 23 (Supp): 311, 1985.
50. Noguchi Y, Hataoka H, Sugimoto S: An estimation method of generating function of heart-rate variability. JJME 24 (Supp): 478, 1986.
51. Ogawa S, Fukuma H, Umayabayashi M, Amamiya T, Nakazima U, Ino U, Morohashi T, Sakamoto S: A fetal growth monitoring system by ultrasonic tomograph and personal computer. JJME 23 (Supp) 310, 1985.
52. Ohta M: Evaluation of fetal movements with ultrasonic Doppler fetal actograph. Acta Obstet Gynaec Jpn 37: 73–82, 1985.
53. Okane M, Shigemitu S, Inaba J, Koresawa N, Kubo T, Iwasaki K: Continuous fetal scalp transcutaneous PO2 monitoring during labor. JJME 23 (Supp): 303, 1985.
54. Okane M, Sjigemitsu S, Inaba J, Koresawa M, Kubo T, Iwasaki K, Kawagoe K: Continuous fetal scalp transcutaneous pCO2 monitoring during labor. JJME 24 (Supp): 476, 1986.
55. Sakao A: In vitro study on relation between the gynecological tumor and the level of the ultrasound reflected waves. Jpn J Med Ultras 11: 155–161, 1984.
56. Shimizu K, Satoh N, Kawano S: Clinical significance of the oxygen saturation in the fetal presenting part during labor. JJME 23 (Supp): 303, 1985.
57. Sugimoto S, Maeda K, Hataoka H: Spectral analysis of fetal

heart rate by linear prediction method. JJME 23 (Supp): 298, 1985.
58. Sumimoto K: Moiré curve evaluation on maternal abdomen in the labor contraction of the uterus. 30th meeting of the study group on medical engineering in perinatal medicine, 1986.
59. Taguchi T: Studies on the periodicity of fetal and neonatal heart rate variability by fast Fourier transform analysis. Acta Obstet Gynaec Jpn 35: 53–60, 1983.
60. Takagi K, Matsuura M, Yamamoto S, Miyake Y, Sakata T, Takagi T: The topographic evaluation of electrical pattern caused by human uterine contraction and its clinical application. Acta Obstet Gynaec Jpn 38 (Supp): 194, 1986.
61. The Committee on Medical Engineering; Guidelines for using diagnostic ultrasound equipment in pregnant women and fetuses. Acta Obstet Gynaec 38: 1011–1012, 1986.
62. Tsujii T, Yagi K, Ohkawa T, Hogaki M, Arai K, Ohkawa K, Yatsugi K, Takeuchi Y: Detection of embryonal heart rate from linear scan ultrasonograph. Jpn J Med Ultras (Proc 46 Meeting) 265–266, 1985.
63. Tsuzaki T, Takeuchi K, Ishihara K, Maeda K: The study of blood flowmetry by pulsed Doppler technique in the placental pores and the umbilical arteries. Jpn J Med Ultras 12: 131–132, 1985.
64. Tsuzaki T, Minagawa Y, Nagata N, Takeuchi Y, Maeda K: The diagnosis of fetal cardiac failure by pulsed-Doppler flowmetry in the fetal vessels. Jpn J Med Ultras 13 (Supp): 165–166, 1986.
65. Tsuzaki T, Morishita K, Nakajima K: Studies on the changes of perinatal statistics after the introduction of full intrapartum fetal monitoring in 11 years. Acta Obstet Gynaec Jpn 38 (Supp): 177, 1986.
66. Tsuzaki T, Minagawa Y, Nagata N, Takeuchi Y, Maeda K: The diagnosis of fetal cardiac failure by pulsed Doppler flowmetry in the fetal vessels. Jpn J Med Ultras 13 (Supp) 165–166, 1986.
67. Watanabe T, Ishii T, Kobayashi N: Development of real time automatic analyzer for movement-voice synchronization in communication. JJME 24 (Supp): 108, 1986.
68. Yagi I, Isobe Y, Fujibayashi H, Ohkawa T, Hogaki M, Arai K, Takeuchi Y: Detection error of conventional auto-correlation fetal heart rate meter in scalp lead FECG. Acta Obstet Gynaec Jpn 12 (Supp): 113, 1985a.
69. Yagi K, Ohkawa T, Hogaki M, Takeuchi Y: Detection error of instantaneous fetal heart rate meter of 1 MHz Doppler signal. JJME 23 (Supp): 296, 1985b.
70. Yoneda T: Fetal mechanocardiogram studied by systolic time intervals in ultrasonic Doppler fetal heart valve signals using new multistylus recorder system. Acta Obstet Gynaec Jpn 33: 1209–1218, 1981.

Address for offprints:
Prof. K. Maeda
Dept. Obstetrics and Gynecology
Tottori University School of Medicine
Yonago 683, Japan

Medical Progress through Technology 12: 213–220 (1987)

Sintered hydroxyapatite for a percutaneous device and its clinical application

Hideki Aoki, Masaru Akao, Yoshiharu Shin, Takayuki Tsuzi & Tatsuo Togawa
Institute for Medical and Dental Engineering, Tokyo Medical and Dental University, 2-3-10 Kanda Surugadai, Chiyoda, Tokyo 101, Japan

Key words: hydroxyapatite, percutaneous device, animal testing, tissue reaction, amino acid composition

Summary

The sintered hydroxyapatite was designed to be utilized as a percutaneous device. The device was percutaneously fixed through the back skin of mongrel dogs. The tissue reaction around the implants was examined histologically. At 1 month the sintered hydroxyapatite was closely contacted with the skin tissue and downgrowth of epidermis was not observed. The long-term implantation ranging from 3 to 17 months showed that the depth of epidermis downgrowth was limited to only 1 mm. The amino acid composition of fibrous capsule formed around the hydroxyapatite showed close resemblance to vertebrate periosteum. It was confirmed that the sintered hydroxyapatite had good compatibility and long-term stability with skin tissue.

Introduction

In the last 10 years, various materials [4] such as polyethlene, silicone rubber, polytetrafluoroethylene and carbon, have been used as percutaneous devices for measurement of internal body information. However, these devices have serious problems such as bacterial infection and downgrowth of epidermis, which make gaps between the device and skin tissue. It has been impossible to retain these percutaneous devices in the skin tissue for the long-term.

In the present study, the sintered hydroxyapatite (HAp), which has superior compatibility with bone tissue, has been utilized for a percutaneous device, and was implanted through the skin of mongrel dogs [2]. The compatibility of the sintered HAp with skin tissue was examined histologically. The amino acid composition of fibrous capsule formed around the HAp was determined. Continuous and long-term blood pressure and deep body temperature were successfully measured without infection using the HAp percutaneous device.

Reaction of sintered hydroxyapatite to skin tissue

Experimental

Hydroxyapatite was prepared by wet method* and sintered at a temperature of 1250° C for 1 h [1]. The relative density was approximately 98%. Fig. 1 shows a schematic illustration of a button shaped percutaneous implant made of sintered HAp. 'A' is called the neck part, and 'C' is the bottom part. A commercial silicone rubber for medical use served as a control.

* A suspension of 0.5 M $Ca(OH)_2$ in 1000 ml distilled water was vigorously stirred and a solution of 0.3 M H_3PO_4 in 1000 ml distilled water was slowly added as drops over 1 to 2 h under a condition of pH >7 to produce a gelatinous precipitate.

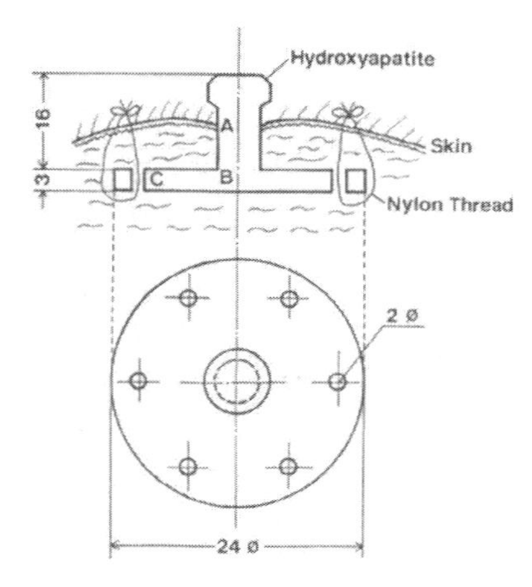

Fig. 1. Schematic representation of sintered hydroxyapatite for percutaneous device through the back skin of a mongrel dog.

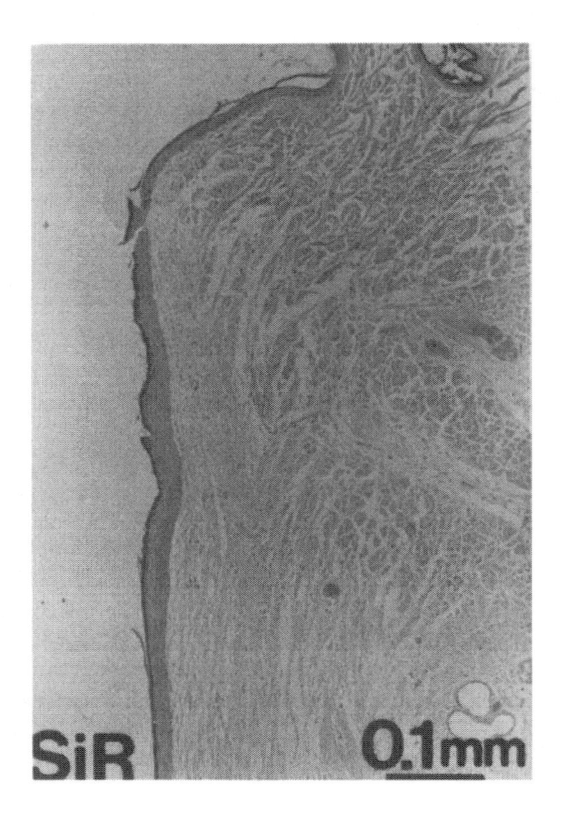

Fig. 2. Histological section of the tissue surrounding silicone rubber 1 month after implantation. The serious downgrowth of epidermis was observed along the surface of the silicone rubber.

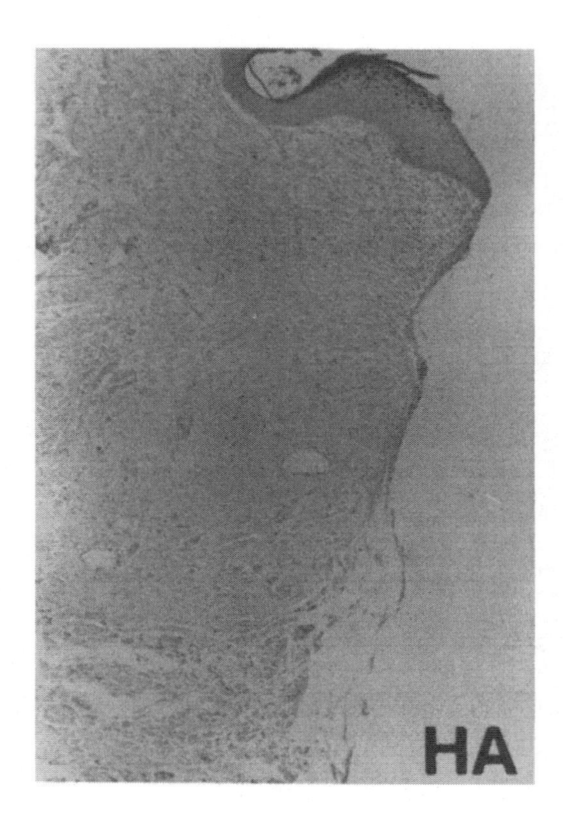

Fig. 3. Histological section of the tissue surrounding sintered hydroxyapatite at 1 month. Neither downgrowth nor inflammation were observed.

The hydroxyapatite and silicone rubber were percutaneously implanted in the back skin of mongrel dogs. The implants were fixed with threads passing through the holes of the lower disks and the skin was then closed with sutures (Fig. 1). The distances among the surgical sites were ranging from 5 to 10 cm. The sutures were removed at 10 days and then the implants were allowed to stand free. Penicillin group antibiotics were subcutaneously injected for 3 days after the surgery.

At 1, 3, 4, 7, 9, and 17 months after implantation, the tissues surrounding the implants were removed, fixed with 10% neutral formalin, embedded in paraffin and stained with hematoxylin and eosin for light microscopic observation.

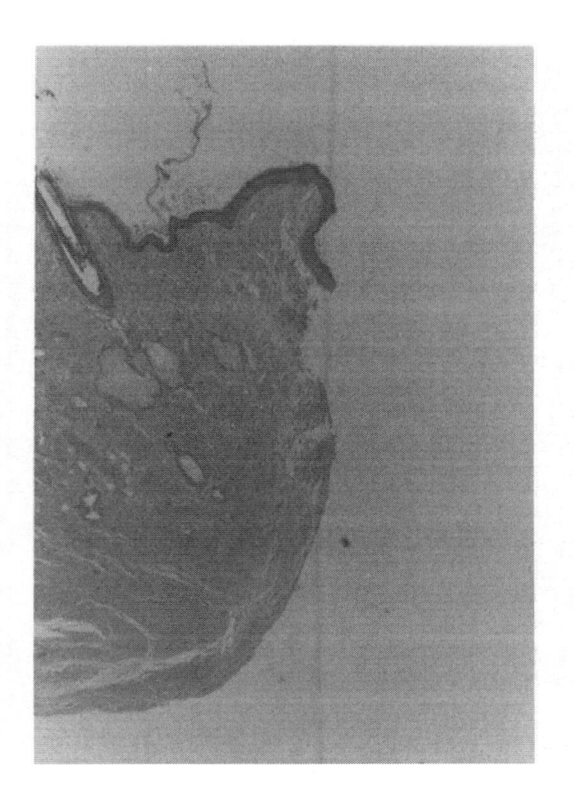

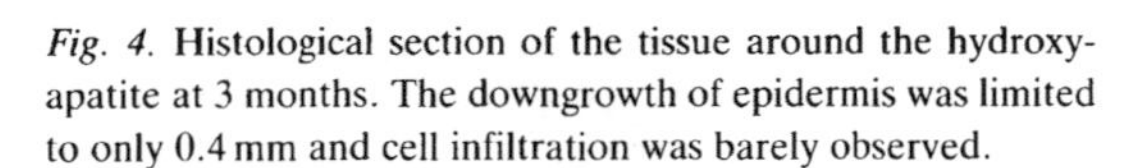

Fig. 4. Histological section of the tissue around the hydroxyapatite at 3 months. The downgrowth of epidermis was limited to only 0.4 mm and cell infiltration was barely observed.

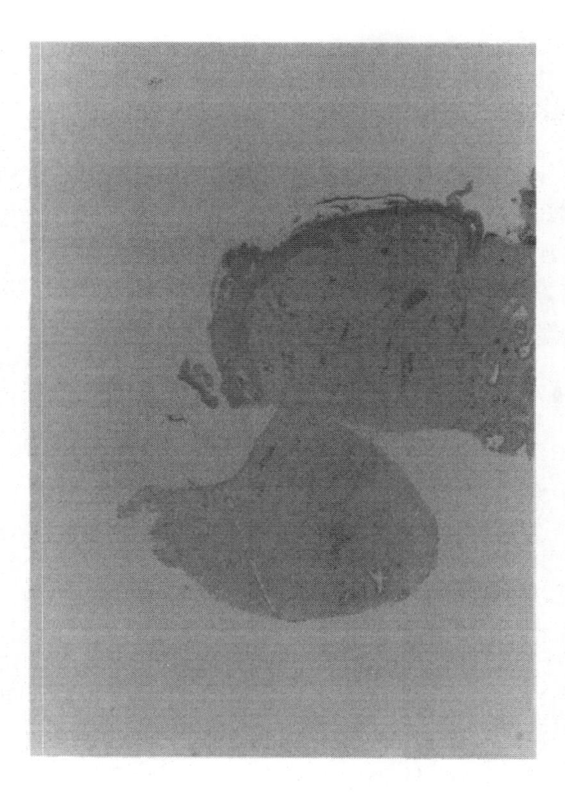

Fig. 5. Histological section of the tissue around the hydroxyapatite at 17 months. The downgrowth was limited to about 0.8 mm. Inflammation and infection were mild.

Histological observation

Fig. 2 shows the histological section of the tissue surrounding silicone rubber at 1 month. The serious downgrowth of epidermis (depth about 2.5 mm) was clearly observed along the neck part of silicone rubber. The fibrous connective tissue was formed at the bottom surface and the thickness was approximately 400 μm. In the connective tissue, inflammatory cells and proliferative capillary vessels were observed.

On the other hand, in the case of sintered HAp at 1 month (Fig. 3), neither epidermis downgrowth nor inflammatory cells were observed at the neck part. The thickness of mature connective tissue formed on the bottom surface was approximately 50 μm. In the connective tissue, cell infiltration was less for the HAp implant than for the silicone rubber.

Downgrowth of epidermis

After 3 months the downgrowth of epidermis was limited to only 0.4 mm for the HAp device, and cell infiltration was barely observed (Fig. 4). For silicone rubber, the downgrowth reached to the bottom part of disk. Some dogs showed high degree of erosion due to inflammation and infection around silicone rubber. Finally the silicone rubber was expelled from the skin tissue in less than 3 months.

At 4 months downgrowth of epidermis of the HAp device was about 0.8 mm. The tissue surrounding was stable without inflammation. As macroscopically observed, at 7 months hemocyte infiltration was seen near the epidermis. However, downgrowth of epidermis was limited (about 1 mm) and no infection was observed. At 9 months downgrowth of epidermis was only about 1 mm.

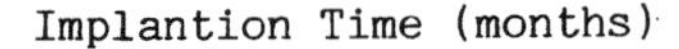

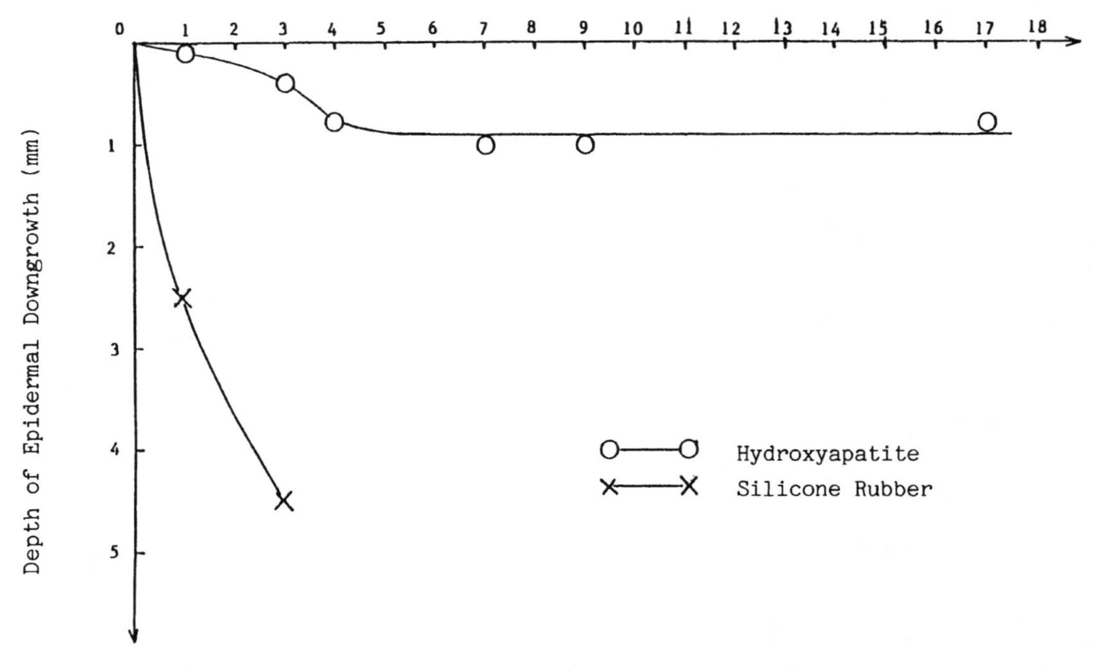

Fig. 6. Depth of epidermis downgrowth for each implantation period.

There were some incidences of inflammation in the course of long-term follow up. In every case they healed with disinfection and a single subcutaneous injection of antibiotics. At 17 months the downgrowth of epidermis was limited to about 0.8 mm. Inflammation and infection were mild. As a whole, it was considered that the tissue reaction of the HAp device was favorable (Fig. 5).

The depth of epidermis downgrowth of both HAp and silicone rubber were plotted for each duration of implantation (Fig. 6). The downgrowth of epidermis is significantly smaller for apatite than for silicone rubber.

Success rate

Data of the basic experiments on HAp percutaneous device were summarized in Fig. 7, based on grading system for condition of implants proposed by Glazener [3]. A condition, which is sealed, dry and clean, no weeping of body fluid or blood, is identified as 'success' and other conditions as 'failure'. Data on a dense polyethylene percutaneous device [3] is shown as reference.

Based on these data it can be concluded that the success rate of hydroxyapatite is quite high in comparison to silicone and other materials. As to the 'failure' cases of apatite, they were caused by physical impact on the electrode itself such as being struck against an obstacle and for other reasons. Several of the failures were recovered by disinfection and other appropriate measures. From these results it becomes clear that HAp device has long-term subcutaneous stability without serious downgrowth of epidermis, inflammation or exudate. It has excellent properties suited for actual application.

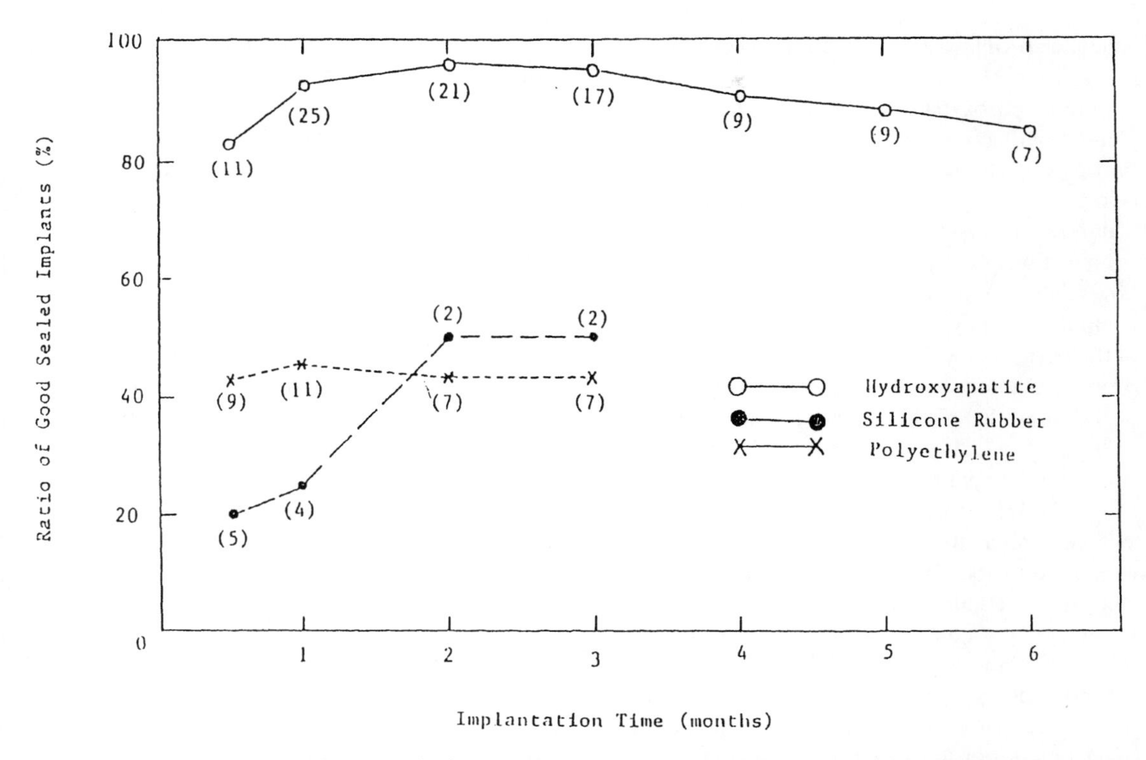

Fig. 7. Success rate of percutaneous implants. The data of polyethylene was calculated from Reference [3]. The number of samples are given in parentheses.

Table 1. Amino acid composition of periosteum and fibrous capsule formed around the hydroxyapatite 23 months after subcutaneous implantation in mongrel dog.

Amino acid	Periosteum	Capsule (skin side)	Capsule (fascia side)
Aspartic acid	41	47	44
Threonine	21	24	24
Serine	33	38	37
Glutamic acid	73	77	71
Proline	156	154	150
Glycine	287	282	282
Alanine	103	96	91
Valine	23	26	25
Methionine	8	9	9
Isoleucine	13	15	15
Leucine	27	33	31
Tyrosine	6	8	7
Phenylalanine	16	18	23
Histidine	6	7	7
Lysine	21	25	24
Arginine	45	26	43
Cystine	2	4	3
4-Hydroxyproline	112	103	107

Amino acid composition of the fibrous capsule

Sintered hydroxypatite was subcutaneously implanted in dogs. After 23 months the surrounding fibrous capsule was sampled to study the amino acid composition according to standard procedures. This was compared to the amino acid composition of periosteum of femur of the same dog (Table 1). It was clarified that amino acid composition of the capsule was very similar to that of the periosteum. The protein was rich in glycine, proline, alanine and hydroxyproline. This study also showed that histidinoalanine which is peculiar to hard tissue collagen existed in the capsule surrounding the apatite.

The fibrous capsule surrounding the HAp and silicone rubber after 3 months of implantation were compared (Table 2). The results showed that the capsule surrounding HAp was composed of collagen with more than 90% purity. However, more than 50% of the capsule around the silicone rubber was non-collagen protein. This is acid protein rich in glutamic acid and frequently observed in pathological tissues or in foreign body reaction.

From these results, it can be stated that the HAp implant is surrounded by a collagen layer the composition of which is similar to that of periosteum. There should be some kind of bonding at the interfacae of sample and layer which eliminates the space between the two. This fact contributes greatly to the prevention of infection.

Application to continuous blood pressure measurement

We made a prototype of a percutaneous connector for the continuous measurement of blood pressure and deep body temperature. HAp device was implanted in the back skin of mature dog, blood pressure transducer in the femoral artery and thermocouple near it. Data from the device were transmitted from connector to receiving monitor 5 meters apart from the site. Fig. 8 is an example of continuous measurement of blood pressure and deep body temperature 2 weeks after implantation. Curve 'A' represents the continuous systolic blood pressure, 'B' the continuous diastolic blood pressure and 'C' the deep body temperature. These long-term measurements of internal variables were established without infection.

Blood pressure and body temperature increased

Table 2. Amino acid composition of capsule surrounding the hydroxyapatite and silicone rubber 3 months after subcutaneous implantation.

Amino acid	Hydroxyapatite	Silicone Rubber
Aspartic acid	52	66
Threonine	27	36
Serine	44	49
Glutamic acid	84	106
Proline	104	89
Glycine	281	226
Alanine	99	98
Valine	25	34
Methionine	11	14
Isoleucine	15	25
Leucine	38	54
Tyrosine	9	15
Phenylalanine	17	23
Histidine	8	12
Lysine	36	52
Arginine	49	50
4-Hydroxyproline	99	52

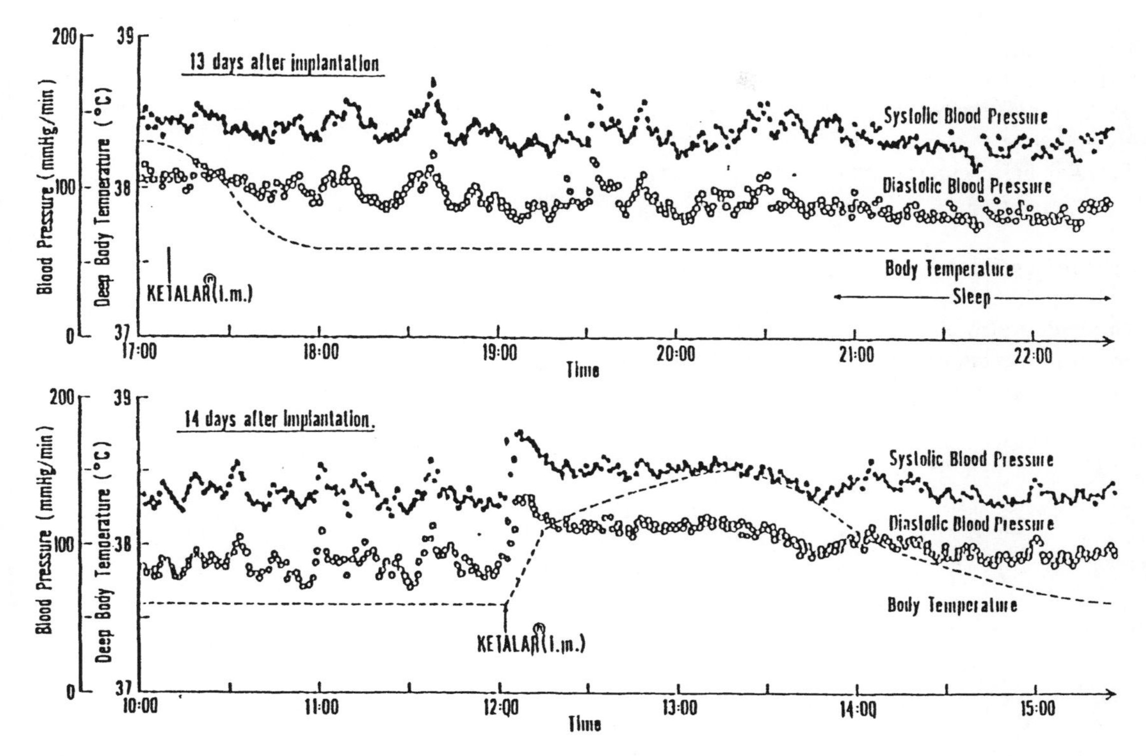

Fig. 8. Direct arterial blood pressure and deep body temperature measured continuously by using hydroxyapatite percutaneous device.

immediately after injection of ketamine hydrochloride. For this dog, systolic and diastolic blood pressure ranged from 120 to 150, and 80 to 100 mmHg, respectively. This example shows a significant long-term stability in blood pressure and deep body temperature measurements.

Future perspective of the percutaneous device

Infection around the percutaneous tunnel is the major problem in the delivery of drug solutions in the body. Especially for CAPD, this is a problem which requires urgent solution. By using HAp percutaneous device, physical transportation and electrical input from outside to inside of the body and output from inside to outside, were possible for long-term without inflammation of infection.

The following are possible applications of the HAp device.

a) Physical input transportation: It can be applied to the continuous administration of various kinds of drugs such as insulin for diabetes patients.
b) Physical output transportation: It may become possible to eliminate waste material from the body as enteroprotia. Or blood can be taken as required through the device.
c) Electrical input: By providing electric stimulus, it may become possible to enhance bone growth, to activate disconnected neutral systems or relieve pain for terminal cancer patients. It is also possible to provide a power source for artificial organs.
d) Electrical output: By the use of sensors, it becomes possible to continuously monitor biological information such as blood pressure, hemodynamics, blood sugar level, hormone volume, ion concentration, pH and deep body temperature.

Thus, it can be applied to the control of the body and detect heart problems before attack. With a single application or combinations of applications, it is possible to cover a wider area of medicine including basic, clinical and prophylactic research.

Acknowledgement

The amino acid analysis was kindly provided by Professor Yoshinori Kuboki, Faculty of Dentistry, Hokkaido University.

References

1. Akao M, Aoki H, Kato K: J Mater Sci 16: 809–812, 1981.
2. Aoki H, Shin Y, Akao M, Tsuji T, Ukegawa Y, Togawa T, Kikuchi R: Advances in biomaterials, Vol. 7. Duheyne P et al. (eds) Elsevier, New York, 1985, p 1–4.
3. Glazener WB, MS Thesis : Clemson University, 1975.
4. Park JB: Biomaterials an introduction, Plenum Press, New York, 1979, p 152–157.

Address for offprints:
Hideki Aoki
Institute for Medical and Dental Engineering
Tokyo Medical and Dental University
2-3-10 Kanda Surugadai, Chiyoda
Tokyo 101, Japan

Medical Progress through Technology 12: 221–232 (1987)

Recent advances in thromboresistant materials

Nobuhiko Yui, Kazunori Kataoka & Yasuhisa Sakurai
Institute of Biomedical Engineering, Tokyo Women's Medical College, 8-1 Kawada-cho, Shinjuku-ku, Tokyo 162, Japan

Key words: surface characterization, antithrombogenic materials, X-ray photoelectron spectroscopy, segmented polyamide

Summary

There are strong demands for innovative antithrombogenic materials, because of their necessity in fabricating artificial organs and progressive surgical prostheses. This paper reviews the recent advances in thromboresistant materials. Special emphasis is placed on the novel feature of the surface characterization of thromboresistant materials by X-ray photoelectron spectroscopy and its biomedical implications. Essential role of crystalline-amorphous microstructured surface in thromboresistant property of semicrystalline segmented copolymer is also discussed in detail.

1. Introduction

Recent progress in 'materials science' has lent a great impetus to today's advanced technology concerned with electronics, aerospace, and life sciences. Especially, intensive biomaterials research for artificial organs has been facilitated in life science fields [2, 9, 33]. Many artificial organs and prosthetic devices are being utilized in contact with blood to fulfill various functions such as circulation, apheresis, and gas exchange. Since artificial materials generally suffer serious foreign body reaction, i.e., thrombus formation, in blood stream, biomaterials for medical purposes must have reliable antithrombogenicity. Therefore, development of highly-functionated artificial organs depends greatly upon the innovation in antithrombogenic materials [42].

Throughout the intensive research on antithrombogenic materials over the last decade, several biomaterials with good antithrombogenicity have been developed for fabricating artificial organs and prosthetic devices. Also, these researches have got insight into blood-materials interaction from the aspects of both biology and materials science to facilitate the molecular design of superior antithrombogenic materials. Further, it is noteworthy to recall the progress in methods estimating the complicated interactions of blood with biomaterial surfaces. These are such methods as the dynamic in vitro simulation test of thrombosis on the material surfaces, and the arteriovenous (AV) shunt test in vivo in which the patency time of the shunt represents the thromboresistant index of shunt materials.

With an increasing interest in the interfacial phenomena of materials with blood, the characterization of outermost surfaces of biomaterials has been actively carried out [27]. Many advanced techniques for surface chemical analysis are presently available [8], and some of them have been intensively applied in surface characterization of antithrombogenic materials. This article reviews the recent advances in surface characterization of antithrombogenic materials with a special emphasis in X-ray photoelectron spectroscopy (XPS). The XPS highlights the material surfaces from their interior, and therefore, enables one to obtain a correlation

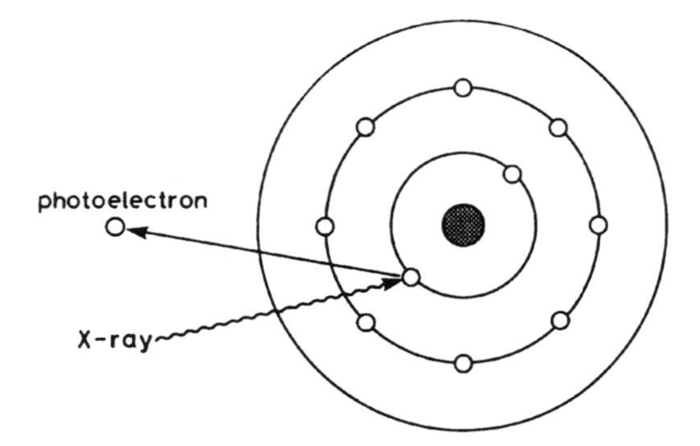

Fig. 1. Emission of photoelectron by bombardment with X-ray.

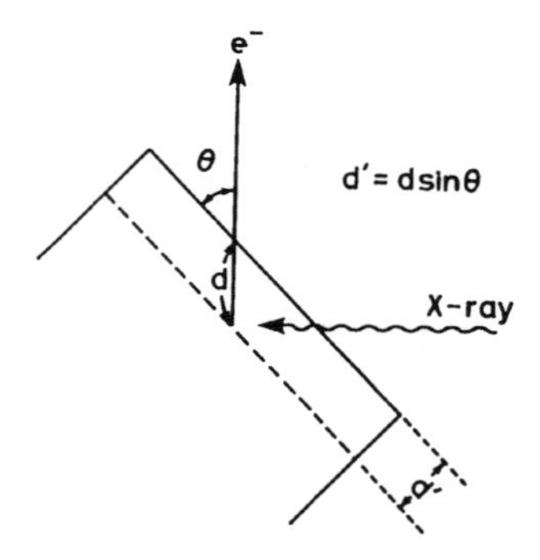

Fig. 2. Principle of angular dependent X-ray photoelectron spectroscopy

of the material surface structure with their antithrombogenicity.

2. Surface characterization by XPS

XPS has its principle in the photo-electron effect discovered by Hert in 1887 [32]. However, the XPS as a surface analytical technique was established by Siegbahn in 1950s. His group observed the chemical shift effect on core-level binding energies and utilized this effect to the electron spectroscopy, first Auger electron spectroscopy (AES), followed by XPS. It was also Siegbahn who coined the acronym ESCA (electron spectroscopy for chemical analysis).

The photoelectron effect is expressed by following equation:

$$E_k = h\nu - E_b$$

where E_k is the kinetic energy of photoelectrons, $h\upsilon$ the incident photon energy, and E_b the electron binding energy. Materials bombarded with X-ray will emit photoelectrons with E_k (Fig. 1). Thus we can estimate E_b of the ejected electron by measuring E_k by XPS. Elemental analysis is accomplished based on the fact that each element has its own E_b. Further, from the energy distribution of photoelectrons, we can estimate the binding state of each atom.

XPS enables us to characterize the material surfaces differentiating from their interior because of the very short mean free path length of electrons. For conventional polymeric materials, the mean free path length of photoelectrons is several nanometers, thus photoelectrons detected by a scintillator located normal to the material surface will come from the depth of ~10nm. Here, the result obtained is the average value of the effective sampling depth of 10nm. From antithrombogenic materials perspective, the characteristics of uppermost surface of 1~2nm are of great interest because it is thin surface structure which blood components including platelets and proteins might recognize. Recently, a new method of angular dependent XPS has been established for estimating depth profiles of atomic composition. By this method, it is capable of detecting the photoelectrons emitted from the depth of ~1nm to ~10nm depending on the tilt angle of the sample. The relation of the effective sampling depth with the tilt angle is schematically shown in Fig. 2, where θ is a tilt or emission angle, d a sampling depth, and d′ an effective sampling depth, to be explained by following equation:

$$d' = d\sin\theta \quad (\text{conventionally } \theta = 15\sim 90°)$$

Considering the magnitude of d of ~10nm, d′ of approximately 1~2.5nm could be realized at low emission angles [28, 41].

3. Classification of antithrombogenic materials

Antithrombogenic materials are generally classified into three categories based on their thromboresistant mechanisms. They are the materials: 1) promoting pseudointima formation on their surfaces; 2) conjugating bioactive agents such as heparin, prostaglandin, and urokinase; and 3) with physicochemical properties favorable for eliminating thrombosis [12]. The materials of both types 1) and 2) retain their antithrombogenic properties through biological mechanisms, namely, by the self-repairing property of the living body (type 1) or by biological reactions against thrombosis (type 2) whereas the materials of type 3) work without any use of biological reagents. This, no requirement of biological reagents, lends the materials of type 3 the wide applications in artificial organs and many other prosthetic devices, requiring a long term implantation.

Platelet adhesion, subsequent activation, and aggregation on foreign surfaces are the major events which facilitate the catastrophic thrombosis. This interaction of platelets with material surface consists of two distinct but serial stages. First one is physicochemical adsorption of platelets where the driving force of platelet adsorption is only physicochemical interaction independent of metabolic action of platelets. One may assure that material surfaces eliminating or minimizing the platelet adsorption could be non-thrombogenic. A promising example for such surface is so-called hydrogel. Its antithrombogenicity is theoretically predicted by Andrade et al. [1], known as minimum interfacial free energy hypothesis. The second stage subsequent to the physicochemical adsorption is defined by the term 'contact-induced activation' where reorganization of intracellular cytoskeletal components such as microfilaments and microtubules occurs through the change in energy-metabolism of platelets [13]. Development of materials eliminating this contact-induced activation of platelets is an alternative approach to achieve non-thrombogenic surfaces. A representative of this type of materials is a microdomain structured material.

4. Antithrombogenicity of hydrogels and its surface characterization

The biomedical investigation of hydrogels began with the development of cross-linked poly(2-hydroxyethyl methacrylate) (PHEMA). The hydrogel would be expected to have a low interfacial free energy which would prevent adsorption and denaturation of blood components. Recently, the hydrogelled surfaces with long-chain hydrophilic macromolecules such as polyacrylamide (PAAm) and poly(ethylene oxide) (PEO) were prepared by grafting these macromolecules on mechanically strong support materials. These materials have the advantages of good mechanical properties and easy fabrication [20]. Since hydrogels have, however, been reported to have a possibility of embolization, calcification, and a consumption of circulating platelets, their antithrombogenicity are still doubtful, especially for relatively long term applications [25].

It has been well known that contact angle and surface tension measurements are useful for characterizing the hydrophilic nature of solid surfaces [6]. Recently, the spectroscopic analyses have been applied to characterize the hydrogel surfaces in an aqueous environment. The XPS study by Ratner et al. revealed that PAAm-grafted silicone rubber drastically changes its surface chemical compositions with the degree of hydration, indicating that the orientation of PAAm chains could be reversibly altered in response to change in the surrounding environment [24]. Similar result was obtained for poly(vinyl alcohol)/poly(dimethylsiloxane) graft copolymers characterized by means of the contact angle measurement [40].

5. Surface structures of multiphase segmented copolymers and the relations to their antithrombogenicity

XPS has been found to be available for characterizing material surfaces with microdomain structure. Since the microdomain structure is a feature of block or graft copolymer composed of chemically dissimilar segments with mutual immiscibility,

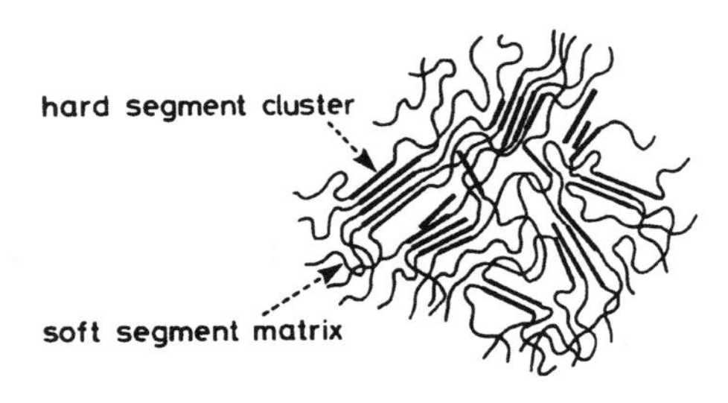

Fig. 3. Microdomain structure for segmented polyether poly(urethaneurea).

there is a feasibility of difference in structure and chemistry between the surfaces and bulk or interior of these materials. A famous example of this type materials is Biomer, which is a family of segmented polyether poly(urethaneurea) (PEUU)s. Biomer was first evaluated as to its biomedical property by Pierce et al. [3]. Since then, Biomer and similar kinds of segmented copolymers have been evaluated for biomedical applications and applied for fabricating various prosthetic devices used in contact with blood. As well-known, pneumatic artificial hearts made from Biomer(Jarvik-7 type) have been implanted in several human patients in the United States [11]. Antithrombogenicity of this type of materials is considered due to the formation of the microdomain structure: clusters of hard segments are dispersed into the continuous matrix of soft segments to form the microdomains (Fig. 3). First study on the effect of molecular structure of PEUU on protein adsorption and platelet adhesion was done by Lyman et al. [17]. They revealed that molecular weight of soft segments in PEUU had a definite effect on platelet adhesion as well as composition of adsorbed proteins. Then they assumed such copolymers with excellent antithrombogenicity to have two phase morphology with microdomains of 3~10nm in size, which approximates the size of globular proteins. Further, they examined surface chemical composition of these copolymers by XPS, and found out the enrichment effect of poly(propylene oxide) (PPO) on the air facing side (AFS) of PEUU films compared to the substrate facing side (SFS) of them. However, the relation of such polyether enrichment with biological response was not argued at that time. For the past 10 years, in order to examine relation between PEUU surface chemical composition and its antithrombogenicity, diverse spectroscopic techniques such as XPS, AES, and attenuated total reflection infrared spectroscopy (ATR-IR) has been successively introduced by a number of investigators. Subsequent to the above-mentioned Lyman's report, Stupp et al. characterized PEUU surfaces through ATR-IR analysis to clarify that chemical composition of these PEUU surfaces were sensitively altered with the casting substrate [34], and, further, many other studies concerning with PEUU surfaces revealed that AFS of PEUU films had a higher content of hydrophobic polyether (generally PPO or poly(tetramethylene oxide) (PTMO) segments whereas SFS of those contained a higher concentration of hard segments [5, 35]. These results clearly demonstrate the concentration of soft segments at AFS during solvent casting and verify that the surface chemical composition of PEUU is sensitive to fabricating conditions such as solution concentration, casting temperature, and kinds of substrate [29]. Moreover, Paynter et al. suggested that a significant excess of polyether segment is commonly present within ~2nm of AFS of PEUU films [31]. Such concentrating effect of soft segments on AFS of these PEUU films can be mainly explained on the basis of minimizing interfacial free energy. Some contentions over this explanation lent an impetus to the further investigations on such phenomena, and Matsuda et al. clarified that the PEUU film in wet state was varied in the surface localization of polyether segments from that in air, and that this variation was reversible [18].

Takahara et al. and Ratner et al. demonstrated the close relationship of the facilitation in microphase separation with the surface concentrating effect of hydrophobic polyether segment from the studies of PEUUs having different diamine units [37, 43].

With the advance in the surface characterization of PEUUs as mentioned above, many investigators have forcefully tried to reconsider antithrombogenicity of PEUUs in relation to their surface chemical compositions. Their reports contain three different opinions concerned with surface-antithrombogenicity of PEUUs; 1) polyether enrichment on PEUU surface leads to good antithrombogenicity; 2) depletion of polyether on PEUU surface causes good antithrombogenicity; and 3) antithrombogenicity of PEUU surface is optimized at a certain compositional balance of soft and hard segments. Merill et al. reported that platelet retention on PEO-based PEUU surfaces decreased linearly with decreasing their ratios of the neutral carbon intensity to the ethereal carbon intensity, suggesting that a surface covered with amorphous PEO would be remarkably inactive toward platelets [4, 19]. Cooper et al. also showed that in the ex vivo AV shunt test the decrease in platelet consumption on PTMO-based PEUU surfaces correlates with increasing concentration of polyether segments on their surfaces, suggesting a feasible correlation of thromboresistance of PEUU surfaces with the magnitude of their surface free energy [15, 16]. Hanson et al., however, revealed that platelet consumption on polyester-based PEUUs as well as polyether-based ones correlated strongly with the concentration of ethereal carbon at their surfaces [7, 26]. In addition, Takahara et al. reported that platelet adhesion on PEO-, PPO-, and PTMO-based PEUU surfaces were influenced by three major factors: 1) the mode of microphase separation; 2) the surface chemical composition; and 3) the surface free energy of each segment. They also pointed out the optimum of surface microphase-separated structure for antithrombogenicity [38, 39]. These inconsistencies among researchers are considered due to the difference in evaluation methods for thromboresistant property, and in sample environments during surface characterization. It is to be noted that polyether segments are liable to change reversibly in their location at the interface with a change in environments [18] and that surface-located PEO segments in an aqueous environment might eliminate similar to hydrogel, physicochemical adsorption of platelets, but initiate embolization in a long term implantation. In addition, Ratner et al. and Cooper et al. demonstrated that a series of PTMO-based PEUUs including a commercial lot was contaminated with a polyether-rich low molecular weight material. This could lead to a significant enrichment of polyether on AFS resulting in the variation of antithrombogenicity [10, 22, 30]. Thus, we should be reminded that the surface chemical composition of PEUUs could be readily affected by many factors such as method of purification and/or fabrication and prolonged implantation in a physiological environment.

Avcothane (Cardiothane) has also been used for fabricating many blood-containing devices such as chambers for total artificial heart and assist devices, owing to its good antithrombogenicity as well as excellent mechanical properties. Avcothane is a polymer blend consisting of poly(dimethylsiloxane) (PDMS) and PEUU segments, and was developed principally by Nyilas who exhibited Avcothane to have the optimum surface composition of PDMS and PEUU segments for antithrombogenicity [21]. Such surface of polymer-blend as Avcothane would be more sensitive to fabrication, preparation and physiological environment compared with ordinary PEUUs. Originally Nyilas et al. examined the surface characterization by ATR-IR to show its multiphase separated surface composed of PDMS and PEUU regions [21]. However, from the XPS study by Sung et al., it was found that AFS of Avcothane film was covered mostly with PDMS, and that PEUU component was hidden beneath the surface [35]. Their further investigation by AES revealed that a deeper sampling depth (over 20nm) was required for both AFS and SFS of the film to show the comparable PDMS and PEUU compositions [36]. Then, there may be an issue on the thromboresistant mechanism of Avcothane surface if it is entirely covered with PDMS segments. One possibility is that the concentration of siloxane groups on the AFS might be greater than ordinary silicone rubber to have a distinct behavior toward the interaction with blood, since the localization of PDMS segments on AFS of Avcothane film would be driven through the immiscibility between PDMS and PEUU segments.

Recently, Kira et al. developed PDMS-based segmented polyurethane for prosthetic devices and then characterized their surface in relation to their antithrombogenicity [14]. They reported that the copolymers with soft segments of PEO-PDMS-PEO triblocks exhibited a small anisotropic dis-

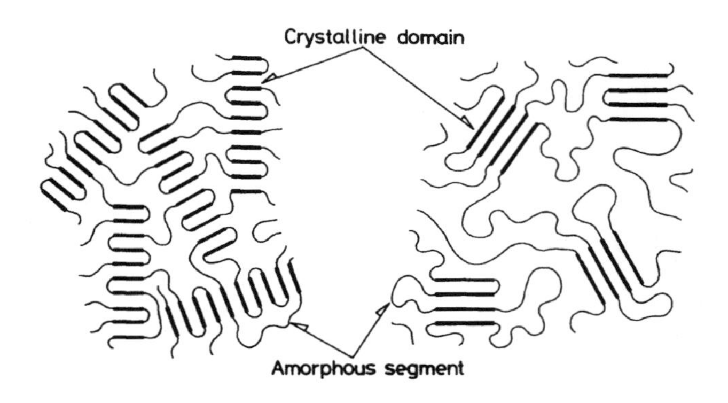

Fig. 4. Microstructure composed of crystalline and amorphous phases.

tribution of hard and soft segments. Moreover, these copolymers were found to show better antithrombogenicity than both Biomer and Avcothane.

Quite recently, Ratner et al. investigated the surface structure of PEUUs with various perfluoro chain extenders [42]. They demonstrated that limited amounts of additional fluorine in the hard segment would not alter the migration of the soft segment to the surface, because of the localization of fluorine atoms in the highly polar hard-segment regions.

The relation of PEUU surface structure with its antithrombogenicity has not been fully understood yet, despite the stepwise clarification of the surface structure of PEUU films. Therefore, more systematic studies done to clarify many factors determining the PEUU surface structure are required to get the close relationship between the surface structure of segmented copolymers and its thromboresistant property.

6. Antithrombogenic segmented polyamides and their surface microstructure

Linear polyamides are well known to undergo a limited crystallization since sections of their chain molecules are capable of packing together closely in parallel arrays. Such crystallization yields formations of microstructure composed of ordered crystalline and disordered amorphous phases, as schematically illustrated in Fig. 4, which is morphologically similar to the microphase separated structure of PEUU. The authors have carried out a series of studies concerned with molecular design of antithrombogenic polyamides because their antithrombogenicity is considered to be closely coupled to such a morphological specific of ordered structure [22, 44, 45]. In particular, the authors prepared various types of segmented copolymers based on PPO and aliphatic polyamide segments to confirm the above consideration (Fig. 5) [6]. Since PPO segment is wholly amorphous and a polyamide one is partially crystallized, these types of copolymers have a characteristic of crystalline-amorphous type microstructure, typical of which is the formation of spherulitic structure. This microstructure is quantitatively characterized by crystallite thickness and long period, which are estimated by wide-angle X-ray diffraction and small-angle X-ray scattering, respectively. With these copolymers, the authors estimated platelet adhesion on the copolymer surfaces, and then examined the results in relation to the copolymer microstructure. Worthy of interest, every type of copolymer took minimum platelet adhesion at the copolymer surfaces having a crystallite thickness of 6.0~6.5nm and a long period of 12~13nm, although the polyamide segment of these copolymers had different chemical structures (Figs. 6 and 7) [47–49]. Moreover, in order to discuss the feasibility of these copolymers for novel antithrombogenic materials, the modified microsphere col-

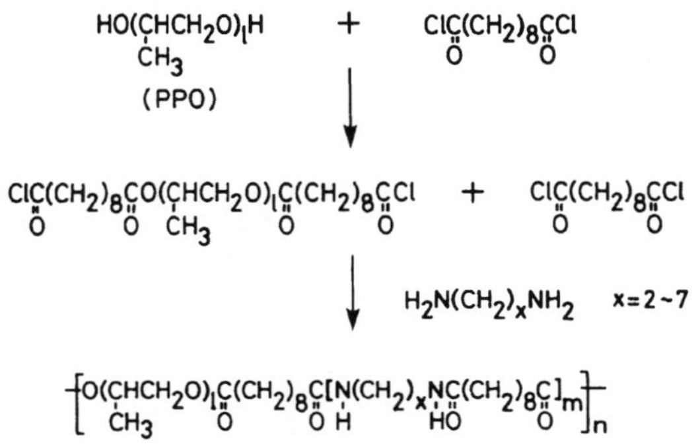

HO(CHCH2O)lH
CH3
(PPO)
ClC(CH2)8CCl
O O
ClC(CH2)8CO(CHCH2O)lC(CH2)8CCl
O O CH3 O O
ClC(CH2)8CCl
O O
H2N(CH2)xNH2 x=2~7
O(CHCH2O)lC(CH2)8C[N(CH2)xNC(CH2)8C]m
CH3 O O H HO O n

Fig. 5. Synthetic route of PPO-segmented aliphatic polyamides.

umn method simulating thrombosis on polymer surface was carried out [50]. Here the in vitro thrombosis time of the copolymers was evaluated by passing Ca^{2+}-readded platelet-rich plasma of white rabbit through the column packed with polymer-precoated glass beads until the column was occluded. The copolymers having the particular microstructure mentioned above were found to exhibit stably longer patency than any other copolymers. The example of such results is shown in Fig. 8. These results suggest that a particular size and distribution of crystalline and amorphous phases in the copolymer are the most essential factors for antithrombogenicity of these copolymers.

21P
31P
41P
61P
71P
Amount of adhering platelets (%)
Long period (nm)
10
12
14
16
18
10
20
30
40
50

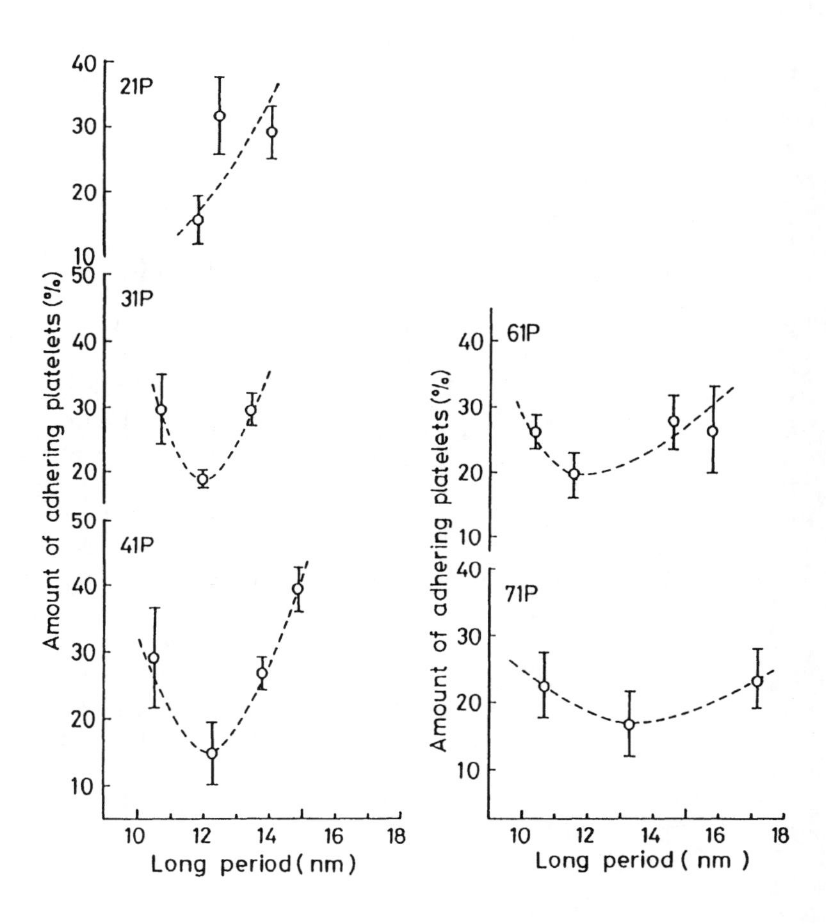

Fig. 6. Relationship between platelet adhesion and long period of PPO-segmented aliphatic polyamides (± S.E.M.).

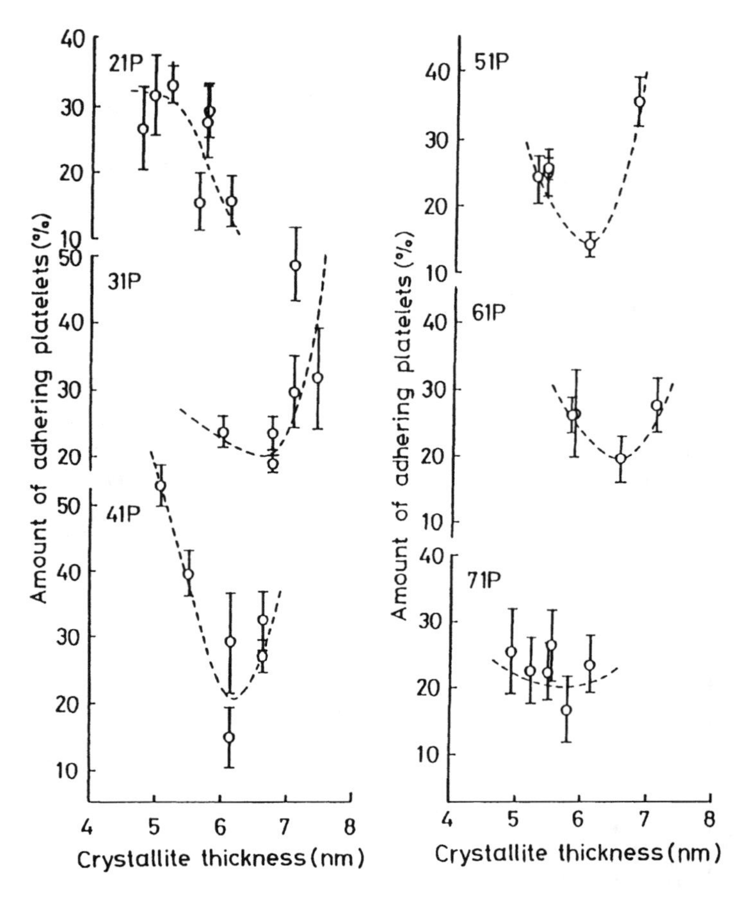

Fig. 7. Relationship between platelet adhesion and crystallite thickness of PPO-segmented aliphatic polyamides (± S.E.M.).

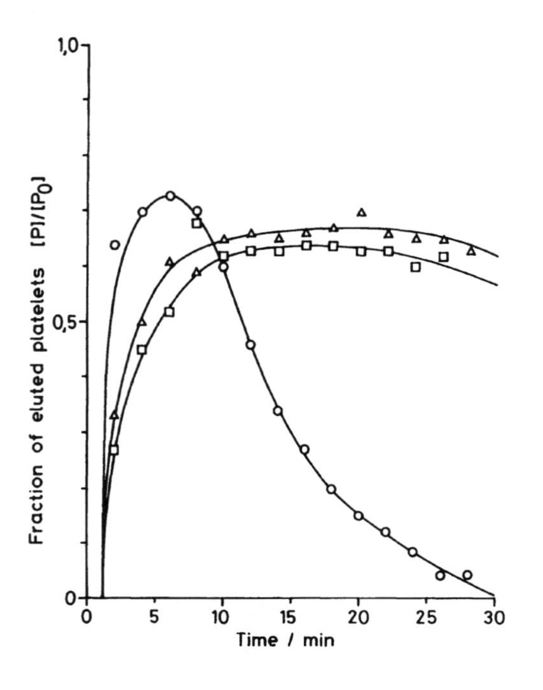

Since the above material characterization is featured by the bulk microstructure of the copolymer, however, there may be an issue whether the surfaces have the same chemical composition and microstructure as their interior. The transmission electron microscopic observation for the cross section of the copolymer surface elucidated this issue to find the continuity of the microstructure composed of crystalline and amorphous phases having width of ~10nm from the interior to the surface of the copolymer, as shown in Fig. 9, being consistent with the preceding results of X-ray analyses with respect to size of these phases. Further, the authors employed XPS for investigating the surface chemical composition of these copolymers and clarified

Fig. 8. Representative results of *in vitro* simulation for thrombosis on PPO-segmented nylon 610 surfaces: (○) nylon 610; (△)61P3-25; (□)61P3-47. The three-sequence code 61P3- represents the weight percentage of PPO in the copolymer.

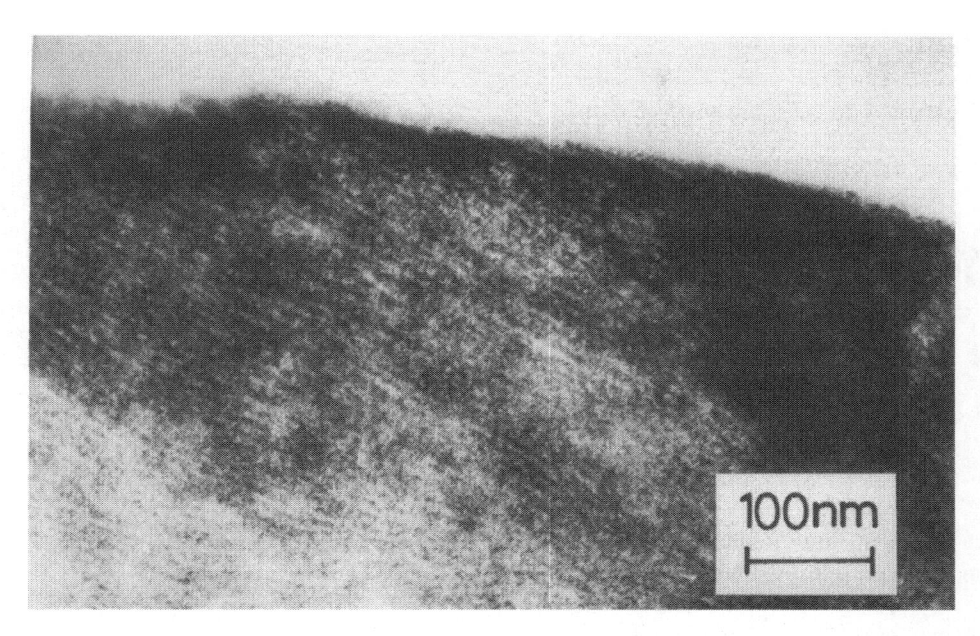

Fig. 9. TEM view of cross section of PPO-segmented nylon 610 (PPO weight percentage of 56%) film stained with RuO_4. This micrograph is presented by courtesy of Prof. Dr. T. Hashimoto and Dr. H. Hasegawa of Kyoto University.

in more detail the relation between the surface chemical composition of the copolymers and the platelet adhesion on the copolymer surfaces [51]. Considering the results obtained for PEUU surfaces, the concentrating effect of the component with lower surface free energy on the AFS may be expected. However, the enrichment of PPO component on the outermost surface of the copolymers was not always varied in the case of our copolymers, an example of which is shown in Fig. 10. This result will be attributed to the polyamide crystallization as a driving force for microstructure formation. Subsequently, the examination of the XPS result in relation to the platelet adhesion suggests that isotropic distribution of PPO component was indispensable, or at least unnecessary, for reducing platelet adhesion (Fig. 11). Therefore, these results support our concept for molecular design of a sur-

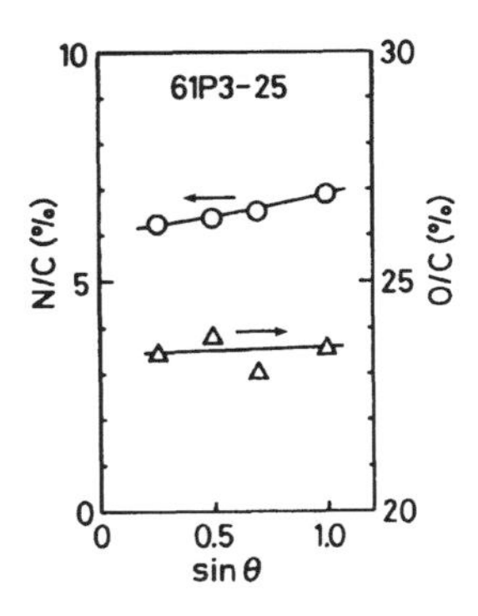

Fig. 10. Change in number ratio of nitrogen to carbon atoms (N/C) and of oxygen to carbon atoms (O/C) with sin θ for air-facing side of PPO-segmented nylon 610 (PPO weight percentage of 25%).

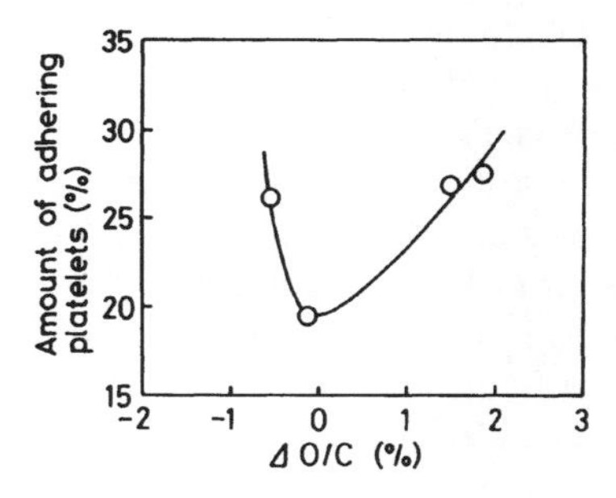

Fig. 11. Variation of ΔO/C for PPO-segmented nylon 610 with platelet adhesion on the copolymer surface. ΔO/C represents the differential of O/C at θ = 15° with that at θ = 90°, which can be used as a parameter of anisotropic distribution of PPO segments.

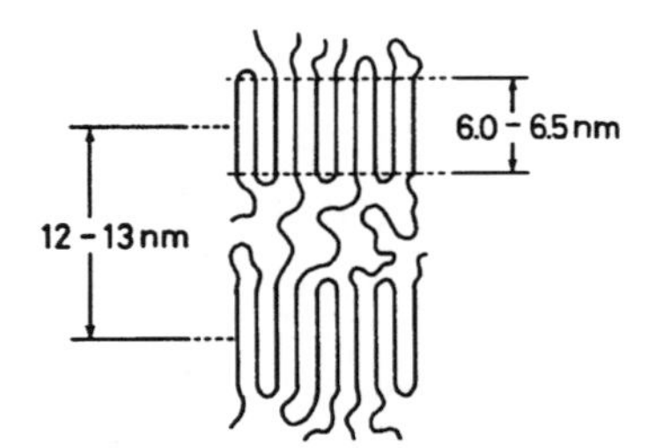

Fig. 12. New design concept of antithrombogenic segmented copolymer with semicrystalline state.

face with excellent antithrombogenicity through regulating the size and distribution of crystalline and amorphous phases on the surface as well as the interior of such segmented polyamides (Fig. 12).

7. Concluding remarks

This article reviewed the surface characterization of diverse antithrombogenic materials mainly by XPS. Though XPS study is preferable to characterize the nature of such surfaces with high reliability, however, present status of characterization in relation to the antithrombogenicity is not enough for fully explaining various phenomena of blood-materials interactions such as protein adsorption and subsequent sequences of events leading to thrombosis or embolization. AES, secondary ion mass spectrometry, and ion scattering spectroscopy as well as XPS could become leading techniques for further extensive research of such surfaces. By facilitating the surface characterization of these materials in physiological environment and making interpretations for their biological responses, it is in the near future that the advent of ideal antithrombogenic materials will enable innovative artificial organs and prosthetic devices to be in clinical service.

References

1. Andrade JD: Interfacial phenomena and biomaterials. Med Instrum 7: 110–120, 1973.
2. Atsumi K: Past, present, and future of artificial organs. Igaku No Ayumi 134: 852–859, 1985.
3. Boretos JW, Pierce WS, Baire RE, LeRoy AF, Donachy HJ: Surface and bulk characteristics of a polyether urethane for artificial hearts. J Biomed Mater Res 9: 327–340, 1975.
4. Costa VSD, Russel DB, Salzman EW, Merrill EW: ESCA studies of polyurethanes: Blood platelet activation in relation to surface composition. J Coll Interf Sci 80: 445–452, 1981.
5. Graham SW, Hercules DM: Surface spectroscopic studies of Biomer. J Biomed Mater Res 15: 465–477, 1981.
6. Hamilton WC: A technique for the characterization of hydrophilic solid surfaces. J Coll Interf Sci 10: 219–222, 1972.
7. Hanson SR, Harker LA, Ratner BD, Hoffman AS: In vivo evaluation of artificial surfaces with a nonhuman primate model of arterial thrombosis. J Lab Clin Med 95: 289–304, 1980.
8. Hercules DM, Hercules SM: Analytical chemistry of surfaces. Part I. General aspects. J Chem Ed 61: 402–409, 1984.
9. Hoffman AS: Medical applications of polymeric fibers. J Appl Polym Sci, Appl Polym Symp 31: 313–334, 1977.
10. Hu CB, Sung CSP: Surface chemical composition – depth profile of polyether polyethaneureas as studied by FT-IR and ESCA. Am Chem Soc, Div Polym Chem, Polym Prepr 21: 156–158, 1980.
11. Joyce LD, DeVries MC, Hastings WS, Olsen DB, Jarvik RK, Kolff WJ: Response of the human body to the first permanent implant of the Jarvik-7 total artificial heart. Trans ASAIO 29: 81–87, 1983.
12. Kataoka K, Yui N: Molecular design of bloodcompatible materials. J Syn Org Chem Jpn 43: 1048–1059, 1985.
13. Kataoka K, Sakurai S, Tsuruta T: Microphase separated polymer surfaces for separation of B and T lymphocytes. Makromol Chem, Suppl 9: 53–67, 1985.
14. Kira K, Minokami T, Yamamoto N, Hayashi K, Yamashita I: Synthesis and evaluation for antithrombogenic materials of polyurethane containing polydimethylsiloxane in the main chain. J Jpn Soc Biomater 1: 29–34, 1983.
15. Lelah MD, Lambrecht LK, Young BR, Cooper SL: Physicochemical characterization and in vivo blood tolerability of cast and extruded Biomer. J Biomed Mater Res 17: 1–22, 1983.
16. Lelah MD, Cooper SL: Polyurethanes in medicine. CRC Press, Florida, 1986.
17. Lyman DJ, Knutson K, McNeill B, Shibatani K: The effects of chemical structure and surface properties of synthetic polymers on the coagulation of blood. IV. The relation between polymer morphology and protein adsorption. Trans ASAIO 21: 49–54, 1975.
18. Matsuda T, Iwata H, Akutsu T: Surface chemical composition & blood compatibility in hydrophobic & hydrophilic segmented polyurethane systems. Polym Prepr Jpn 32: 2003–2006, 1983.

19. Merrill EW, Costa VSD, Salzman EW, Russell DB, Kirchner L, Wangh DF, Trudel G, Stopper S, Vital V: A critical study of segmented polyurethanes. In: Cooper SL, Peppas NA (eds) Biomaterials: Interfacial phenomena and applications. Adv Chem Ser 199, Am Chem Soc, Washington DC, 1982, pp 95–107.
20. Mori Y, Nagaoka S, Takiuchi H, Tanzawa H, Kikuchi T, Noishiki Y: The effect of the long polyethylene oxide chains grafted to the polymer on antithrombogenicity. Jpn J Artif Organs 10: 993–996, 1981.
21. Nyilas E, Ward Jr RS: Development of blood-compatible elastomers V Surface structure and blood compatibility of Avcothane elastomers. J Biomed Mater Res Symp 8: 69–84, 1977.
22. Ogata N, Sanui K, Tanaka H, Takahashi Y, Kitamura E, Sakurai Y, Okano T, Kataoka T, Akaike T: Effect of crystallinity of condensation polymers on platelet adhesion. J Appl Polym Sci 26: 4207–4216, 1981.
23. Paynter RW, Ratner BD, Thomas HR: Polyurethane surfaces: An XPS study. Am Chem Soc Div Polym Prepr 24: 13–14, 1983.
24. Ratner BD, Weathersby P, Hoffman AS: Radiation-grafted hydrogels for biomedical applications as studied by the ESCA technique. J Appl Polym Sci 22: 643–664, 1978.
25. Ratner BD, Hoffman AS, Hanson SR, Harker LA, Whiffen JD: Blood-compatibility-water-content relationships for radiationgrafted hydrogels. J Polym Sci Polym Symp 66: 363–375, 1979.
26. Ratner BD: ESCA and SEM studies on polyurethanes for biomedical applications. In: Dwight DW, Fabish TJ, Thomas HR (eds) Photon, electron, and ion probes of polymer structure and properties. ACS Symp Ser 162, Am Chem Soc, Washington DC, 1981, pp 371–382.
27. Ratner BD: Surface characterization of materials for blood contact applications. In: Cooper SL, Peppas NA (eds) Biomaterials: Interfacial phenomena and applications. Adv Chem Ser 199, Am Chem Soc, Washington DC, 1982, pp 9–23.
28. Ratner BD: Surface characterization of biomaterials by eectron spectroscopy for chemical analysis. Ann Biomed Eng 11: 313–336, 1983.
29. Ratner BD: ESCA studies of extracted polyurethanes and polyurethane extracts: Biomedical implications. In: Mittal KL (ed) Physicochemical aspects of polymer science 2. Plenum Press, New York, 1983, pp 969–983.
30. Ratner BD, Paynter RW, Thomas HR: Polyurethane surfaces: An XPS study. Trans Soc Biomater 6: 21, 1983.
31. Ratner BD, Paynter RW, Thomas HR: An XPS and SEM study of polyurethane surfaces: Experimental considerations. In: Shalaby SW, Hoffman AS, Ratner BD, Horbett TA (eds) Polymers as biomaterials. Plenum Press, New York, 1984, pp 121–134.
32. Seah MP, Briggs D: A perspective on the analysis of surfaces and interfaces. In: Briggs D, Seah MP (eds) Practical surface analysis by Auger and X-ray photoelectron spectroscopy. Joh Wiley & Sons, Chichester, 1983, pp 1–16.
33. Shalaby SW, Hoffman AS, Ratner BD, Horbett TA (eds): Polymers as biomaterials. Plenum Press, New York, 1984.
34. Stupp SI, Kauffman JW, Carr SH: Interactions between segmented polyurethane surfaces and the plasma protein fibrinogen. Biomed Mater Res 11: 237–250, 1977.
35. Sung CSP, Hu CB: ESCA stuies of surface chemical composition of segmented polyurethanes. J Biomed Mater Res 13: 161–171, 1979.
36. Sung CSP, Hu CB: Application of Auger electron spectroscopy for surface chemical analysis of Avcothane. J Biomed Mater Res 13: 45–55, 1979.
37. Takahara A, Tashita J, Kajiyama T, Takayanagi M: Surface depth profiles of polyether in segmented poly(urethaneureas) with various polyether components. Rep Prog Polym Phys Jpn 27: 229–232, 1984.
38. Takahara A, Tashita J, Kajiyama T, Takayanagi M, MacKnight WJ: Microphase separated structure and blood compatibility of segmented poly(urethaneureas) with diferent diamines in the hard segment. Polymer 26: 978–986, 1985.
39. Takahara A, Kajiyama T: Effect of polyether components on surface composition and blood compatibility of segmented polyurethaneureas. J Chem Soc Jpn: 1293–1301, 1985.
40. Tezuka Y, Matsui S, Fukushima A, Miya M, Imai K, Kataoka K, Sakurai Y: Surface structure and blood compatibility of poly(vinyl alcohol)/poly(dimethylsiloxane) graft copolymers. Kobunshi Ronbunshu 42: 629–634, 1985.
41. Thomas HR, O'Malley JJ: Surface studies on multicomponent polymer systems by X-ray photoelectron spectroscopy. Polystyrene/poly(ethylene oxide) diblock copolymers. Macromolecules 12: 323–329, 1979.
42. Tsuruta T, Sakurai Y (eds): Biomaterials Science 1 and 2. Nankodo, Tokyo, 1982.
43. Yoon SC, Ratner BD: Surface structure of segmented poly(ether urethanes) and poly(ether urethane ureas) with various perfluoro chain extenders. An X-ray photoelectron spectroscopic investigation. Macromolecules 19: 1068–1079, 1986.
44. Yui N, Takahashi Y, Sanui K, Ogata N, Kataoka K, Okano T, Sakurai Y: Effect of crystallinity of polymeric materials on antithrombogenicity. Jpn J Artif Organ 10: 1070–1073, 1981.
45. Yui N, Sanui K, Ogata N, Kataoka K, Okano T, Sakurai Y: Effect of crystallinity of polyamides on adhesion-separation behavior of granulocytes. J Biomed Mater Res 17: 383–388, 1983.
46. Yui N, Tanaka J, Sanui K, Ogata N: Polyether-segmented polyamides as a new designed antithrombogenicmaterial: Microstructure of poly(propylene oxide)-segmented nylon 610. Makromol Chem 185: 2259–2267, 1984.
47. Yui N, Tanaka J, Sanui K, Ogata N, Kataoka K, Okano T, Sakurai Y: Characterization of the microstructure of poly(propylene oxide)-segmented polyamide and its suppression of platelet adhesion. Polym J 16: 119–128, 1984.
48. Yui N, Oomiyama T, Sanui K, Ogata N, Kataoka K, Okano T, Sakuai Y: Polyether-segmented polyamide as a new

antithrombogenic material: Relationship between platelet adhesion and microstructure of poly(propylene oxide)-segmented aliphatic polyamides. Makromol Chem Rapid Commun 5: 805–809, 1984.

49. Yui N, Sanui K, Ogata N, Kataoka K, Okano T, Sakurai Y: Effct of microstructure of poly(propylene oxide)-segmented polyamides on platelet adhesion. J Biomed Mater Res 20: 929–943, 1986.
50. Yui N, Kataoka K, Sakurai Y, Aoki T, Sanui K, Ogata N: In vitro and in vivo studies on antithrombogenicity of poly(propylene oxide)-segmented nylon 610 in relation to its crystalline-amorphous microstructure. Biomaterials, submitted.
51. Yui N, Kataoka K, Sakurai Y, Sanui K. Ogata N, Takahara A, Kajiyama T: ESCA study of new antithrombogenic materials: Surface composition of poly(propylene oxide)-segmented nylon 610 and its blood compatibility Makromol Chem 187: 943–953, 1986.

Address for offprints:
Kazunori Kataoka
Institute of Biomedical Engineering
Tokyo Women's Medical College
8–1 Kawada-cho, Shinjuku-ku
Tokyo 162, Japan

Medical Progress through Technology 12: 233–242 (1987)

Biomagnetism in Japan

M. Kotani[1], H. Mori[2], S. Kuriki[3], Y. Uchikawa[4], K. Chiyotani[5] & I. Nemoto[6]
[1] *Department of Electronic Engineering, Tokyo Denki University;* [2] *Department of Internal Medicine, School of Medicine, The University of Tokushima;* [3] *Research Institute of Applied Electricity, Hokkaido University;* [4] *Department of Applied Electronic Engineering, Tokyo Denki University;* [5] *Rosai Hospital for Silicosis;* [6] *Department of Mathematical Science, Tokyo Denki University, Japan*

Abstract

The study of biomagnetic fields originating in a biological body is called biomagnetism. Among various fields of biomagnetism, this paper reviews the research and clinical works in magnetocardiogram, neuromagnetism, magneto-oculogram, magnetopneumogram and magnetic measurement for cell motility carried out in Japan.

1. Introduction

The study of biomagnetic fields originating in a biological body is called biomagnetism. Biomagnetic fields are due either to electric currents or to magnetic materials. The fields emanating from the heart, arms, and brain are examples of magnetic fields produced by currents flowing within the body. These are the action currents arising when nerves or muscles are excited. On the other hand, in the lungs, particular magnetic materials may be unintentionally inhaled and accumulated. Such materials may also be ingested and thereby enter the stomach and intestines. When these materials are magnetized by the magnetic field of the earth or by other external magnetic fields, they become small magnets and in turn generate magnetic field outside the body.

The strongest field, produced by the lungs, is 10^{-9}T (Tesla), equivalent to about one ten-thousandth of the field of the earth (Fig. 1). The fields produced by the heart and brain are smaller. Although conventional flux-gate magnetometers would barely suffice for measurement of such minute fields, the rapid advance of superconduction technologies has made extremely sensitive magnetometers available, which are called 'SQUID' (Superconducting Quantum Interference Device) magnetometers and exploit the 'Josephson effect' occurring in the superconducting state (Fig. 2).

However, it is extremely difficult to measure the weak biomagnetic fields in the midst of the magnetic noise in cities and the strong magnetic field of the earth. If we compare this to ordinary sound, it would be like trying to measure the whine of a mosquito under a railway overpass. The chief causes of magnetic noise are (1) disturbances in the magnetic field of the earth due to the movements of large objects constructed of ferromagnetic materials such as trains, cars, and elevators, and (2) other kinds of machinery used in metropolitan areas. As shown in Figure 1, such magnetic noise amounts to about 10^{-7}T in cities and 10^{-9}T elsewhere. There are two approaches to overcome this difficulty. In the first, the measurement is made in a shielded room which eliminates the outside noise. The second approach called 'canceling method' is a less costly method without a shielded room in which two oppositely oriented magnetic pick up coils are connected in series (Fig. 3). Since magnetic fields produced by relatively distant sources (such as the earth) are parallel, they are canceled, and only fields emanating from sources close to the patient's body are measured.

Being stimulated by the development of extremely sensitive SQUID magnetometers and a

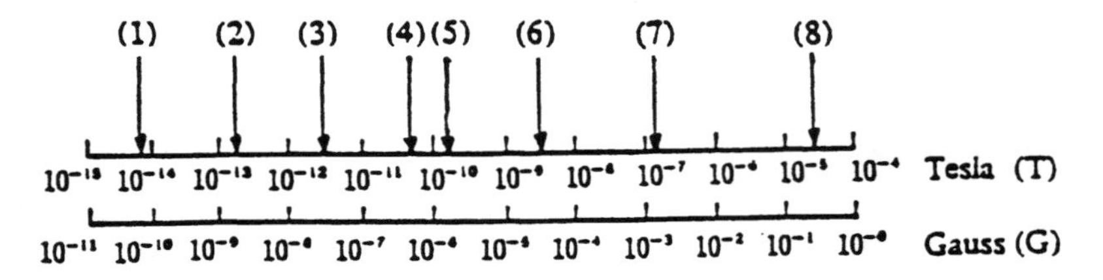

Fig. 1. Comparison of magnetic field intensities: (1) sensitivity of SQUID magnetometer; (2) brain; (3) arm; (4) heart; (5) sensitivity of flux-gate magnetometer; (7) city noise; (8) earth's magnetic field.

newly-risen theory of the biomagnetism, which was originated by Cohen and his colleagues of M.I.T., a number of researchers in Japan took their first step to apply biomagnetism to their own fields of specialities such as heart, brain, muscle, lung and so forth, by the very beginning of 1980s.

This review is written by the leader of each group: Mori for magnetocardiogram, Kuriki for neuromagnetism, Uchikawa for magneto-oculogram, Chiyotani for magnetopneumogram and Nemoto for cell motility.

2. Magnetocardiogram (MCG)

Baule and McFee [1] first recorded the magnetic field produced by the electromotive forces of the human heart and named this record a magnetocardiogram (MCG). Introduction of SQUID magnetometer and a second-derivative gradiometer pickup coil assembly enabled us to obtain a good MCG record relatively easily without using magnetically shielded room.

MCG has been studied by Cohen et al. [2], Lepeschkin [3], Wikswo et al. [4] and Saarinen et al. [5]. It has been studied by Awano et al. [6] and Ohmichi et al. [7] in Japan. The clinical application of MCG has been done since 1980.

Saito and Nakaya [8] recorded MCG in 50 healthy subjects. They noticed that the distribution of the pattern of QRS wave on the anterior chest wall was relatively consistent in normal subjects, and it corresponded well with the intraventricular excitation process. Tall R wave recorded at the middle lower portion (D, E, F-2, 3) and deep S wave at the left upper portion of the anterior chest wall (B, C-4) were considered to reflect the magnetic field produced by the large electromotive forces of the left ventricle directing inferiorly to the left. And the small Q wave recorded at the lower portion of the anterior chest wall was considered to reflect the magnetic field produced by the electromotive forces of the interventricular septum.

Fujino et al. [9, 10] recorded MCG in 60 normal subjects and 95 patients with left ventricular overloading, and clarified the clinical usefulness of the MCG for the diagnosis of the left ventricular overloading. MCG recorded at 36 points of the anterior chest wall at the intersections of each six longitudinal and transverse lines. Vertical lines pass through V_{3R} to V_4 and the midpoint between V_4 and V_5 of the ECG leads (0,1, ... 4,4′). Transverse lines at the level of the first to the sixth intercostal spaces at the sternal margin were named as A to F (Fig. 4). Characteristic pattern of MCG in left ventricular overloading was deep S and positive T waves in upper anterior chest wall. Amplitude of the Q wave in the lower anterior chest wall decreased in systolic overloading of the left ventricle indicating a decreased septal vector.

Diagnostic reliability of MCG and ECG was compared on the basis of echocardiographic findings of left ventricular hypertrophy and dilatation (thickness of the left ventricular posterior wall $\geqslant$11 mm and/or end-diastolic dimension of the left ventricle $\geqslant$50 mm). $S_{B-3} + R_{E-3} \geqslant 4.0 \times 10^{-11}$T in MCG and $R_{V5(6)} + S_{V1} \geqslant 3/5$ mV and/or $R_{V5(6)} \geqslant 2.5$ mV in ECG were used as parameters indicating left ventricular overloading. Sensitivities of the ECG and MCG were 44.3% and 48.6%; specifities were 97.5% and 88.9%; and the predictive values were 93.9% and 79.1% respectively. Thus MCG was found to have higher specificity and predictive value than ECG.

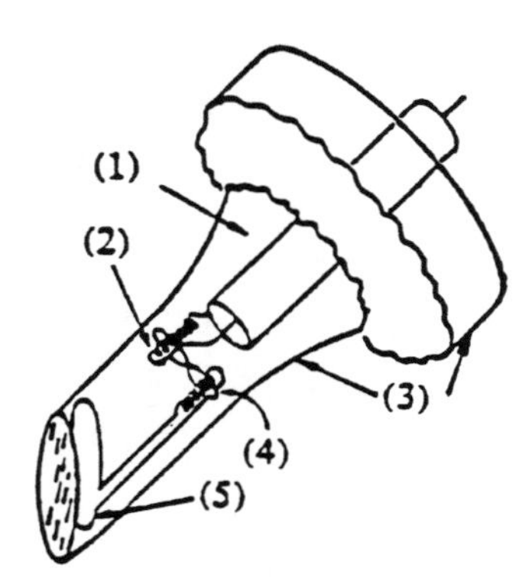

Fig. 2. Detection component of SQUID magnetometer: (1) Liquid helium; (2) coupling coil; (3) dewar; (4) SQUID; (5) detection coil.

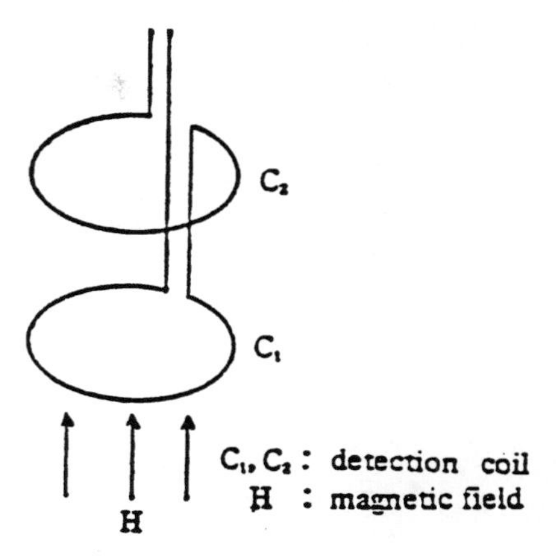

Fig. 3. Magnetic flux detection coil using differential probe. C1, C2; detection coils. H: magnetic field.

Abnormality of repolarization is frequently observed in left ventricular overloading. T wave was normal both in MCG and ECG in 29 cases (35.8%) and was abnormal in 34 cases (42.0%). Repolarization abnormality was diagnosed only by MCG in 18 cases (22.2%), but there was no case in whom repolarization abnormality was diagnosed only by ECG. Fig. 4 shows standard 12 lead ECG, MCG, isopotential map, isomagnetic map and vector arrow map at the time coincident with the peak of the T wave of lead II of the ECG in a case with hypertension of stage I of WHO classification. T wave was normal in standard lead ECG, but was abnormal in MCG, showing inverted T wave in F-3 and flat T waves in E-3 and F-1, 2. Single dipole directing leftwards inferiorly was observed in isoelectric map. Isomagnetic map and vector arrow map showed an additional dipole which located downwards and directs rightwards. This additional dipole was considered to be accounted for the repolarization abnormality expressed in MCG. Such multiple dipoles are more easily expressed on MCG than ECG.

Nakaya [11] examined the ECG and MCG in 50 healthy subjects and 29 patients with right ventricular overloading to compare the diagnostic reliability. Right ventricular overloading was diagnosed in MCG when one of the following criteria was filled: (i) $R_{B-2} \geqslant 15 \times 10^{-12}$T; (ii) $S_{F-3} \geqslant 4 \times 10^{-12}$T and $R/S \leqslant 4$. Roman's criteria modified by the author based on the normal data was used for the electrocardiographic diagnosis. Sensitivities of the MCG and ECG were 75.9% and 37.0%; specificities were 94.0% and 92.0%; and the predictive values were 82.3% and 72.1%, respectively. Thus it was shown that the MCG had higher sensitivity and predictive value than ECG.

Morikawa et al. [12] pointed out that the MCG was diagnostic for right ventricular overloading even in cases whose conventional ECG was not diagnostic.

Murakami and Nakaya [13] examined the MCG in 31 cases of myocardial infarction (MI). They noticed that the QRS wave showed characteristic pattern distribution corresponding to the localization of the MI. They presented a case with anterolateral MI diagnosed by Thallium-201 myocardial imaging whose conventional ECG was not diagnostic, but MCG was diagnostic.

3. Neuromagnetism

Measurements of neuromagnetic fields using SQUID sensors have been proved to be particularly successful in localizing the cerebral sources of the activities elicited by stimulation, and the activities involved in voluntary movement. The ability is also useful in clinical application to determine the position of the epileptic focus. Works in progress by many groups over the world are referred to in former reviews [14, 18, 21].

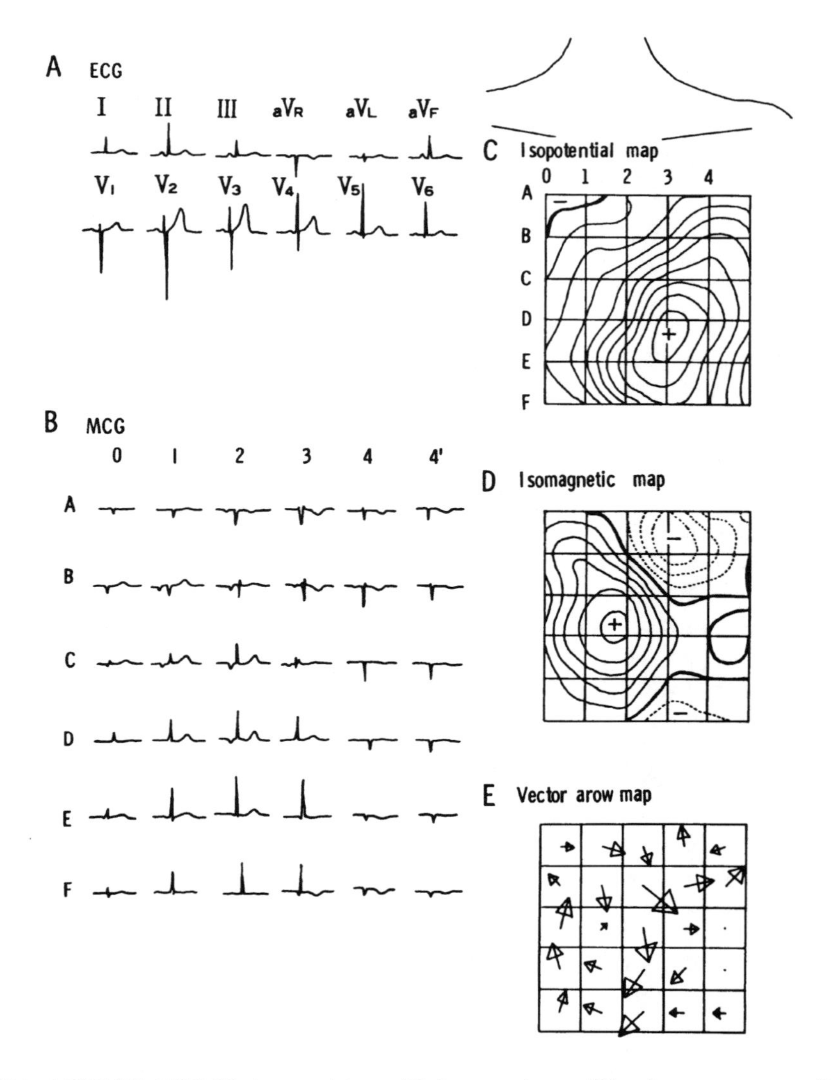

Fig. 4. Standard 12 lead ECG (A), MCG (B), isopotential map (C), isomagnetic map (D) and vector arrow map (E) of a case with hypertension of stage I of WHO classification.

Several groups are working on the neuromagnetism in Japan. Theoretical studies at Kyushu University, Fukuoka, are concerned with computation of the spatial distribution of MEG and EEG, which are associated with pathological situations such as edema, calcification and tumor. Multiple current dipoles are assumed around the tumor as the source of abnormal neural activity [20]. Effects of the variation of the conductivity, which determines the distribution of volume current within the skull, are taken into account [19].

Electrotechnical Laboratory (ETL) group, Ibaraki, is fabricating planar dc-SQUIDs coupled to a magnetometer. The SQUIDs are made of all hard metal (NbN) junctions by microlithography techniques. They detect α rhythms in a magnetically shielded room.

Magnetic fields elicited by visual stimulus (VEF) and the fields associated with eye movement (MOG) are measured and analyzed by Tokyo Denki University group, Tokyo. An rf-SQUID is used in the magnetically shielded room at the ETL. For

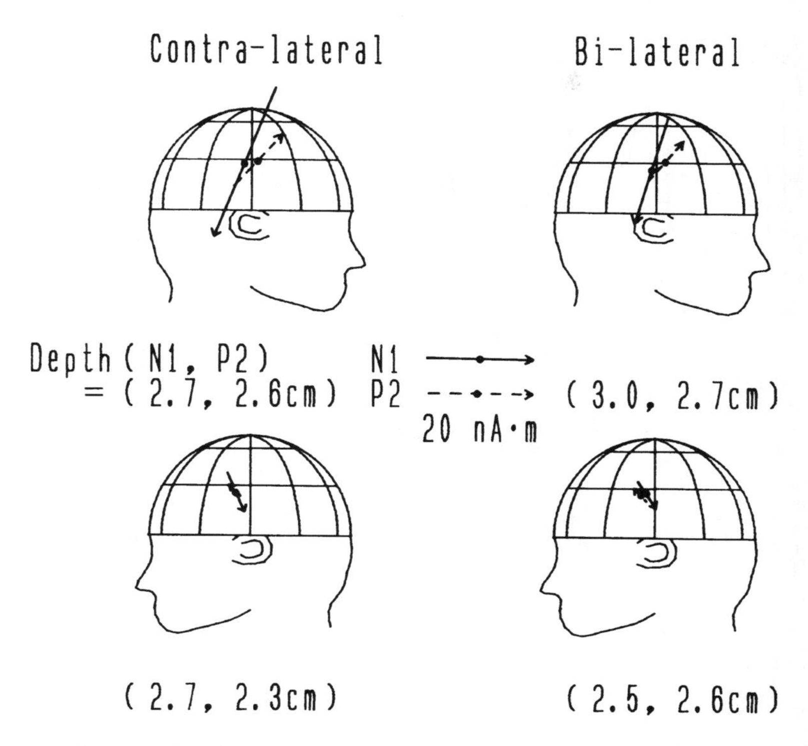

Fig. 5. Estimated current dipoes at right and left hemispheres for contra- and bilateral stimuli of 1 kHz 800 ms tone burst. The strength and the direction are indicated by an arrow.

the MOG a current dipole of 10^{-7}A is estimated at the retina [18].

Somatically evoked fields (SEF) are measured at Hokkaido University, Sapporo, using an rf-SQUID with a second derivative gradiometer in a normal laboratory [16]. Electrical stimulus is given to the ulnar nerve of the wrist. At the hemisphere contralateral to the stimulus, the responses appear in two main peaks at latencies of 65–80 and 130–180 ms. From an isofield contour map measured, the location of an equivalent current dipole is estimated near the somatosensory area at the Rolandic fissure. At the hemisphere ipsilateral to the stimulus, no clear responses are observed.

The SEFs are observed not only at the head but also at the back of the neck [17]. Three to five peaks appear in 50–150 ms after stimulus depending on the peripheral nerves of the wrist stimulated. The responses at various points over the neck showed a polarity reversal of the peaks across the midline of the neck. Isofield patterns show a dipolar feature indicating an equivalent source beneath the spinous process C6. It is suggested that the postsynaptic process in the activity of the spinal cord is responsible for the SEF.

A pure tone burst is used to elicit auditory evoked fields (AEF). Ipsi- and contralateral stimuli to the measuring hemisphere and bilateral stimuli are given to the subject at 1 KHz for 200 or 800 ms with an interval of 1.5–3 s. For the long tone burst (800 ms), two main peaks of N1 at 100 ms and P2 at 180 ms appear, being followed by a negative shift for about 500 ms, at the posterior temporal area of the right hemisphere. For the short tone burst (200 ms), similar response but without the negative shift are observed. A least-square fit is performed for the mapped field data to find parameters of the equivalent curret dipole. The estimated depth and the location of the dipole (Fig. 5) appear to correspond to the primary auditory cortex. For both the contra- and bilateral stimuli, the dipole strength is larger at the right hemisphere than at the left hemisphere.

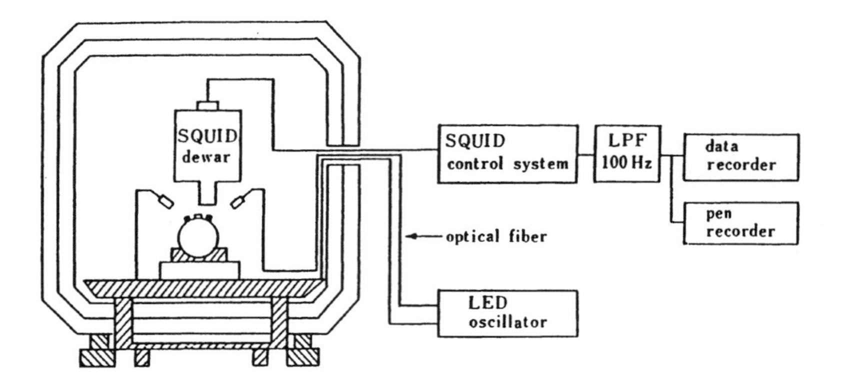

Fig. 6. Block diagram of the measurement system on MOG.

The Hokkaido University group also develops planar dc SQUIDs with NbN junctions aiming at achieving a lower noise level than the rf-SQUID [15]. Planar gradiometers applicable to the neuromagnetic measurement are studied.

4. Magneto-oculogram (MOG)

The recordings of the magnetic field associated with eye movement are called magneto-oculogram (MOG) [22–24]. MOG has several advantages over electric-oculogram (EOG) in the non-invasive and contactless measurements. The first measurement of MOG was performed by Katila et al. [23]. In Japan, Uchikawa, et al., Tokyo Denki University, Tokyo measured EOG of normal subjects in the magnetically shielded room with a SQUID magnetometer connected to a second-order gradiometer.

The measurements were performed in the magnetically shielded room with a SQUID (Superconducting Quantum Interference Devices) connected to a second-order gradiometer with a baseline of 3.2 cm and a coil of 2.48 cm diameter. Fig. 6 shows the experimental system to measure the magnetic field of eye movement. In order to avoid the magnetic noise the optical fibers were used to lead the indicating signal of eye movement. Magnetic signals in the band width of DC to 100 Hz with 50 Hz filter were stored on tape recorder for further data processing.

The strength of magnetic fields, in general, can be observed on the order of 10 pT when the eyeball moves. It is also possible to investigate the smooth pursuit, saccade, adaption, etc. by using MOG in the similar way as EOG. Figure 7 shows the magnetic recordings of different eye movements; (A) shows the case of rapid movement in the displacement of 50 degrees to the left from the eye center; (B) shows the slow movement for 4 seconds with the same degrees and (C) shows the result of fixation of long period with rotation of eyeball. These results indicate that the noninvasive magnetic approach for opthalmology will be useful for a diagnostic measure.

The further investigation is to identify the electrical sources in the human eye as the similar problem of the other biomagnetic fields such MCGs and MEGs [18, 25]. In order to calculate the source localization with the equivalent current dipole (ECD), which has been widely used to account for bio-electric activity [25, 26]. The authors measured the distribution of magnetic fields at different positions on the eye and calculated the isofield contour maps. The calculation of the ECD was made with the comparison between experimental isofields contour maps and theoretical ones. A typical example of the calculated ECD was 200 to 300 nA-m in the intensity and located at 2.5 cm in the depth from eyeball surface corresponding to the retina. This result is in rough agreement with empirical expectation.

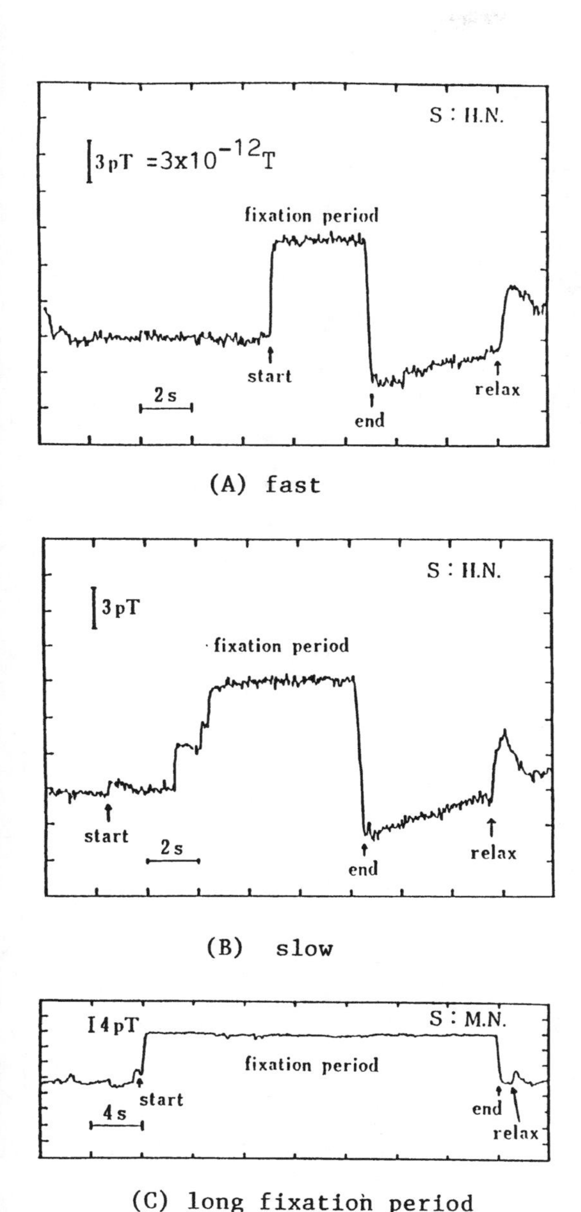

Fig. 7. Magnetic recordings associated with different eye movements.

5. Magnetopneumograms [29]

The measurement of the magnetic field of the lung, magnetopneumogram, provides a good tool for researchers in this field. The research of this field in Japan has progressed after the return of Kotani back to his home country. He was one of the Cohen's colleagues at M.I.T. At a very early phase, Kotani joined with a group of the Rosai Hospital for Silicosis (Director: Chiyotani), a very specialized hospital in Japan. They organized a co-operative working group (K.C. group) and began the preliminary work in the beginning of 1980s. The work of this group was initially focused on the following items; 1) to produce a device which will be suited for measuring magnetic field of the human lung, and 2) to settle the standard technique for magnetization and measurement.

With the purpose of producing a measuring device, several types of magnetizing and measuring apparatus were designed on a experimental basis, mainly for the convenient use in the factories and hospitals. After several improvements were made, the final measuring device, which could be run automatically by using a built-in microcomputer, was established and put on the trade market, bearing the mark of 'K.C. 800 Model', in 1983. The standard technique for measuring, another main purpose at this phase, was also settled in the meantime.

Then the group tried to apply the technique to the practical use in the factories where the labors were exposed to the environmental dust at working places. In this series of trials, the lung magnetic field of workers was actually measured in several kinds of factories such as welders, foundry workers and of hospitalized patients having pneumoconioses such as silicosis, asbestosis, welder's lung, foundry worker's lung and so on.

To meet the request of factories more practically, a movable measuring instrument is strongly desired. As a matter of fact, most of factory owners have a wish to monitor the accurate amount of dust deposit in the lungs of their individual workers, because this monitoring may warn of a prospective or probable risk of dust disease and also indicate the standard of total preventive practices carried on by factory owners themselves. After several months of trials, Kotani completed successfully the special car (Fig. 8) in 1984, on which the measuring apparatus was fully equipped. By introducing this car, the measurements of the lung magnetic field of the workers have been easily made at any time.

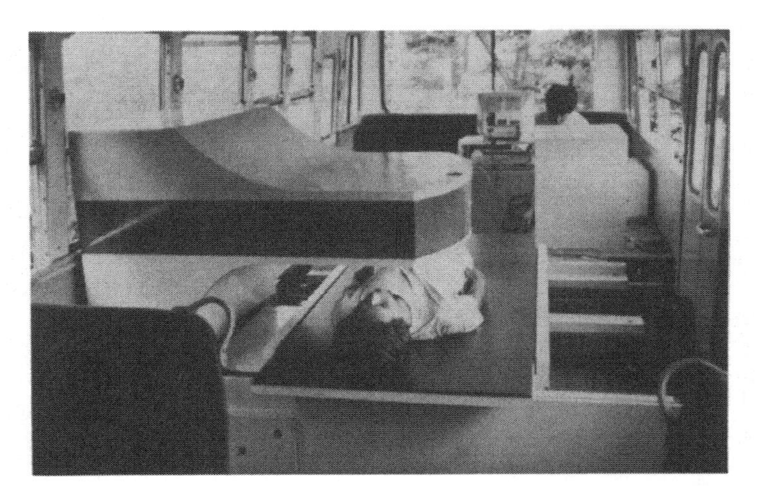

Fig. 8. Inside view of the bus. Measurement system for magnetopneumogram is installed at the center of the bus.

Chiyotani focused on his interest in the relationship between amount of dust deposit and degree of resulting pathological changes in the human lungs, i.e. whether or not more dust actually resulted in more advanced pathological change. This was because the positive relationship might prove the magnetopneumogram to be an ideal examination measure in preventive practice, perhaps in place of x-ray radiographs. In his series of experiments using macrosections of human autopsied lungs, Chiyotani found a considerable positive dose-effect relationship.

Then two major working groups other than K.C. group have newly entered this research field, Professor Takishima and his colleagues of Tohoku University and associate Professor Aizawa and his colleague of Kitazato University.

Takishima, replying to the request of municipal corporations, carried out a field survey to investigate the influences of environmental floating dust, caused by scrubbing of road surfaces by spike tire, on the health condition of dwellers in Sendai City where the dwellers had been expected to inhale a certain amount of dust in winter and early spring seasons. According to his report, Takishima recognized that the measurement of lung magnetic fields played a very important role in his epidemiological survey. Aizawa and his colleagues focused their interest on the bronchial clearance mechanism. In their series of experiments, Aizawa recognized that the measurement of magnetic field also could be an ideal method to monitor the clearance and the retention of ferromagnetic dust injected to the bronchial tree of experimental animals.

The research of magnetopneumogram and its practical application in related fields particularly in industrial sites is expected undoubtedly to grow steadily in the future, in Japan. To boost this magnetopneumogram to be widespread practice for prevention of dust hazard in the industries, an urgent problem is how to improve the quantitative accuracy of measured amount of the dust deposit in practically usable standard.

6. Magnetometric measurement of cell motility

The study of lung magnetism has recently opened up a new field, namely, magnetometric measurement of intracellular movements of the microstructures in the cell. The principle is quite simple. Cells which have ingested ferrimagnetic particles are exposed to an external magnetic field which mangetizes the particles within. The weak field from the cells decay with time (called relaxation) due to the misalignment of the magnetic moments caused most likely by mechanical motions of the intracellular structures. Therefore, magnetic measurement will yield data reflecting the intracellular movements of the microstructures of the cells and it is expected to provide a new approach to cellular motility for which the conventional methodology is to a large degree of biochemistry. The magnetic method makes it possible to investigate the motion in real time and thus to contribute to understanding of mechanical aspects of cellular motility.

Magnetometric measurement of cell motility is being studied at Tokyo Denki University and Research and Development Corporation in Japan. At Harvard School of Public Health, U.S.A., and Universitat Bern, Switzerland, relevant investigations are in progress. Hamster pulmonary macrophages have been mainly used for these investigations because they are easy to harvest and they engage themselves in active phagocytosis even under in vitro conditions. It is also natural that they should be a good target for investigation of cellular motility. Below is a summary of the works done at the institutions in Japan described above [28–32].

If the relaxation is caused by the intracellular movements, then it should be energy dependent. To see this, relaxation was measured at various temperatures. The results showed a clear dependence on temperature. The relationship between incubation temperature and the rate of relaxation has been studied in detail [30]. Another thing studied closely is the effects of inhibiting the ATP synthesis [31]. The source of energy for intracellular movements is ATP which is synthesized in two pathways in the cell; namely, glycolysis and oxydative phosphorylation. MIA (monoiodoacetic acid) is known to inhibit the former pathway and KCN the latter. These inhibitors were used to change the intracellular ATP concentration. The results yielded a clear relationship between the intracellular ATP concentration and the rate of relaxation. This, in turn, is considered to represent the relationship between the ATP concentration and the intracellular motility of the cells.

Other chemicals such as cytochalasine B and colchicin are being tested too. These are known to destroy microfilaments and microtubules which play an important role in motility. In this and the above experiments, relaxation measurement alone does not give enough information to estimate the energy responsible for randomizing the orientation of the particles. Secondary magnetization using a weak magnetic field which aligns the particles after enough relaxation takes place makes it possible to relatively estimate the energy [32].

The magnetic method to investigate the intracellular motility of cells is yet to be evaluated for validity and effectiveness. However, it is expected to provide a new approach to cellular motility. Cell motility is one of the most important factors in the life of a living body. Yet its mechanisms are not well understood. The conventional approaches are not suitable for observing the motions themselves whereas the magnetic method provides an easy way to estimate the degree of intracellular motility and possibly of its energy.

References

1. Baule G, McFee R: Detection of the magnetic field of the heart. Am Heart J 66: 95–96, 1963.
2. Cohen D, Edelsack EA, Zimmerman J: Magnetocardiogram taken inside a shielded room with a superconducting point-contact magnetometer. Appl Phys Letters 16: 278–280, 1970.
3. Lepeschkin E: Progress in magnetocardiography. J Electrocardiol 12:1–2, 1979.
4. Wikswo JP Jr, Fairbank WM: Application of superconducting magnetometers to the measurement of the vector magnetocardiogram. IREE Trans Magnetics MAG-13: 354–357, 1977.
5. Saarinen M, Siltanen P, Karp PJ, Katila TE: The normal magnetocardiogram. I. Morphology. Ann Clin Res 10 (suppl 21): 1–43, 1978.
6. Awano I, Muramoto A, Awona N, Koga S: Application of superconductivity and magnetocardiogram. Low Temp Med 4: 89–100, 1978.
7. Ohmichi H, Ibuka M: Medical applications of SQUID. Appl Phys 48: 361–365, 1975.
8. Saito K, Nakaya Y: QRS wave of the magnetocardiogram of the normal subjects. Jpn J Appl Physiol 13: 191–201, 1983.
9. Fujino K, Sumi M, Saito K, Murakami M, Higuchi T, Nakaya Y, Mori H: Magnetocardiogram of patients with left ventricular overloading recorded with second-derivative SQUID gradiometer. J Electrocardiol 17: 219–228, 1984.
10. Fujino K, Nakaya Y: Studies on magnetocardiogram in left ventricular overloading. Jpn J Appl Physiol 13: 202–214, 1983.
11. Nakaya Y: Magnetocardiography. A comparison with elec-

trocardiography. J Cardiography 14 (suppl III): 31–40, 1984.
12. Morikawa M, Saito K, Takahashi M, Nakaya Y, Bando S, Mori H: Magnetocardiogram in right ventricular hypertrophy. Jpn Heart 23 (suppl): 725–727, 1982.
13. Murakami M, Nakaya Y: Studies on the QRS wave of the magnetocardiogram in myocardial infarction. Jpn J Appl Physiol 14: 14–25, 1984.
14. Clarke J: SQUIDs, brains and gravity waves. Phys Today 39: No. 3, 36–44, 1986.
15. Matsuda M, Kuriki S, Nagano Y: Fabrication of NbN Josephson tunnel junctions and their application to dc-SQUIDs. Jpn J Appl Physiol 25: 1986 (in press).
16. Mizutani Y, Kuriki S: Measurements of somatically evoked magnetic fields at head and neck. Med Biol Eng Comput 23 (suppl): 32–33, 1985.
17. Mizutani Y, Kuriki S: Somatically evoked magnetic fields in the vicinity of the neck. IEEE Trans Biomed Eng BME-33: 510–516, 1986.
18. Romani GL: Biomagnetism: An application of SQUID sensors to medicine and physiology. Physica 126B: 70–81, 1984.
19. Ueno S, Wakisako H, Matsuoka S: Determination of the spatial distribution of abnormal EEG and MEG from current dipole in inhomogeneous volume conductor. IL Nuovo Cimento 2D: 558–566, 1983.
20. Ueno S, Iramina K, Ozaki H, Harada K: The MEG topography and the source model of abnomal neural activities associated with brain lessions. IEEE Trans Magn Mag-22: 1986 to be published.
21. Williamsom SJ, Kaufman L: Application of SQUID sensors to the investigation of neural activity in the human brain. IEEE Trans Magn Mag-19: 835–844, 1983.
22. Williamson SJ, Kaufman L: Biomagnetism. J. of Magnetism and Magnetic Materials, 22: 129–202, 1981.
23. Katila K, Maniewski R, Poutanen T, Varpula T, Karp P: Magnetic fields produced by the human eye. J Appl Phys 52: 2565–2571, 1981.
24. Noguchi H, Aihara K, Kotani M: Measurement of magnetic field associated with eye movement. Jpn J Med Elect & Bio Eng 24: 163–168, 1986.
25. Cuffin N, Cohen D: Magnetic fields of a dipole in special volume conductor shapes. IEEE Trans Biomed Eng BME-24: 372–381, 1976.
26. Geselwitz DB: An overview. IEEE Trans Biomed Eng BME-26: 497–504, 1979.
27. Kotani M, Chiyotani K: A new system for measurement of weak magnetic fields emanating from the human body: Development and clinical applications. International J. of Precision Machinery 1: 57–94, 1985.
28. Nemoto I, Kojima K, Toyotama H: Possibility of estimating the activities of alveolar macrophages by magnetic measurement. Paper of Technical Group, TGMBE, 82–101, IECE Japan, 1983.
29. Nemoto I, Toyotama H, Brain JD, Gehr P: In vivo and in vitro measurements of magnetic relaxation in hamster pulmonary macrophages. In: Weinberg H et al. (Eds) Biomagnetism: Application and Theory. Pergamon Press, 1985, pp 433–437.
30. Nemoto I, Toyotama H, Brain JD, Gehr P. Submitted for publication.
31. Nemoto I, Ogura K, Toyotama H: Magnetometric estimation of intracellular motility of pulmonary macrophages under the influence of inhibitors of ATP synthesis. Med Biol Eng Comput 23 (suppl Part I): 54–55, 1985.
32. Nemoto I: A model of magnetization and relaxation of ferrimagnetic particles in the lungs. IEEE Trans Biomed Eng BME-29: 745–752, 1982.

Address for offprints:
Makoto Kotani
Department of Electronic Engineering
Tokyo Denki University
Kanda, Nishikicho, Chiyodaku,
Tokyo 101, Japan

Medical Progress through Technology 12: 243–257 (1987)

Automatic radiologic reporting system using speech recognition

T. Matumoto, T.A. Iinuma, Y. Tateno, H. Ikehira, T. Yamasaki, K. Fukuhisa, H. Tsunemoto, F. Shishido, Y. Kubo[1] & K. Inamura[1]
National Institute of Radiological Sciences; [1]Nippon Electric corporation, Japan

Key words: reporting system, speech recognition, image reading, diagnosis

Abstract

A radiograph report is usually made from an oral dictation by a radiologist, which is then typed. Typing Japanese is rather inconvenient and consumes many hours. In this paper we introduce a computer-assisted reporting system for radiologic images using speech recognition. The hardware of the reporting system consists of a speech recognizer DP-200(NEC) and a personal computer PC-8801 or PC-9801. The DP-200 has the capability of storing 500 different words spoken by a radiologist. At present, three application programs have been designed. These are for the interpretation of a liver scintigram, a bone scintigram and a chest radiograph. Data entry is done by the radiologist at a CRT display terminal in a conversational manner with predefined and predetermined branching. The time required to make a normal report using the liver or bone scintigram system was within one minute. The reporting time was several minutes in the case of an abnormality report. It is suggested that the system is useful for making an imaging report, for constructing the data base for the interpretation of medical images and for the picture archiving and communication system.

1. Introduction

Medical information recorded at a hospital is usually composed of data which have been entered by either general staff or an expert such as a radiologist. A general purpose computer is widely used for input of data by the former, and helps to create a good hospital information system. However, there are various problems in the latter case and a computer is not necessarily useful. One of the reasons is that a considerable amount of medical information is illogical and also, an interface unit which connects a machine with a human is technically imperfect. Generally speaking, Japanese people have little experience with a typewriter and it is therefore thought that the work burden will be substantialy alleviated if data are input by voice instead of by a typewriter. Recently, a voice entry unit that is able to recognize a word or a clause out of several hundred has been developed. We have been attempting to apply this unit to the medical field since 1982 [2]. Since the performance of a voice entry unit is not perfect at present, the medical information to be entered must comply with the following guidelines: (1) The number of words or clauses should be limited; (2) The method of presenting the medical information must be logical. Examples of medical information which have these characteristics are as follows; history data of a patient, laboratory data, report data of an image reading by a radiologist, and report data of the pathological anatomy and results of an operation. One of the purposes of this paper is to introduce a system which can automatically make a diagnostic report of a medical image by using a computer and a voice entry unit.

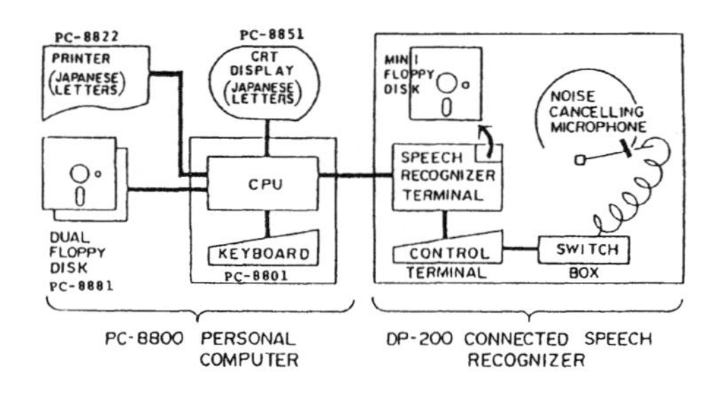

Fig. 1. Block diagram of the reporting system for liver and bone scintigrams. In the case of the system for chest radiographs, the personal computer PC-9801 is substituted for the PC-8801 system.

2. Design and construction of the system

A radiograph report is usually made from an oral dictation by a radiologist, which is then typed. Typing Japanese is rather inconvenient and consumes many hours. In this chapter we will outline a reporting system for radiologic images which we designed.

Objectives of the system. With the development of a computer-assisted radiologic reporting system we aimed at the following objectives: to enhance the readability of an imaging report, to reduce secretarial and related costs, to possibly decrease (and not increase) the workload of a radiologist, and to promote effects of education in radiologic reporting.

Features of the system. The reporting system was developed with the following main features. The report entry is done by the radiologist at a CRT display terminal in a conversational manner with predefined and predetermined branching. Entry of report data is done through a personal computer equipped with a keyboard or in a voice entry mode using a speech recognizer.

Hardware of the system. The hardware is shown in Fig. 1. The system consists of a speech recognizer DP-200(NEC) and a personal computer PC-8801 (or PC-9801). The DP-200 has the capability of storing 500 different words spoken by a radiologist. A personal computer is composed of a central processing unit of 184 KB (or 256 KB for PC-9801), a keyboard, a CRT display terminal, a Japanese character printer, and a floppy disk unit for eight inch disks. The speech recognizer consists of a speech recognition terminal with a five-inch mini-floppy disk unit, a control terminal with a visual display and a noise cancelling microphone with an earphone.

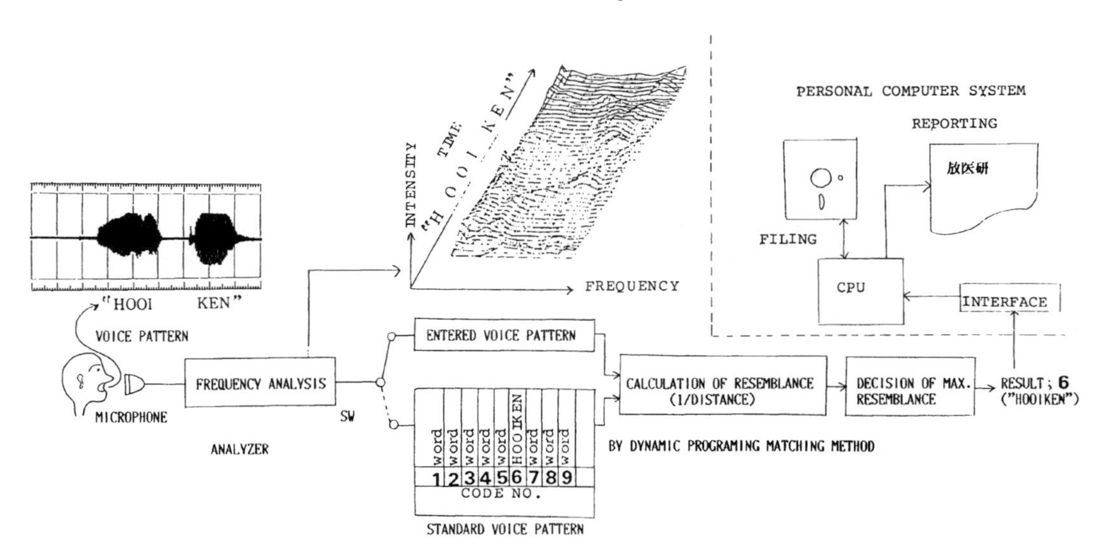

Fig. 2. The principles of the operation of the speech recognizer (DP-200) adopted for the reporting system.

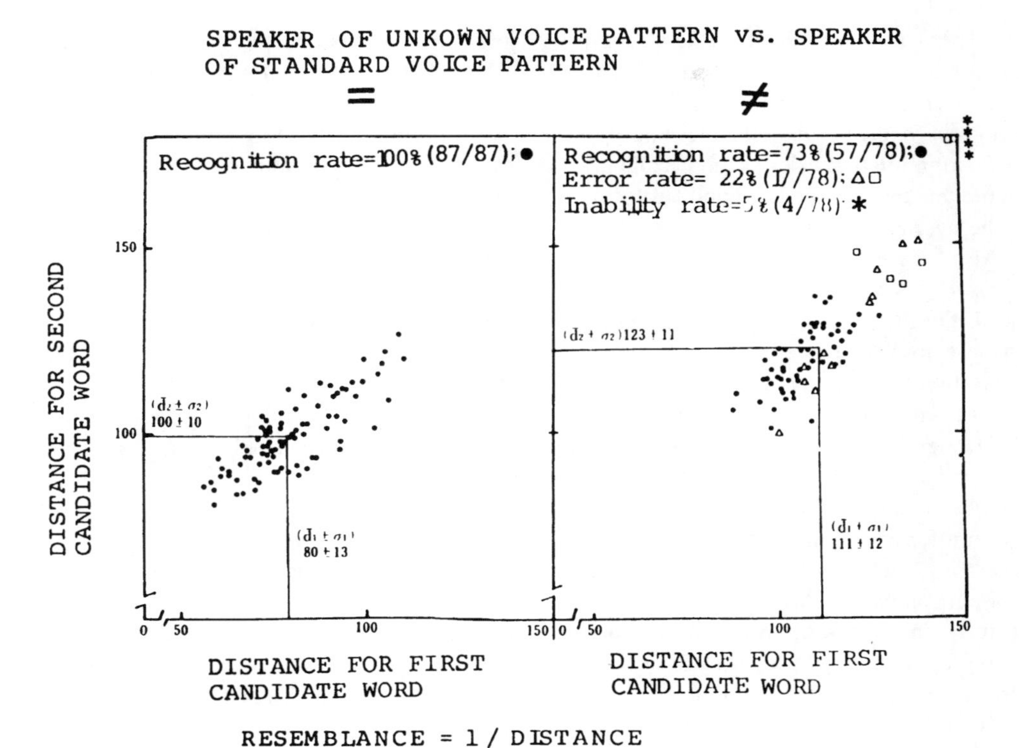

Fig. 3. Test results of the recognition rate of words input by voice entry.

Principle of speech recognition. The principle of speech recognition used by the system is shown in Fig. 2. At first, the radiologist must register his/her own standard voice patterns (which correspond to the frequency spectrum analyzed and digitized by the frequency analyzer) into the memory of the speech recognizer DP-200. Next, these must be transferred from the DP-200 memory into a minifloppy disk as digital data. When a radiologist operates the reporting system, he/she must transfer this standard voice pattern data from the minifloppy disk into the memory of the speech recognizer. When a radiologist speaks into the microphone, the frequency distribution of his/her voice is measured by the frequency analyzer and is compared with that of the standard voice patterns by the comparator. The degree of resemblance (inverse of a distance) between the unknown voice pattern and each standard voice pattern registered in the DP-200 memory is calculated by a dynamic programming matching method. A word which has the maximum degree of resemblance is selected. The data output to the personal computer is a code number assigned to the word.

Fig. 3 shows the results of a test when a person utters a certain word and speech recognition is carried out repeatedly. The value for the word given the greatest degree of resemblance is plotted on the x-axis and that of the another word given the next greatest degree of resemblance is plotted on the y-axis. The left-hand-side of Fig. 3 shows the results of a test when a person uttered a certain word repeatedly using the standard voice patterns registered on his/her own minifloppy disk. The greatest and the next greatest degree of resemblance calculated for each utterance is distributed with a variation. The word given the greatest degree of resemblance corresponds to the word that was intended to be entered in every case (this is represented by: ●). That is, the recognition rate was 100%. The right-hand-side of the figure shows the results of a test when the person uttered a certain word repeatedly using the standard voice patterns registered on another person's minifloppy disk. The distribution of the degree of resemblance has the same tendency as the left-hand-side of figure, but the average of degree of resemblance is smaller. Also, the figure includes several cases where a word given the greatest degree of resemblance is not the word that was intended to be entered (these are represented by: □△). That is, the recognition error rate was 22% and the recognition rate was reduced to 73%. Furthermore, the cases of extremely small degree of resemblance which are represented by: * (recognition inability rate) was 5%. Generally, the voice pattern of a certain person for a word is different from that of another person. Accordingly, when a voice pattern of another person, which is different from the pattern registered in the voice entry unit, is spoken into the microphone, the recognition rate is reduced. In the case of ordinary use (corresponding to the left figure), the recognition rate of the speech recognizer is 95% to 100% depending on the radiologist, and the recognition speed is within 0.3 s for each utterance, which is fast enough for practical use.

Software of the system. The programs of the reporting system are divided into two components which run on the personal computer and the voice entry unit (DP-200). At first, let us briefly explain the programs which run on the DP-200.

(a) Program for registering standard voice patterns. When a voice entry unit is to be used in practice, a radiologist first needs to register into the DP-200 memory his/her standard voice patterns for all the words he/she will possibly use. This program is used at that time. For example, three hundred and four words were chosen as the candidate words in the case of the interpretation of a liver scintigram. To register the standard voice patterns for each of these words, it would take about from 10 to 15 minutes for a person who is familiar with the reporting system and about 25 minutes for one who is not. This registration procedure only needs to be executed once, because if the standard voice patterns are recorded on his/her own minifloppy disk once, they can be used repeatedly for registering the contents into the DP-200 memory.

(b) Program for testing standard voice patterns. In this test the operator utters each word corresponding to the standard voice patterns registered on his/her own minifloppy disk and this program tests the recognition rate of each word.

(c) Program for the renewal of standard voice patterns. This is used to renew the standard voice patterns registered when the voice pattern has changed, for example due to a cold.

(d) On line recognition program. This is a program to transmit the results of speech recognition to a personal computer.

Now, let us discuss the application programs which run on the personal computer. At present, three such programs have been designed. These are for the interpretation of a liver scintigram, a bone scintigram and a chest radiograph. The program for a liver scintigram is written in BASIC and the others in PASCAL. These programs are independent of each other and contain the above mentioned programs related to the speech recognizer DP-200, together with the operating system of the personal computer. Each program is composed of three parts, which have the following common functions.

(a) Program for data input. This is used in order to enter data of an image reading by a radiologist in conversation form. That is, the radiologist replies by speaking when a questionnaire is displayed on the CRT screen. When the voice entered through the microphone is not correctly recognized, a signal tone is emitted to the radiologist through an earphone. When the result is mistakenly recognized, if a word of meaning of 'before' is uttered, the previous question reappears on the screen. The words to control changing of the CRT screen (these are commands of 'next', 'delete', 'up' etc.) are also available. The questionnaire and the candidate words to be entered by voice are displayed on the CRT screen. The candidate words are displayed under or at the right of the questionnaire. After data input by voice entry is finished, the control of the system is passed onto the next program automatically.

(b) Program for composing and printing a report. The voice entry data are edited and grammatically correct sentences are constructed by the program. Finally, the report is printed out, and any number of copies can be printed according to demand.

(c) Program for filing report data. This is a program to transfer the code numbers generated as a result of speech recognition from the DP-200 memory to the floppy disk of the personal computer. A report can be reprinted by reading out these files from the floppy disk and also processing of statistics by the personal computer can be carried out.

3. Flowchart and features of reporting system

System for liver scintigram. As the first attempt at a reporting system, we selected the interpretation of liver scintigrams because these interpretations are rather simple compared to that of X-ray images, such as of the chest or GI-tract, and require a smaller number of words for a report [5]. The words to be spoken (noun, verb, modifier etc.) consist of information relating to patient identification, findings and diagnoses etc. The number of words to be spoken is 304 in all. The questionnaire format is based on past experiences of image reading. For example, the format of interpretation is made with reference to the worksheet for reporting to the Efficacy Group for Liver Scintigraphy (the sub-committee on efficacy of the medical & pharmaceutical committee of the Japan Radioisotope Association) in Japan [4].

The stepwise procedure used is illustrated by a flowchart in Fig. 4. The flowchart also shows the items of the report to be entered. Data entry is done with predefined and predetermined branching. The principal reporting process consists of five parts; (1) the heading with patient identification; (2) specific findings and descriptive findings; (3) diagnostic classification; (4) instruction to a clinician; (5) output of report and file.

The operation of the system is as follows; first, a radiologist must enter the program for interpreting a liver scintigram from the eight-inch floppy disks and transfer his/her own standard voice patterns of the candidate words from the minifloppy disk to the memory of the speech recognizer DP-200. Next, the radiologist must say his/her name as the password, which will be identified by the system. Then, questions and the possible answers are displayed on the CRT screen one by one, which the radiologist responds to by saying one of these answers. Fig. 5 (A) shows an example of a CRT display for data input concerning patient identification. The items with a question mark are; 1. user's name, 2. patient's name, 3. clinical diagnosis, 4. patient's number, 5. age, 6. sex, 7. date of study, 8. radiopharmaceutical used and 9. administered dose. In this part only, answering is performed with the keyboard of the personal computer because the key entry mode is more efficient than voice entry for data such as administrative information. At the end (item 10.) of this CRT screen, the radiologist must answer three questions; whether there are any findings, whether it is normal, and whether the image quality is poor. The radiologit replies using one of the candidate words. If he/she replies that it was normal, the program proceeds to the CRT screen for diagnosis. If the image quality of the liver scintigram is poor, the radiologist replies that the image is uninterpretable, states the cause of the poor study and proceeds to the CRT screen for instructions to a clinician. If there is an abnormal finding, the radiologist states the existence of an abnormal finding. The screen which follows this is shown in the figure (B). This screen is used for entering the state of radioisotope uptake and distribution, whether there is an abnormality of the liver-location, whether there is a deformation of the liver, and whether there is a hypertrophy or atrophy etc. The next frame (C) is for describing the location, size and number of space occupying lesions. Frame (D) is for entering the diagnoses corresponding to each finding. The findings and diagnoses are entered for each view of the gamma camera (anterior, posterior, right lateral, left lateral etc.). Then, in frames (C) and (D), the radiologist subjectively assigns a probability to each finding and diagnosis. These probabilities are used to express a grade of confidence in each finding or diagnosis when the report is printed. That is, typical modifiers used to express these probabilities are 'definitely', 'probably', 'possibly', etc.

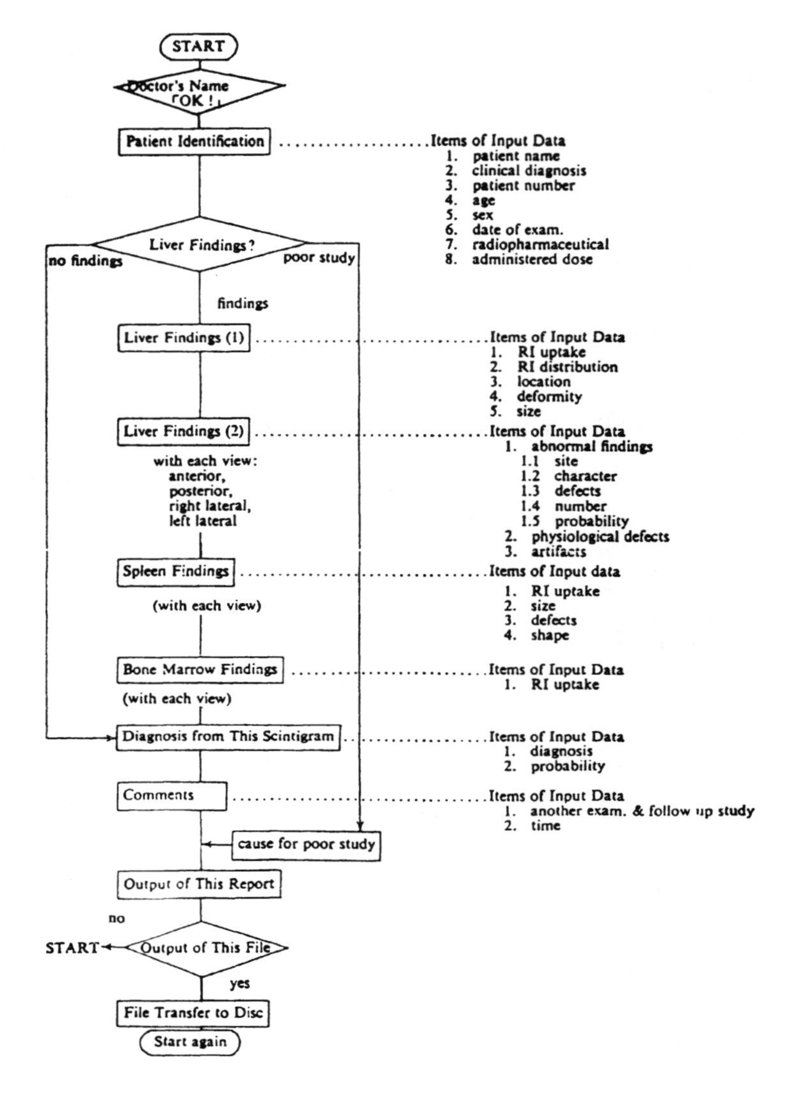

Fig. 4. A flowchart of the input data program for the interpretation of a liver scintigram.

When information is input by voice entry, a radiologist can choose one of three modes. The first mode is shown in Fig. 5. The screen has several questionnaires with a group of candidate words assembled for voice entry. A radiologist is able to input the desired word by voice entry while seeing what he/she may choose from on the CRT screen. Accordingly, this mode is useful for comprehending how to enter data. The second mode does not display the answer to be selected, but only displays the questionnaires. This can be used by a radiologist who has become familiar with the program. Report information can be input by voice entry faster in this mode than in the former. The third mode displays the candidate words only when a radiologist enters a word which has not been registered beforehand in mode No. 2. This is useful in the case where a radiologist forgets the word to be selected.

Finally, the important task of the reporting system is to construct descriptive statements. The entry data are compiled, edited, and sentences are automatically constructed by the program. Fig. 6 shows an example of the final report of a liver scintigram. It is also possible to add comments in a free format by using the keyboard of the personal computer.

Data filed in the eight-inch floppy disk is transmitted to a general purpose computer with a large memory capacity after it is transformed from the data format of N-BASIC to IBM format by a file converter program. In this way, a data base of interpretation of liver scintigrams is constructed.

A main feature of the report system for a liver scintigram is that the questionnaire and the procedure for data input is predetermined by the program. In other words, since the operator must comply with this procedure of data input, he/she may feel that is not a flexible system. However, it is convenient when the operator is not familiar with this system.

System for bone scintigram. A reporting system for a bone scintigram was developed following the system for a liver scintigram. A flowchart of the program is shown in Fig. 7. The bone scintigram system is composed of a data input module, a file converter module and a module for searching for and outputting previous data. The last module is useful to state whether the previous clinical conditions of a patient regressed or progressed when repeat examinations happened. The data input module follows the typical logic-pattern of image reading used among doctor who have experience of nuclear medicine. The flow of the program is analogous to the liver scintigram system previously developed. The system contains a thesaurus for the interpretation of bone scintigrams which is composed of 360 words and was edited by three experts in the field of nuclear medicine. Although a radiologist must report the findings and diagnoses for every camera view in the case of the liver system, he/she reads the plural images together and only enters overall judgements in this program. The structure of the flowchart was made simple by adopting this method and the time required to make a report was reduced from that of the liver system. The manner in which a sentence is automatically made from data by the program is analogous to the liver system.

System for chest radiographs. Objects for interpreting are the direct chest X-ray film of a right lateral view and an anterior view. A thesaurus to record the information was compiled, after four experts in the field of chest diagnosis discussed the standardization of interpreting chest X-ray film. The number of words necessary for the system is large in comparison with the liver and bone systems, and reaches a total of 973 in all. There are 420 candidate words just to describe findings. This number is close to the limit (500) which can be registered in a voice entry unit. Due to this reason, voice entry is only used for entering findings and the input of a diagnosis and other information is carried out through the keyboard of the personal computer. Furthermore, the system is designed so that it is possible to switch it to either a voice or a key entry mode when a finding is entered. The system also has the function of allowing additions or modifications to be made to information entered previously by voice or key entry. Comments can be recorded freely by using the word processor connected to the system. A flowchart of the system is shown in Fig. 8. Since the amount of information to be entered is enormous, the procedure for data input seems very complicated. But the manipulation of input data is easier than for the previous systems for liver and bone scintigrams because the hardware is composed of a PC-9801, a 16 bit-machine, and peripheral equipment, instead of the PC-8801 system, a 8 bit-machine. Also, the data input program is designed so that it is possible to directly move to any CRT-screen desired by using a function key or the key entry mode.

4. Results

The time required to make a normal report using the liver or bone scintigram system was within one minute. The reporting time is several minutes in the case of an abnormality report (at present, the system for chest radiographs is not yet used clini-

(A)

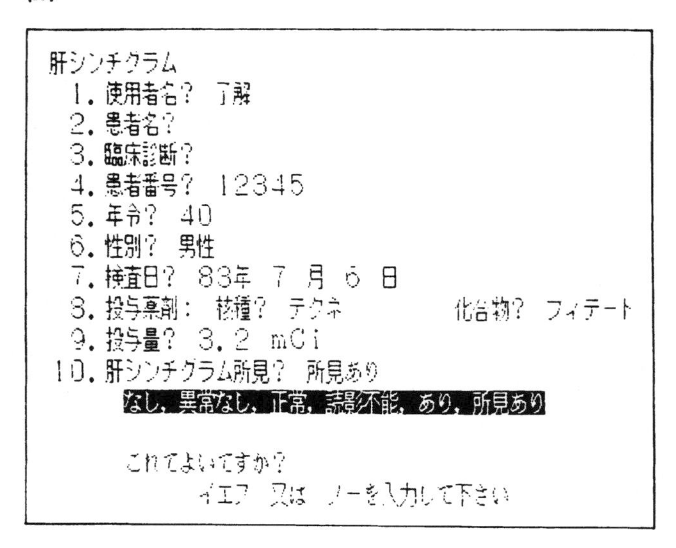

(B)

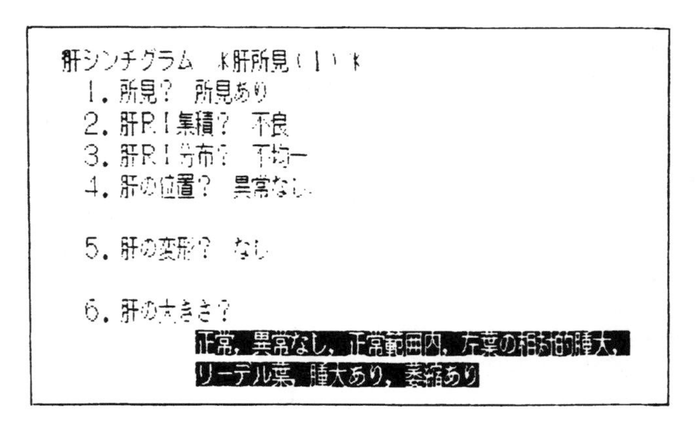

Fig. 5. Example questionnaire, and answers by voice entry of the candidate words displayed on the CRT screen. (A) Patient identification; (B) Liver findings (1); (C) Liver finding (2); (D) Diagnosis from this scintigram.

cally due to modification of the program). This time is dependent on the number of findings interpreted by a radiologist. A radiologist can produce a report within the same time that it takes to handwrite one in the case of a normal report, although it is difficult to compare the performance of voice entry with that of handwriting. In the case of an abnormality report, the system has a tendency to require more time to produce a report than it takes to handwrite one. However, if a radiologist must take medical information from a handwritten report and input it by means of an intermediary, such as an IBM-card reader, OCR or MCR, to a computer for the purpose of education or research, then this system is far more efficient in comparison with it. This is because standardized information is di-

(C)

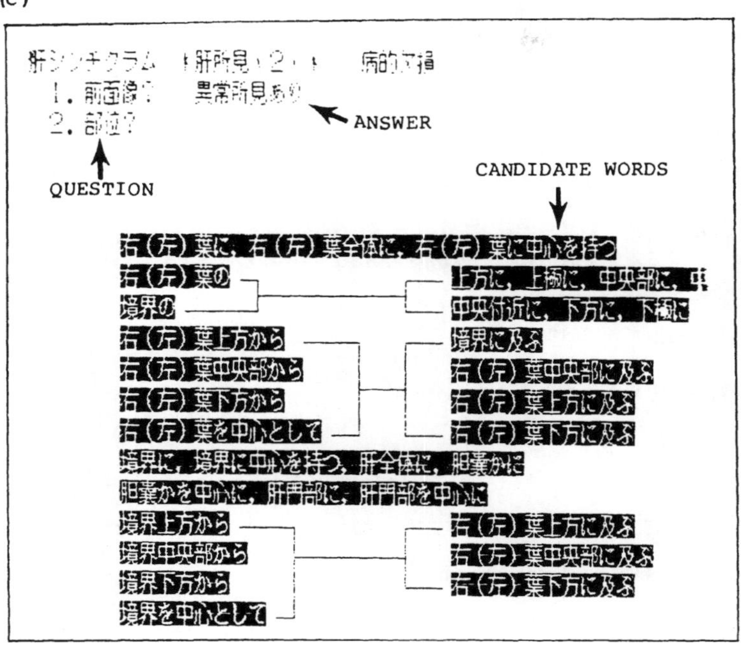

(D)

肝シンチグラム 「診断」 後面像
異常所見あり 境界の 上方に
小さな 欠損 2 個 95%
1. 診断？
異常なし、正常、正常範囲内
局在性病変、び慢性肝疾患、肝硬変、胆道系異常
肝外性病変、全身性疾患、形態異常、その他、ツギ

rectly recorded in a computer without an intermediary when a report is made.

Recently, bone scintigrams have become widely used in Japan and are now more common than liver scintigrams. Next we will show the results which statistically analyzed report data produced using the system.

It is important as a foundation of optimizing the system, to study the frequency with which a word intended to be entered by voice was actually used for reporting. The utilization rate of various types of words is shown in Fig. 9. (A) shows the number of words in eight groups of words from which candidate words for voice entry (360) are selected. These words were entered in accordance with the flowchart in Fig. 7. In Fig. 9 (B), the report is

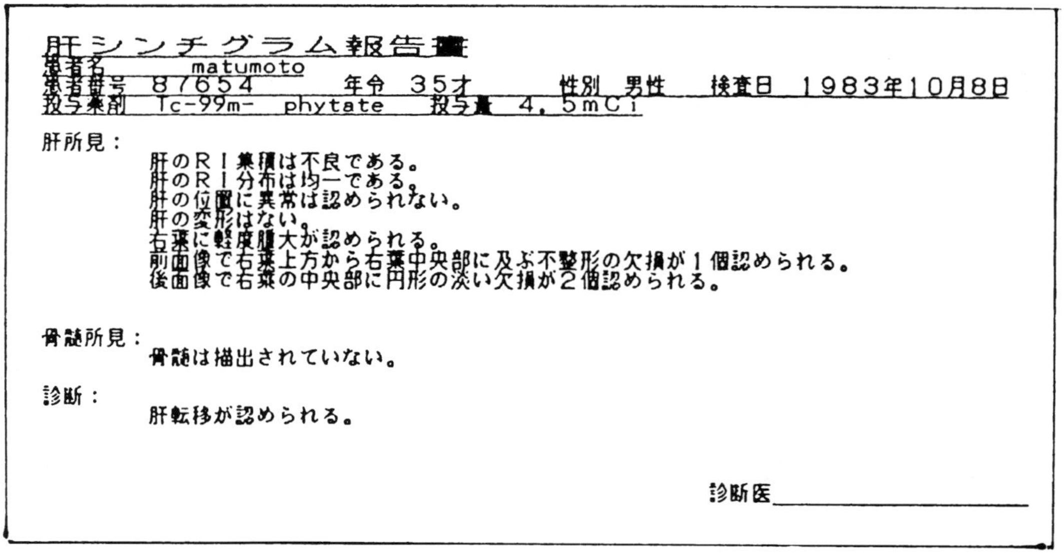

肝シンチグラム報告書
患者名 matumoto
患者番号 87654 年令 35才 性別 男性 検査日 1983年10月8日
投与薬剤 Tc-99m- phytate 投与量 4．5mCi

肝所見：
肝のＲＩ集積は不良である。
肝のＲＩ分布は均一である。
肝の位置に異常は認められない。
肝の変形はない。
右葉に軽度腫大が認められる。
前面像で右葉上方から右葉中央部に及ぶ不整形の欠損が１個認められる。
後面像で右葉の中央部に円形の淡い欠損が２個認められる。

骨髄所見：
骨髄は描出されていない。

診断：
肝転移が認められる。

診断医＿＿＿＿＿＿＿＿

Fig. 6. An example of the final report of a liver scintigram.

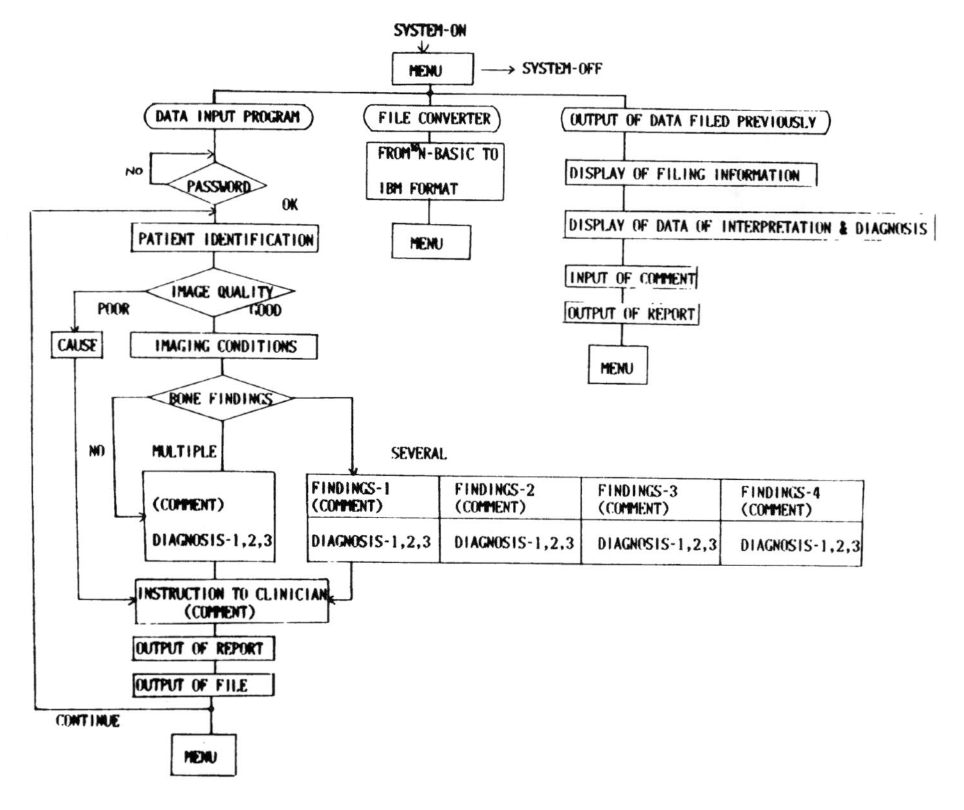

Fig. 7. A flowchart of the input data program for a bone scintigram.

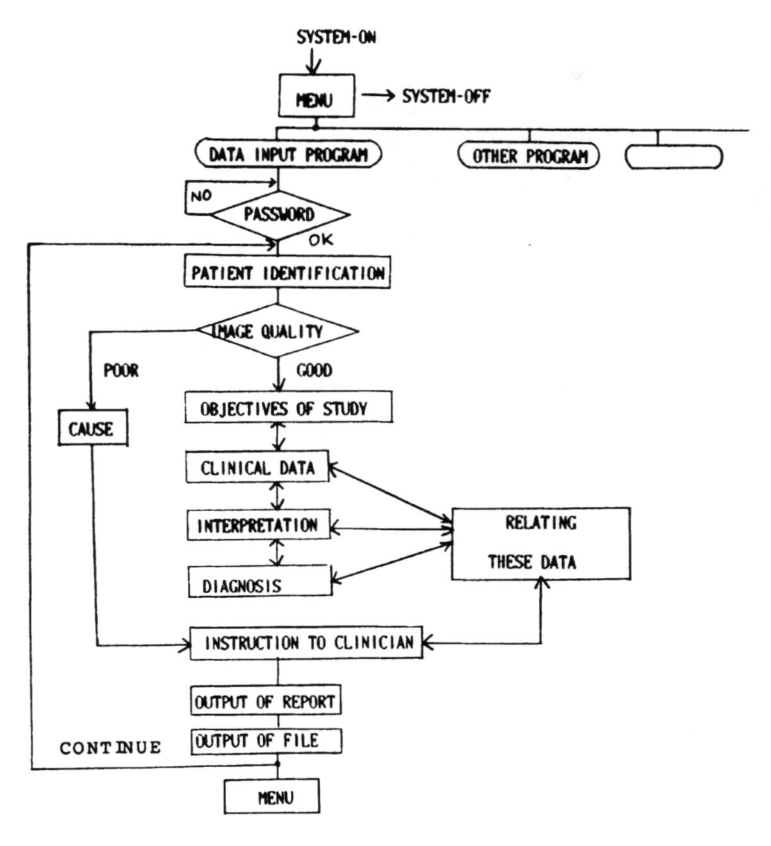

Fig. 8. A flowchart of the input data program for a chest radiograph.

classified into being either a normal report, an abnormality report with multiple findings, or an abnormality report with several findings. Among 310 reports written from 1984 through to 1985, normal reports were 35% of the whole, and abnormality ones 65% (which consists of those with several findings (58%)) and those with multiple findings (7%). Fig. 9 (C) shows that the total number of words used to make the reports was 6326. This means that an average of about twenty words were used for each report. Among these, words describing imaging conditions took up 34% of the whole. The remining 66% were words regarding the findings, diagnoses, and instructions to a clinician. If the words used to express the imaging conditions are not included, an average of 13.4 words was used for each report. Four, eighteen and ten words were entered for a normal report, an abnormality report with several findings and an abnormality report with multiple fidings, respectively. Information on imaging conditions and patient identification is indispensable to constructing a data base of the interpretations of medical images. However, these are data which are already known before imaging and a radiologist does not necessarily need to enter them. This implies that the system should be reconstructed so that a radiologist or even another person is able to enter this part more efficiently in order to reduce the time preparing a report. Fig. 9(D) shows the utilization rate of words for abnormality reports with several findings. It indicates that decriptive terms (the nature and the location) for findings occupied 65% of the words used in reporting. Fig. 10 depicts the distribution of the number of words as a function of the number of times they had been used. Words which had never

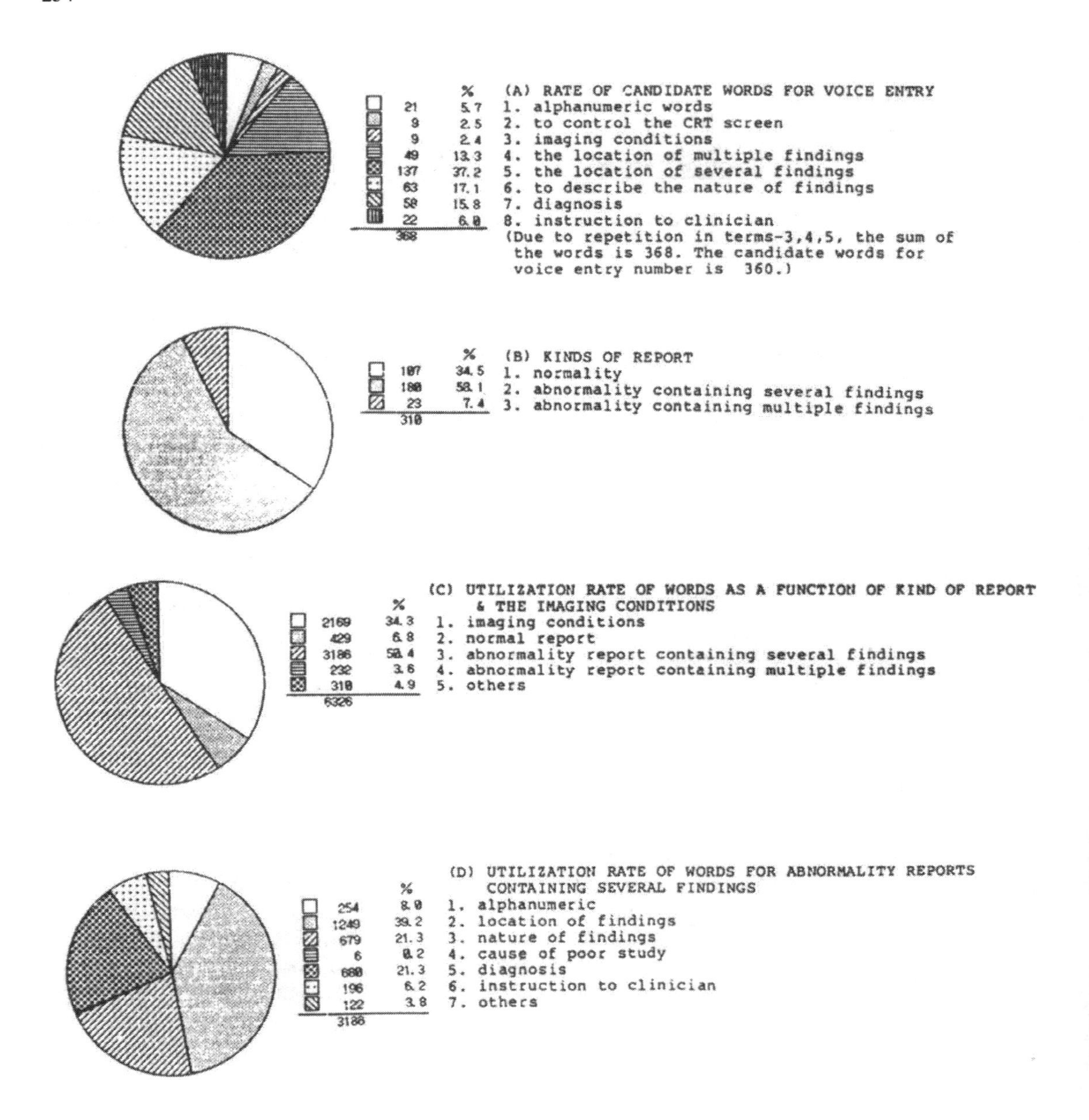

Fig. 9. Utilization rate of the candidate words for voice entry.

been used in the past year among the 360 words assembled as candidate words for voice entry, occupied 41% of the total. Also, words used once, twice or three times made up for 10%, 8% and 5%, respectively. These data show the need for investigating why voice entry of these words was not carried out. Words with no prospect of use should be excluded from the thesaurus. On the other hand, there were a few words which were used extremely frequenly. The entering of words which are always entered when a report is made should be made unnecesary and their use should be preset in

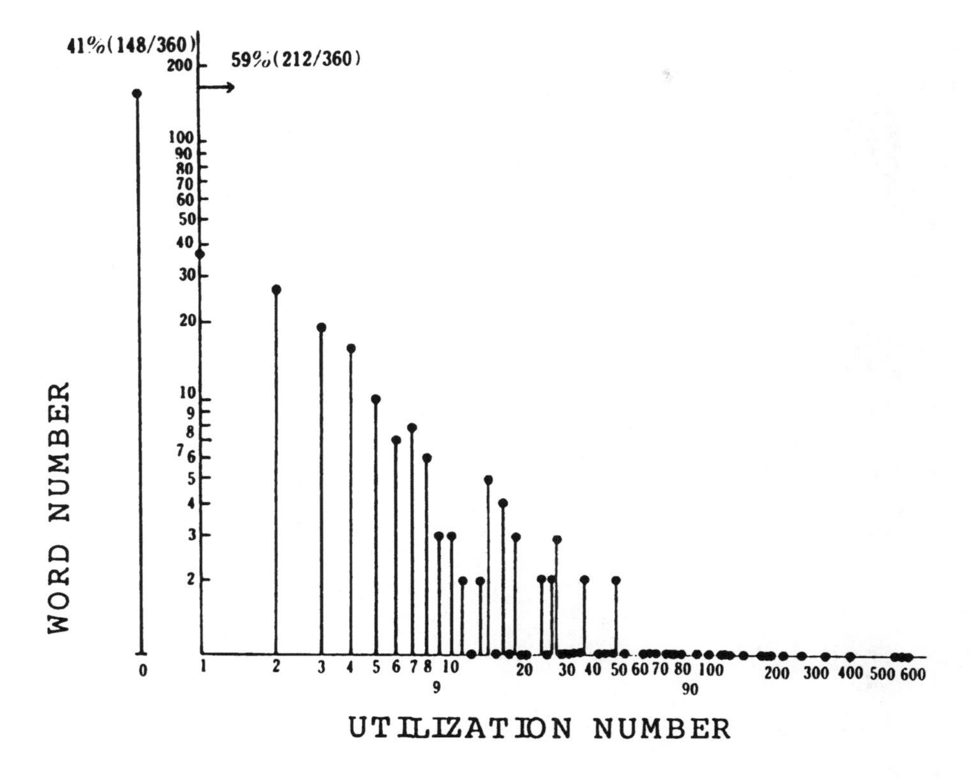

Fig. 10. Number of the candidate word for voice entry as a function of the number of times it was used.

the program. Furthermore, it was found that there were several words which radiologists felt were necessary when preparing a report. These words should obviously be added to the thesaurus. A modification of the system is now being undertaken as a result of the above findings.

An example of analysis of the diagnostic terms used is shown in Fig. 11. Fig. 11 (A) classifies diseases by calculating the frequency of their IRD code number, which is determined by the clinician and represents a confirmed diagnosis. It is reported that in the case of breast cancer (Fig. 11 (B)), most patients have metastasis of the cancer to the chest or head and in the case of the uterine cancer (Fig. 11 (C)) the metastasis principally occurs in the chest and pelvis.

5. Discussion

In 1973 Brolin [1] extensively reviewed past research of radiologic reporting. He classified reporting systems into two kinds, an automatic typewriter system and a computer assisted system. The former unit automatically types standardized words, phrases and texts which are used frequently in ordinary reporting. At present, it has been developed so that it is possible to make a report by connecting the standardized terms and to make modifications such as additions, renewals and deletions etc., by means of a word processor unit.

The computer system defined by Brolin is divided into a free text system and a standardized input system. In the case of the former, results of interpretations and diagnoses of medical images are recored into a computer, letter by letter. Accordingly, as Brolin indicated, these systems do not interfere with the usual method of dictation, and the communication function of the report of transmitting information to a clinician is not affected. However, the computer facilities are only used for case finding, statistical tabulation and for docu-

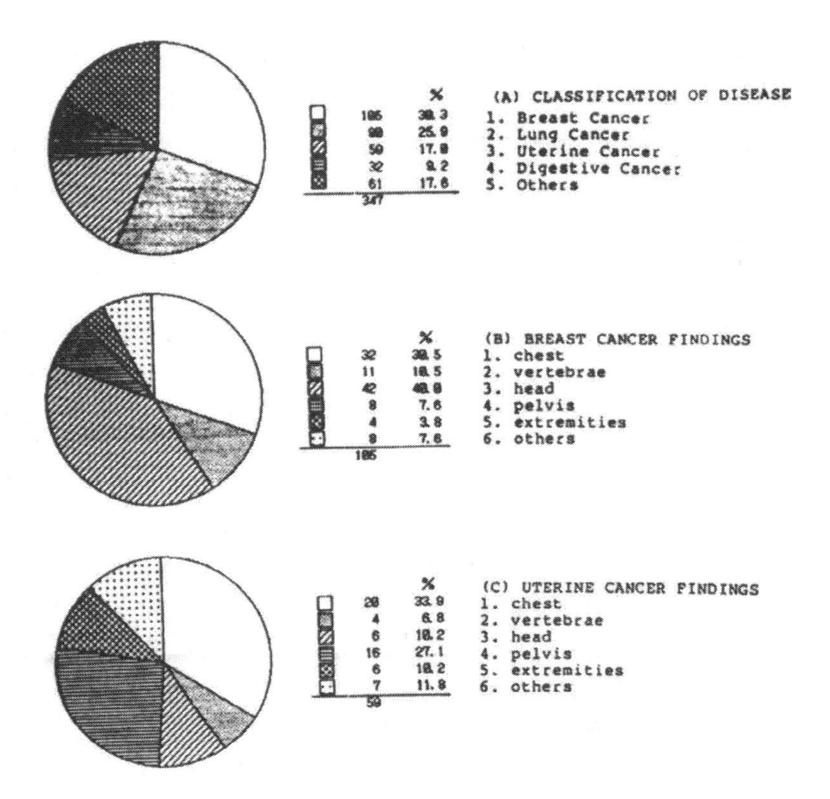

Fig. 11. Statistics of the diagnostic term. Frequency of (A) confirmed diagnosis, (B) anatomic term reported for the case of breast cancer, (C) anatomic term reported for the case of uterine cancer.

mentation. If it is intended to construct a data base of the reporting of medical images, a word or a phrase from the reports must be recognized so that medically valuable information can be extracted. Also, attention should be paid to the need for a standardized thesaurus for constructing a data base of the interpreting of medical images.

On the other hand, the main principle of a standardized input system is that only informative words and phrases shall be entered. This structured, standardized input has an effect on the vocabulary and the communication function of the reporting. However, if a thesaurus is carefully edited by experts and effectively used, it is relatively easier to construct a data base for reporting than by the free text system. Due to these reasons, we selected the standardized input systems for radiologic reporting and edited the thesauruses for the liver scintigram, bone scintigram, and chest radiograph. Furthermore, in order to increase the usability of these thesauruses and the ease in finding relevant words and phrases, we developed a reporting system which was implemented by a voice entry mode in addition to the key entry mode.

It is obvious that voice entry is more efficient than handwriting or typewriting. However, the recognition rate and the recognition speed of a speech recognizer must be sufficiently high for the system to be used in practice. It is necessary to learn the operation of the unit in order to execute voice entry with a sufficiently high recognition rate using the speech recognizer (DP-200) adopted in our system. A high recognition rate can be achieved after a little practice, although individual differences in adaptability to the unit are recognized.

A paper regarding a reporting system using the

voice entry mode was reported by Leeming et al. in 1982 [3]. In the system reported, a radiologist using his voice entered a code consisting of a combination of letters and numbers. As our system allows the entry of words and phrases in every day use, it can be considered to have advanced one step more than the Leeming system.

We tried reporting systems for the interpretation of liver and bone scintigrams first, because a standardization of image reading and diagnoses for these scintigrams is more advanced and simple than those for X-ray images such as a chest and GI-tract radiographs. As less terms are used for images in nuclear medicine than are for X-ray images, it was easy to design the program which is able to print out grammatically correct sentences. The system for chest X-ray images, which contains enormous quantities of information, was difficult to design so that the program automatcally made a sentence. Therefore, in the system for chest radiographs, a radiologist need to enter a series of words or phrases that all resembles a grammatically correct sentence as closely as possible.

In the chest radiograph system, in order to resolve the problem of difficulty in finding the correct term, the implementation of a program which retrieves the IRD code for the diagnostic term has been attempted.

6. Conclusion

Although the system is far from complete (at present, the system requires more time from the radiologist than the old manual system for output of a report), we feel that it is useful for making an imaging report, data acquisition, making an efficacy study of various methods of medical imaging and for the picture archiving and communication system (PACS). The method studied here is relatively easy to apply to the reporting of other medical images. In the near future this system will be expanded for the interpretation of GI tract X-ray images from mass screening.

Acknowledgement

This work was supported in part by the Grant-in-Aid for Cancer Research (61–13) from the Ministry of Health and Welfare.
The author thanks T. Nobechi, O. Doi, S. Sone and F. Ogawa for help in designing the system for chest radiographs and T. Yoshida and Y. Seki for their advice and technical assistance.

References

1. Brolin I: Radiologic reporting. ACTA RADIOLOGICA Suppl 323, 1973.
2. Iinuma TA, Tateno Y, Shishido F, Matumoto T, Matsuoka G, Yamada T, Inamura K, Kubo Y: Medical applications of the speech recognition – automatically reporting and filing (in Japanese). Jpn J Med Elect Biol Eng 20: 37–442, 1982.
3. Leeming BW, Porter D, Jackson JD, Bleich HL, Simon M: Computerized radiologic reporting with voice data-entry. Radiology 138: 585–588, 1981.
4. Matumoto T, Iinuma TA, Tateno Y, Machida K: Estimation of clinical efficacy for scintigraphic images of liver (1) Method and ROC analysis for SOL-detection (in Japanese). Jpn J Nucl Med 19: 51–65, 1982.
5. Shishido F, Matumoto T, Tateno Y, Iinuma TA, Yamasaki T, Kubo Y, Seki Y, Inamura K, Matsuoka G, Yamada T: Development of a reporting system with voice entry for radiological imaging and its application for liver scintigraphy (in Japanese). Jpn J Nucl Med 21: 679–686, 1984.

Address for offprints:
T. Matumoto
Division of Clinical Research
National Institute of Radiological Sciences
9-1, 4-chome, Anagawa Chiba-shi, 260 Japan

Volume contents

H. Hutten, Preface 3
K. Atsumi, I. Fujimasa, K. Imachi, M. Nakajima, K. Mabuchi, S. Tsukagoshi, T. Chinzei & Y. Abe, Research and development on total artificial heart in University of Tokyo 5
Z. Yamazaki & N. Inoue, Hepatic assist device, using membrane plasma separator and dialyzer 17
T. Tsuji, Patient monitoring during and after open heart surgery by an improved deep body thermometer 25
N. Shichiri, R. Kawamori & Y. Yamasaki, The development of artificial endocrine pancreas. From bedside-, wearable-type to implantable one 39
Y. Handa & N. Hoshimiya, Functional electrical stimulation for the control of the upper extremities 51
M. Sugawara, Blood flow in the heart and large vessels 65
F. Kajiya, O. Hiramatsu, K. Mito, Y. Ogasawara & K. Tsujioka, An optical-fiber laser Doppler velocimeter and its application to measurements of coronary blood flow velocities 77
A. Kitabatake, H. Ito & M. Inoue, Current development in Doppler echocardiography. The real-time two-dimensional Doppler flow imaging system 87
S. Eiho, M. Kuwahara & N. Asada, Left ventricular image processing 101
K. Doniwa, T. Kawaguchi & M. Okajima, Body surface potential mapping – its application to animal experiments and clinical examinations 117
K. Yamakoshi & A. Kamiya, Noninvasive measurement of arterial blood pressure and elastic properties using photoelectric plethysmography technique 123
M. Esashi & T. Matsuo, Solid-state micro sensors 145
H. Kanai, M. Haeno & K. Sakamoto, Electrical measurement of fluid distribution in legs and arms 159
Y. Yamamoto & T. Yamamoto, Measurement of electrical bio-impedance and its applications 171
T. Shiina, K. Ikeda & M. Saito, Estimation of tissue parameters derived from reflected ultrasound 185
K. Maeda, Recent progress of technology in obstetrics and gynecology, particularly in perinatal medicine in Japan 197
H. Aoki, M. Akao, Y. Shin, T. Tsuzi & T. Togawa, Sintered hydroxyapatite for a percutaneous device and its clinical application 213
N. Yui, K. Kataoka & Y. Sakurai, Recent advances in thromboresistant materials 221
M. Kotani, H. Mori, S. Kuriki, Y. Uchikawa, K. Chiyotani & I. Nemoto, Biomagnetism in Japan 233
T. Matumoto, T.A. Iinuma, Y. Tateno, H. Ikehira, T. Yamasaki, K. Fukuhisa, H. Tsunemoto, F. Shishido, Y. Kubo & K. Inamura, Automatic radiologic reporting system using speech recognition 243
Volume contents 259
List of contributors 261
Instructions to authors 263

List of contributors

Abe, Y., 5
Akao, M., 213
Aoki, H., 213
Asada, N., 101
Atsumi, K., 5
Chinzei, T., 5
Chiyotani, K., 233
Doniwa, K., 117
Eiho, S., 101
Esashi, M., 145
Fujimasa, I., 5
Fukuhisa, K., 243
Haeno, M., 159
Handa, Y., 51
Hiramatsu, O., 77
Hoshimiya, N., 51
Hutten, H., 3
Iinuma, T.A., 243
Ikeda, K., 185
Ikehira, H., 243
Imachi, K., 5
Inamura, K., 243
Inoue, M., 87
Inoue, N., 17
Ito, H., 87
Kajiya, F., 77
Kamiya, A., 123
Kanai, H., 159
Kataoka, K., 221
Kawaguchi, T., 117
Kawamori, R., 39
Katabatake, A., 87
Kotani, M., 233
Kubo, Y., 243
Kuriki, S., 233
Kuwahara, M., 101
Mabuchi, K., 5
Maeda, K., 197
Matsuo, T., 145
Matumoto, T., 243
Mito, K., 77
Mori, H., 233
Nemoto, I., 233
Ogasawara, Y., 77
Okajima, M., 117
Saito, M., 185
Sakamoto, K., 159
Sakurai, Y., 221
Schichiri, N., 39
Shiina, T., 185
Shin, Y., 213
Shishido, F., 243
Sugawara, M., 65
Tateno, Y., 243
Togawa, T., 213
Tsuji, T., 25
Tsujioka, K., 77
Tsukagoshi, S., 5
Tsunemoto, H., 243
Tsuzi, T., 213
Uchikawa, Y., 233
Yamakoshi, Y., 123
Yamamoto, T., 171
Yamamoto, Y., 171
Yamasaki, T., 243
Yamasaki, Y., 39
Yamazaki, Z., 17
Yui, N., 221

Medical Progress through Technology

INSTRUCTIONS TO AUTHORS

Presentation and preparation of the manuscript

Manuscripts should be written in standard English and submitted in triplicate. The author should retain the original and send good, clear, legible photocopies. Manuscripts should be typed double-spaced throughout on one side of DIN A4 paper (21 × 29 cm or 8.5 × 11 inch), with sufficiently wide margins (3–5 cm). All pages (including the tables, figures, legends and references) should be numbered consecutively in the upper right-hand corner. Each page should also include the senior author's surname typed in the upper left-hand corner.

The manuscript should be arranged in the following order (typed cap. + lower case):

Title page (page 1)

- Title (the title should be as short as possible, but should contain adequate information regarding the contents).
- Subtitle (this may be used to supplement and thereby shorten an excessively long main title).
- Author's full name (if more than one, use '&' before the last name).
- Affiliation(s)/Address(es).

Key words/Abstract/Abbreviations (page 2)

- Key words (maximum of 6, in alphabetical order, suitable for indexing).
- Abstract (brief and informative, not to exceed 250 words).
  Abbreviations arranged alphabetically, only those which are not familiar and/or commonly used.

Main text

- The relative importance of headings and subheadings should be clear. The approximate location of figures and tables should be indicated in the margin.
  New paragraphs should be indicated by clear indentation.
- The use of footnotes should be avoided. However, if essential, they should be typed on appropriate pages, but clearly separated from the text with a line above them.
- Mathematical formulas should have a clarification of all symbols and an accompanying 'translation' of the meaning, e.g., 'this formula shows that when the highly variable factor λ is found to exceed unity, the viscosity of the medium δ is no longer significant'.
- Acknowledgements (also grants, support etc. if any); should follow the text and precede the references.
- Photographs should be supplied as black-and-white, high contrast glossy prints. Colour plates may be inserted at the author's own expense.
- Figures as well as Legends should be identified by arabic numbers.
  Where multi-part figures are used, each part should be clearly identified in the legend, preferably with (lower case) letters.
- The top of the figure should be indicated on the back. Figures which need to be placed landscape should be avoided if possible.
- Identify each illustration, on the back, by lightly writing author's name and figure number.

Style manuals

The following three books are recommended as guides in writing scientific papers:

- Council of biology editors style manual. A guide for authors, editors, and publishers in the biological sciences 4th edn. Bethesda MD: Council of Biology Editors, 1978.
- O'Connor M, Woodford FP (eds): Writing scientific papers in English. Amsterdam: Elsevier, 1976.
- Reynolds L, Simmonds D: Presentation of data in science. Publications, slides, posters, overhead projections, tape-slides, television. The Hague: Martinus Nijhoff, 1983.

Offprints

- The authors will receive 50 offprints free of charge.
- Ordering information for additional offprints will be sent after acceptance of the manuscript.

Abbreviations and units

Only SI units and abbreviations should be used although some quantities may be used in common units, e.g. mmHg. Abbreviations should be explained when they first appear in the text.
If a non-standard abbreviation is to be used extensively, it should be defined in full on page 2 as mentioned above. Whenever in doubt use SI (Système International) units.

General

To save time and trouble for all concerned, the authors are requested, when preparing manuscripts, to follow the latest issue of the journal in all details not mentioned here. The attention of typists is drawn to the journal's usage of lowercase and capital letters and punctuation style.

References

- References should be cited in numerical order, the number being placed in parentheses. Citations of personal communications and unpublished data should be avoided unless absolutely necessary. When used, such citations should appear in the text only, e.g. '(E.D. Smith, personal communication)', and not in the reference list.
- Abbreviate titles of periodicals according to the style of the Index Medicus.
- Follow the format (arrangement, punctuation) shown below (Vancouver Style):

Chapter in book

1. Bauer RB. Mechanical compression of the vertebral arteries. In: Berguer R, Bauer RD, eds. Vertebrobasilar arterial occlusive disease: medical and surgical management. New York: Raven Press, 1984: 45–71.

Article in periodical

10. du Doulay G, Shah SH, Currie JC, Logue V. The mechanism of hydromyelia in Chiari type 1 malformations. Br J Radiol 1974; 47: 579–87.

Book

14. Cohen J. Statistical power analysis for the behavioral sciences. Revised ed. New York: Academic press, 1977: 217–48.

- Never use italics in titles of articles or books.

Tables

- Each table should be mentioned in the text. Careful thought should be given to the orientation of each table when it is constructed. Tables which can be arranged so that they can be read without rotating the page are preferred. With a little thought, virtually any table can be converted into this type, with increased convenience to the user.
- Tables may be edited by the publisher to permit more compact typesetting.
- Tables should be numbered with arabic numerals, followed by the title. Horizontal rules should be indicated; vertical rules should not be used. Table-footnotes should be marked with superscript letters.

Figures

- Each figure should be mentioned in the text.
- Line drawings should be in a form suitable for reproduction without modification. Extremely small type should be avoided as figures are often reduced in size.